P9-ELG-781

Health Inequities in Canada

Edited by Olena Hankivsky
with Sarah de Leeuw, Jo-Anne Lee,
Bilkis Vissandjée, and Nazilla Khanlou

Health Inequities in Canada: Intersectional Frameworks and Practices

UBCPress · Vancouver · Toronto

© UBC Press 2011

All rights reserved. No part of this publication may be reproduced, stored in a retrieval system, or transmitted, in any form or by any means, without prior written permission of the publisher, or, in Canada, in the case of photocopying or other reprographic copying, a licence from Access Copyright, www.accesscopyright.ca.

20 19 18 17 16 15 14 13 12 11   5 4 3 2 1

Printed in Canada on FSC-certified ancient-forest-free paper
(100% post-consumer recycled) that is processed chlorine- and acid-free.

Library and Archives Canada Cataloguing in Publication

   Health inequities in Canada : intersectional frameworks and practices / edited by Olena Hankivsky.

Includes bibliographical references and index.
ISBN 978-0-7748-1975-6 (bound); ISBN 978-0-7748-1972-5 (pbk)

   1. Health services accessibility – Canada. 2. Health – Social aspects – Canada. 3. Equality – Health aspects – Canada. 4. Health and race – Canada. 5. Health – Sex differences – Canada. 6. Women's health services – Canada. 7. Minorities – Medical care – Canada. 8. Social medicine – Canada. I. Hankivsky, Olena

RA449.H424 2011   362.1'0420971   C2011-900894-7

e-book ISBNs: 978-0-7748-1977-0 (PDF); 978-0-7748-1978-7 (epub)

Canadä

UBC Press gratefully acknowledges the financial support for our publishing program of the Government of Canada (through the Canada Book Fund), the Canada Council for the Arts, and the British Columbia Arts Council.

This book has been published with the help of a grant from the Canadian Federation for the Humanities and Social Sciences, through the Aid to Scholarly Publications Program, using funds provided by the Social Sciences and Humanities Research Council of Canada.

Printed and bound in Canada by Friesens
Set in Stone by Artegraphica Design Co. Ltd.
Copy editor: Deborah Kerr
Proofreader: Tara Tovell
Indexer: Pat Buchanan

UBC Press
The University of British Columbia
2029 West Mall
Vancouver, BC V6T 1Z2
www.ubcpress.ca

I dedicate this book to my colleague and dear friend
  Rita Kaur Dhamoon
and to the conversation that changed everything....

Contents

Figures and Tables

Acknowledgments

The publication of this book was made possible by the financial contributions of the Women's Health Research Network, funded by the Michael Smith Foundation for Health Research, and the University Publications Fund at Simon Fraser University. Every book project of this nature requires a team effort. I would like to thank my amazing co-editors: Sarah de Leeuw, Jo-Anne Lee, Bilkis Vissandjée, and Nazilla Khanlou, who provided invaluable intellectual direction and encouragement throughout all stages of putting together this collection. And to Diego de Merich – grazie mille. Your patience, hard work, attention to detail, editing suggestions and support throughout the process ensured the realization of this important and exciting project.

Health Inequities in Canada

Introduction:
Purpose, Overview, and Contribution

Olena Hankivsky, Sarah de Leeuw, Jo-Anne Lee,
Bilkis Vissandjée, and Nazilla Khanlou

Why This Collection?

Certainly, the transformational promise of intersectionality as a research paradigm for improving the understanding of and response to diversity in health and illness is increasingly recognized by health policy researchers.[1] Moreover, applications of intersectionality in clinical, health services, population health, and even basic science research contexts are beginning to emerge, including in the Canadian context.[2] And recently, a practical guide has been developed for researchers working across all health pillars and for policy makers who are interested in applying an intersectional framework (Hankivsky and Cormier 2009).

At the same time, intersectionality has not made significant strides in transforming mainstream health research and policy. Its slow uptake in health research is perhaps especially worthy of challenge because health is such a complex and multi-dimensional phenomenon, one determined and constituted in such great respect by the social, spatial, and temporal contexts in which people and communities exist. As manifest in people's health status and well-being, identity categories and their relationship to power and states of (dis)empowerment can be understood as embodied and eminently material. Thus, it seems especially urgent – when theorizing and researching health – to apply analytical frameworks that account for and that take seriously the ways in which people's identities, the places they live, and those with whom they engage are constantly affected by power while also interlocking and overlapping in ever-dynamic, always relational, unbounded and unfixed ways. The framework of intersectionality offers excellent potential to do just this. Health research that clearly demonstrates how intersectionality can be deployed offers much-needed examples of how to implement the theory.

To date, however, there has been only one edited collection that has examined the relationship between intersectionality and health: *Gender, Race, Class and Health: Intersectional Approaches* (Schulz and Mullings 2006), which profiles US-based research that has primarily focused on the relationship between gender, race, and class. The present volume is thus a muchneeded contribution to the existing intersectionality and health literature. For the first time, interdisciplinary scholars from nursing, medicine, public health, sociology, anthropology, social work, education, First Nations studies, political science, criminology, women's studies, geography, and health sciences as well as community-based researchers and activists are brought together to highlight exemplary Canadian innovations in intersectional health scholarship, to facilitate dialogue on key issues and tensions within the field, and to produce new knowledge about the concepts and methods of intersectionality research to inform research, policy, and practice.

The goal of this collection is to link theory and practice in a way that is largely absent in mainstream health research and policy. Theoretically, the book draws on cutting-edge social science literature to determine how to best conceptualize and understand intersectionality. The contributions illuminate how to analyze and address simultaneous but distinct axes of subjectification and how the intersectional perspective challenges hegemonic positions within knowledge production. This exercise promotes knowledge exchange between social science and health researchers, analysts, and advocates, an essential process for moving intersectional theoretical constructs to policy and practice. In terms of practice, the chapters demonstrate how researchers who are inspired by and who draw on an intersectionality perspective, albeit using different interpretations and approaches, can develop and execute research designs that include the use of qualitative, quantitative, and mixed methods. Some chapters seek to apply existing theories of intersectionality to concrete cases and practices; others build the theories by drawing on existing practices and lived experiences.

This volume developed out of "Intersectionality and Women's Health: From Theory to Practice," an April 2007 conference held at Simon Fraser University in Vancouver, which received generous support from the Women's Health Research Network funded by the Michael Smith Foundation for Health Research. The conference provided an excellent venue for bringing together, for the first in Canada, researchers who were actively engaged in theoretical and applied aspects of intersectionality. This collection also complements and builds on *Intersectionality: Moving Women's Health Research and Policy Forward* (Hankivsky and Cormier 2009), a step-by-step guide for applying an intersectionality perspective in health research and policy.

The present volume makes no claim to be comprehensive in terms of covering all possible health topics, but it does showcase important intersectionality approaches emerging in the Canadian context for identifying and responding to health inequities in the context of research, health services, policy, and advocacy. To ensure consistency and coherence, all contributing authors grappled with and responded to three key questions in their work:

- What is the approach to/definition of intersectionality used in your chapter?
- What is the value added of using an intersectionality approach to your research? (e.g., what is the transformative potential of an intersectionality-type approach/analysis for identifying and responding to health inequities, especially among traditionally vulnerable and marginalized populations?).
- What are the key challenges for future intersectionality work in your area of research?

The contributors' response to these questions reveals that work in this area is at very different stages of development and that researchers continue to be challenged by the complexities of intersectionality thinking. Nevertheless, the collection as a whole also demonstrates that the idea and promise of intersectionality have indeed taken hold in the Canadian health research community – across all health research pillars – and that they promise to make profound changes to how health disparities are understood and responded to.

The Organization of the Collection

In Chapter 1, Rita Dhamoon and Olena Hankivsky provide the theoretical grounding for the collection. They address conceptual dimensions of intersectionality, offer a critique of the scholarship to date, and suggest avenues for future research. In particular, they engage with current trends and debates in health studies, including important developments in terms of intersectional scholarship, and they demonstrate the significance of intersectionality for health research, especially through its application to the case example of cardiovascular disease. The remainder of the book is organized into four distinct but overlapping and complementary parts, detailed below. A unique feature of this collection is that it is a collaborative effort. Each part is co-edited, allowing for the inclusion of diverse perspectives from health scholars – from a variety of disciplines, a range of intersecting social locations and positions of power – who are united by their passion for and belief in the intellectual and applied project of intersectionality and health.

Part 1: Theoretical and Methodological Innovations
Edited by Sarah de Leeuw and Olena Hankivsky

Part 1 provides examples of new trajectories of thought and new modes of thinking about questions of health within the paradigm of intersectionality. Because many of the ideas explored in the chapters deal with as yet relatively undertheorized applications of intersectionality theory to understandings about health in the Canadian context, the nature of the methodological innovations discussed by the authors is not always straightforward. Still, the essays are all consistent in that they highlight new ways to theorize and to empirically research the multiple factors and processes that ultimately determine people's health and well-being. They concretely demonstrate "putting intersectionality to work" while displaying an inspirational concern for social justice. They grapple with new ways to understand the many factors in people's lives that ultimately constitute health. Each chapter provides a unique example of implementing theories of intersectionality in order to answer specific questions about health or a lack thereof in the Canadian landscape. All the chapters display an abiding concern about how social, cultural, and spatial powers collude and intersect to produce states of health. Implicit in these concerns is methodological innovation, principally because the very act of thinking through questions of health by privileging intersectionality theory requires new theories and methods.

In Chapter 2, Sarah de Leeuw and Margo Greenwood demonstrate that the deep health divides between Indigenous and non-Indigenous people in Canada can never be properly addressed without an intersectional approach that accounts for social determinants such as colonial history, deterritorialization, and (en)forced constructions of socio-cultural identities. It is these, the authors argue, that have left (particularly) Indigenous women vulnerable to shifts in health policies, underscoring the need to think about health in a "complexified" way that accounts for multi-faceted factors (and the ways they interact with each other) that affect the health or well-being of Aboriginal people. In an intersectionality approach about the state of Indigenous people's health, the authors incorporate historical methodologies and analytical frameworks that link health policies to the social production of people's states of being. Like the other contributors, the authors are interested in promoting new ways of understanding Indigenous health in Canada, ways that at every turn carefully and complexly account for systems of socio-cultural power.

In Chapter 3, Jennifer Black and Gerry Veenstra employ theories and methods of intersectionality to explore health outcomes as shaped by the factors of race, gender, and place. Their study thoughtfully combines intersectionality with census and health survey data. This process reminds us that intercategorical approaches to research can be deployed to answer a vast array of questions and that, as a function of how research is undertaken and envisioned, results can be rich and multi-dimensional. Further, the authors illustrate that material space and place, or the sites in which people live, are far from neutral or ambient. Instead, neighbourhood geographies must be conceptualized as active forces alongside race, gender, and class, and then integrated into the methodological ways that health is understood. Black and Veenstra conclude that in order to understand health outcomes and health disparities, it is not sufficient to simply add, or stack, the categories that define people. What must instead be theorized and researched are the interactions between and among the categories (including locational categories) that define people. The principal methodological innovation achieved by Black and Veenstra is precisely that, in answering questions about how to understand health, they employed new ways of asking health-related questions, ways that integrate "the spatial" into more standard race-class-gender triads of intersectional analysis. Black and Veenstra's work corroborates the conclusions of other chapters throughout the text: if the complex array of health disparities in Canada and elsewhere is to be understood, new theoretical and methodological lens and questions must be applied to the topic.

In Chapter 4, Colleen Reid and her colleagues sketch the importance of incorporating intersectionality into the burgeoning field of feminist participatory action research. In an in-depth and highly community-relevant research project, the authors examine linkages between women's employability and their effect on health and well-being. This grounded participant-driven project, which explicitly takes power relations into account, could not have unfolded without the theoretical frameworks and methods afforded by an intersectionality approach, again demonstrating the relevance and importance of a lens that validates complexity and diversity among social subjects. Again, as in other chapters in this part of the book, the methodological innovations explored by the authors are anchored in the research itself. Conceptualizing women's employability through neither a single analytical lens nor a straightforwardly intersectional approach results in new ways to theorize the health and well-being of women whose voices and experiences are not always fully represented in health research.

And in Chapter 5, like Black and Veenstra, who illustrate how new understandings of health come from integrating location into analytical frameworks, Sheryl Reimer-Kirkham and Sonya Sharma add religious orientation to the more standard categories of gender, class, and race. In doing so, and thus by providing another example of how to set intersectionality into the practice of health research, they demonstrate that the nature of care provision, and the ways in which patients engage clinicians and other patients, is an outcome of variable, interrelating, and diverse characteristics. The methodological innovations in this chapter are twofold. First, it draws from a broad range of interviews with subjects not often conceptualized through intersectionality theory. Secondly, it injects ideas of religiosity into intersectional analysis, an innovative methodological approach in itself.

Despite, then, the array of geographies, perspectives, and the different types of health themes addressed in the chapters that comprise Part 1, what remains a consistent and abiding message is that healthier states of being will arise for Canadians only if health research and practice embrace complex and nuanced approaches. A dynamic and pluralized collection of methodologies dealing with questions about health in Canada is ground-breaking.

The authors in this part of the book reinforce the idea that basing an investigation or intervention on a smattering of factors that contribute to people's marginalized health status is not sufficient. Nor is it sufficient to think about health as based on singular or individualized factors. Instead, and fundamentally, the authors propose that if social justice is to be achieved in Canada – health is a crucial component here – intersectionality must be embraced and put to work.

Part 2: Intersectionality Research across the Life Course
Edited by Nazilla Khanlou and Olena Hankivsky

The chapters in Part 2 contribute to our understanding of the intersections of life stages with selected identity markers and with axes of power, privilege, and oppression. This is an important contribution because, as Olena Hankivsky (2007, 81) has argued recently, "the current challenge is how to translate conceptual approaches to intersectionality to inform the practical requirements of lifespan frameworks" and in so doing, determine which factors should be included in this analysis and how multiple factors can be examined to capture the interactive complexity of different experiences (Carter, Sellers, and Squires 2002).

The first three chapters address the experiences of youth, whereas the latter two examine those of mid- to later life. Together, the chapters contribute to centring the lived experiences of those who "occupy multiple locations to advance their own freedoms and own agendas of justice" (this volume, 21). What emerges from the chapters is the voice of strength in diverse settings by diverse individuals and despite challenges. The findings deconstruct our notions of the marginalized Other and caution us to avoid the dichotomy created by our labelling of others.

In Chapter 6, Natalie Clark and Sarah Hunt consider rural young women's health experiences. Applying auto-ethnography as their research method, they link their community-based experiences as researchers and practitioners with those of the young women and with their own perceptions of health while growing up. The chapter contributes to an understudied area by focusing on the perspectives of young rural and Indigenous women. Throughout it, the authors intersperse their own voices, relay their experiences, and provide case studies. As a result, they create a bridge for the reader to experience the text at an intersubjective level, instead of as a distant observer.

In Chapter 7, Jo-Anne Lee and Alison Sum report on a participatory action research study. Using photovoice as their methodology, they examine the health and identity of racialized young women with transnational lives. Transnational and post-colonial feminist theories are integrated into an intersectional feminist analysis of the young women's experiences. The four emerging themes consist of self-understandings of health; mobility, identity, and health (culturally hybrid subjects and situated experiential knowledge); living between worlds (exploring health, identity, and belonging); and finding balance (relational health and intimacy). Through poignant narratives from the young women as they discuss the photos they took for the study (photovoice), Lee and Sum call for a reconsideration of the concept of health in the context of transnational lives.

Chapter 8, by Nazilla Khanlou and Tahira Gonsalves, examines the psychosocial integration of immigrant and second-generation youth. The authors argue that prevailing models of integration do not apply for all immigrant and second-generation youth when considering the intersections of their life stage, gender, racialized status, and their immigrant status or that of their parents. Drawing from two community-based mixed-method studies (including qualitative and quantitative methods), the authors examine youth cultural identities and psychosocial integration and their relevance for youth mental health promotion in pluralistic societies. The authors suggest that an intersectional approach will aid our understanding of positions of oppression and privilege by immigrants and their children, leading to an comprehension of negotiation of their agency across structures.

The healthy immigrant effect (HIE) is considered by Karen Kobayashi and Steven Prus in Chapter 9. The authors utilize intersectionality as their conceptual framework and intercategorical approach as their methodology to examine the HIE. Using data from the 2005 Canadian Community Health Survey, they explore the intersections of age (mid-life, older adult), gender, and visible minority status. The HIE is found to apply to mid-life males, but the differences are less consistent for mid-life women. Gender differences exist for recent visible minority immigrants who are above sixty-five years of age. However, the authors call for policy makers to consider the differential health care needs of immigrant adults, in light of the gender and age differences found in their analysis, pointing to a more complex understanding of how gender interacts with other factors. The authors discuss the implications of applying an intersectional framework and intercategorical approach to future research on immigrant health.

In Chapter 10, Wendy Hulko applies intersectionality and an interlocking oppressions perspective to examine the later life experiences of older people with dementia. Employing grounded theory, she discusses the subjective experiences of dementia and their link to participants' social locations, focusing on experiencing, othering, and theorizing dementia. Her findings lead the author to argue that the extent to which dementia is problematicized is related to the social location of the person with dementia. Specifically, more marginalized persons will resist being considered only in terms of their symptoms, whereas more privileged ones will consider their dementia negatively. Hulko concludes that an intersectional perspective challenges prevailing assumptions on disabling conditions.

Part 3: Social Context, Policy, and Health
Edited by Bilkis Vissandjée and Olena Hankivsky

Part 3 highlights the significance of intersecting social determinants of health such as gender, ethnicity, and migration, and how these evolve over the life trajectory. Discussions with illustrative examples demonstrate the extent to which social determinants of health are intertwined. This part of the book reveals that migration, a gendered experience, is a complex social determinant of health. It is well demonstrated that locality and the temporal nature of the migratory experience interact through changing culturally and socially bound "imperatives" and that situations of vulnerability as well as resilience are progressively constructed and multidirectional. The contributors also lay out with compelling examples the intersecting and dynamic nature of gender as it interacts with other social determinants and relations.

In Chapter 12, Parin Dossa and Isabel Dyck discuss the role of agency in selected "intersectional" theories. They present rich narratives that intensify the requirement to go beyond social relations and political economies to understand the impact of social discrimination on the body. They skilfully build on recognized approaches in health geography to show how daily activities produce meanings and experiences of space as healthy or its converse. The creation of "healthy space" is orchestrated along the complex ways in which health, gender, and place are interrelated. Coordinated processes take place at multiple sites. Dossa and Dyck concur with Anthony Giddens (1984) and Judith Lorber (1994, 1997) as they indicate that there are clusters of rules and resources that are sustained across time and space within and among social systems such as gender, religion, and justice. One of their examples features food preparation and consumption practices along the lines of traditional healing and religious observance; physical, social, and symbolic dimensions of healthy space emerge through overwhelming women's narratives as specifics of migration settlement issues are discussed. Yet, Dossa and Dyck are quite eloquent in their statement of the current "invisibility" of multiple locations that women occupy in the process of migration and resettlement, and in the "cartography" of healthy spaces.

The complex meanings given to food, as illustrated in the women's accounts, attest to the importance associated with food along the migratory trajectory. Dossa and Dyck's statement that the imperative of being a "good citizen" – which may be interpreted as a "good immigrant" – is to take responsibility for eating healthily feeds perfectly into Chapter 13, by Bilkis Vissandjée and Ilene Hyman. In it, the authors describe the importance of an intersectional analysis when deriving, implementing, and evaluating diabetes prevention and management programs. The explanations for the loss of the initial healthy migrant effect point to the lack of visibility in the cartography of healthy spaces as alluded to by Dossa and Dyck; in this regard, the stress of settlement is certainly a contributing factor to sustained changes in dietary habits and lifestyle, which can lead to the potential disruption of metabolic processes and chronic disease precursors, such as obesity and diabetes. Describing the heterogeneity of experiences of women and the need for the analyses of intersecting determinants, Vissandjée and Hyman call for careful consideration of interacting distal mechanisms by which health inequality occurs in a diverse group. Relevant risk factors and selected successful interventions for prevention and management of diabetes are discussed at the end of their chapter while applying an intersectionality lens. Vissandjée and Hyman conclude by highlighting the importance of best policies, programs, and practices – in the case of diabetes prevention and management among migrants – which need to reflect the nuances of differences and heterogeneity of evolving identities.

In Chapter 11, building on the notions of prejudice and discrimination, Jacqueline Oxman-Martinez and Jill Hanley illustrate the potential for discrimination based on sex and ethnocultural characteristics, as gender issues and migration experiences reflect differentiated patterns of social relationships. Their chapter highlights the importance of asking effective questions, especially to vulnerable women, even if time and sensitivity may be at stake. They demonstrate that the process of informing policies sensitive to gender, ethnicity, and migration could easily turn into a messy and entangled legal process. This is particularly true in the case of violence experienced by women with precarious immigration status. The authors plead for an intersectional analysis in order to unravel the simultaneous influences of women's immigration status (systemic factor) and socio-cultural determinants leading – often too quietly – to different forms of violence. Oxman-Martinez and Hanley illustrate the influence of differential power relationships: already vulnerable women may be exposed to systemic and structural risks without adequately knowing their rights or the means to access the appropriate resources.

Though their topics differ, Oxman-Martinez and Hanley concur with Dossa and Dyck in calling for a much-needed debate on the rights of migrants while increasing the visibility of multiple locations that women occupy in the resettlement process and in the cartography of healthy spaces. By providing concrete examples, Oxman-Martinez and Hanley demonstrate that the much-sought option for migrant women – reunification – might in fact increase risk factors of exposure to structural as well as systemic violence. They conclude by reviewing the dimensions of the framework they presented in their chapter. This brings into sharper relief women's structural location within interrelated relationships of power as well as their ability to negotiate multiple markers of difference.

In Chapter 14, building on the capacity of negotiation with an intersectional perspective, Joan Samuels-Dennis, Marilyn Ford-Gilbee, and Annette Bailey present the interconnected fields of trauma, post-traumatic stress disorder (PTSD), and recovery research. The depth of their analysis is quite appealing as they weave together the traumatic experiences of women along with the long-term introspective causes, effects, and consequences of abuse. Their intersectionality model of trauma and PTSD effectively integrates principles of intersectionality and the stress process model (Pearlin 1999). The examples provided make explicit the need to examine how various forms of social disadvantage intersect to influence exposure to violence, the response of self and others, and community and institutional support for women's escape and safety from violence. The authors demonstrate that a single stress-response framework to examine and understand the factors that influence the development and persistence of mental health problems among women simply cannot address the proximal and distal elements in the complex pathways of women's lives. In this regard, the authors concur with Oxman- Martinez and Hanley that an intersectional analysis allows for the disclosure of the numerous (evident and less evident) systems of oppression and exclusion leading to social and health inequalities.

Chapter 14 resonates with other chapters in Part 3 by highlighting the importance of grounding intersectionality in the social determinants of health approach. More specifically, referring to Dossa and Dyck's arguments, Samuels-Dennis, Bailey, and Ford-Gilboe identify women's neighbourhood of residence as one of the most important life contexts that both positively and negatively influence women's lived experiences. They subscribe to the fact that women's multiple social statuses intersect in geographic spaces. Oxman-Martinez and Hanley, as well as Vissandjée and Hyman, overlap with these authors with illustrations of power and privilege associated with these intersections leading to the development and ill-management of selected chronic diseases as well as the persistence of mental health problems through their influence on victimization, trauma-induced interpersonal stressors, and women's access to resources.

Part 4: Disrupting Power and Health Inequities
Edited by Jo-Anne Lee and Olena Hankivsky

The authors in Part 4 speak directly to health researchers who perceive social justice and equity in health as their goals. Because intersectional approaches centre social justice and equality, they hold great potential for more fully understanding the conditions that give rise to injustice and inequality, and how individuals and groups respond. The research studies discussed in Part 4 represent many of the principles the editors of this volume have identified as ideal intersectional-type research. As well as carefully demonstrating how they conceptualize their research, analyze findings, and operationalize methodologies in intersectional analyses, they identify key principles that help bridge the gap between intersectionality theory and practice. This attention to the praxis of intersectional-type research prompts them to ask new and different questions, and to "drive research and policy work to be more responsive to social justice agendas." Authors apply intersectional analyses to reveal previously hidden issues and operations of power in policy making, health services for women, and organizational governance in a national women's organization.

In Chapter 17, Colleen Varcoe, Bernadette Pauly, and Shari Laliberté investigate questions of ethics in policy making; in Chapter 15, Annette Browne, Colleen Varcoe, and Alycia Fridkin take up health services and poverty, trauma, violence, and pain; in Chapter 16, Katherine Rossiter and Marina Morrow examine the implications of intersectionality for mental health research, policy, and practice; and in Chapter 18, Jo-Anne Lee reflects on a Canadian national women's organization that champions the adoption of intersectional feminist frameworks (IFFs) in research while simultaneously confronting challenges of implementation in its practices.

Chapters 15 and 17 demonstrate Leslie McCall's (2005) elaboration of inter- and intracategorical methods in intersectional research. They problematize and challenge popular and scientific constructions of marginalized individual and group social identities. For example, against depictions of abject despair and victimhood, Browne, Varcoe, and Fridkin uncover self-help community networks and individuals who provide support and care for one another. Extending this finding, they question how health researchers and media construct "the problem" in ways that reassert biased assumptions and stereotypes about drug addicts, the poor, and women. They argue that intersectional researchers must perform inter- and intracategorical analysis across multiple levels to reveal which structures of inequality are affecting individuals and limiting possibilities. They challenge how and which categories of analysis are seen as relevant to women's health needs. Instead of asking questions about intersecting identities, they ask how social problems come together to affect poor women's lives and question the paradoxical refusal on the part of policy makers to respond to complex problems with equally nuanced policy responses. They also disrupt normative discourses regarding social and health problems associated with these groups by revealing underlying assumptions and biases reflecting pre-existing and long-standing stereotypes. The baggage that comes with labelling a social problem as a health problem mediates how the problem will be addressed at the policy level and at the level of health service delivery as well as which government ministry, departments, and agencies will be involved. Too often, principles of simplicity and singularity govern policy and program design.

In Chapter 17, Varcoe, Pauly, and Laliberté pose similar questions about policies and programs that are framed and developed in ways that do not reflect the lived reality of those most affected. In their study on ethics and policy making, they draw attention to intersections of multiple problems that produce multiple effects. Turning away from a view of policy making as a rational process in which research findings provide evidence that will prompt a response from policy makers, they suggest that evidence can be used to help mobilize public outcry and, once attention to an issue has been achieved, to use evidence to support the community's preferred response. Policy making is viewed as problem solving, where health problems compete for public and media attention. Furthermore, the authors suggest a critical relational view of social justice that aligns with intersectional approaches as an alternative to the distributive model of social justice. In a critical relational view, health justice entails more than equality of access or even of outcomes. Rather, a critical relational view attends to political, economic, and structural contexts that create ongoing conditions of inequality. Hence, social justice in health is more than simply redistributing resources to provide access to health services: it is also about addressing the historical roots and structural conditions that give rise to the specific social problems confronting those most oppressed – poor, racialized, and Indigenous women.

Mental health continues to be an underscrutinized and undertheorized area of health research. Chapter 16, by Rossiter and Morrow, is an important contribution to discussions about this often invisible part of Canada's health landscape. In efforts to expand and make more responsive mental health services and clinical practices, the authors employ intersectionality inspired methods and theories to push the edges of mental health research. Like the other discussions in Part 4, this chapter addresses the specific issue of power through the explorations of two important developments in the field: programs to address stigma/discrimination against people with mental illnesses, and recovery models of care. The authors conclude that the improvement of people's health, and specifically disparities rooted in mental health, rests both on more nuanced – and thus more accurate – assessments of the experiences of individuals and the recognition of complex and relational needs across diverse populations.

In Chapter 18, hidden structures and mechanisms of power are also revealed in Lee's self-ethnography of her role in the Canadian Research Institute for the Advancement of Women. As Lee states, "although epistemological debates may help to clarify what we mean by feminist intersectional approaches at the level of theory, these debates on their own are insufficient to fully understand and address the overall, multiple, and shifting effects of intersecting structures of inequality" (this volume, 360). She cautions against being overly optimistic about the efficacy of intersectional analyses: "If one is working within an established organization that is struggling to understand gender discrimination, whose governance structure does not reflect principles underlying IFFs, whose research staff might not have the necessary training in IFFs, and where the most marginalized women are not at the decision-making table, then IFFs will not only meet considerable resistance and foot dragging, but any conceptual contributions [to advancing social justice and equity] will be moot" (this volume, 360).

Some feminists, including a number of contributors to this volume, do not adopt any specific terms to address the interwoven relationship between modes of difference. Therefore, the term "intersectionality" is not universally deployed. Alternative language and terminology describing the relationship between distinct axes of differences does appear, such as "interactions," to punctuate the dynamic nature of the relationship. Contestability around how to describe relationships of difference reflects the flexibility and multiplicity of approaches that exist both within the United States (where the term first gained prominence among feminists) and beyond. Debates about discursive and conceptual boundaries are not unique to this field of study; indeed, there may be utility in maintaining "intersectionality" as a broad umbrella term rather than a definitive description of how difference, power, or identity operate. At the same time, intersectionality has gained widespread usage, and it is a recognizable term that delineates the broad body of scholarship that emphasizes the ways in which differences work through one another to produce something unique and distinct from any single form of difference standing alone. As the reader will note, several general patterns of this paradigm or framework are consistently present in the chapters of this book and the analytic insights they produce advance novel and fresh perspectives on health inequities.

First, the authors identify that an intersectionality framework not only challenges the primacy of a singular category (such as "women" or gender), but it also transcends an additive approach because of its emphasis on simultaneity and mutuality of differences. Second, this research paradigm provides a way to address the complexities of othering – namely, the ways in which difference is produced so as to (re)assert standards of normalcy. Thus, rather than thinking in terms of single binaries of man-woman, black-white, straight-gay, an intersectionality framework addresses variations within and between such binaries. Third, it places the focus of analysis on the social nature of difference – namely, the inseparability of the self and the social – and as such, it moves away from the individualization of difference. Fourth, this framework pays attention to lived experiences that are often constant aspects of the analysis. Fifth, it attends to both the variation between and among social collectivities, and the relationality that exists between social collectives; in other words, an intersectionality framework challenges the homogenization that often occurs in the study of social groups, and it shows that differences exist not in isolation but in relation to other socially produced differences. Sixth, this framework places context at its centre, thereby highlighting the significance of socio-political patterns and the particularities of time and space, as well as the implications of these commonalities and differences for social life. Finally, power is a central theme of the analysis, not only in terms of multi-constitutive axes of oppression, but also in terms of interacting modes of productive power and resistance.

Notes

1   On intersectionality as a research paradigm in the study of health and illness, refer to Hankivsky and Cormier (2009), Bates, Hankivsky, and Springer (2009), Doyal (2009), Warner (2008), Collins, von Unger, and Armbrister (2008), Schulz and Mullings (2006), Weber (2006), Weber and Parra-Medina (2003), Vinz and Dören (2007).

2   On applications of intersectionality in clinical, health services, population health, and basic science research, refer to Bredström (2006), Burman (2004), Chuback et al. (2007), Cummings and Jackson (2008), Deeb-Sossa (2007), Rowland Hogue (2000), Schulz and Mullings (2006), Steinbugler, Press, and Johnson Dias (2006), Greenwood and Christian (2008), Kelly (2009), Reid and Herbert (2005), Meyer, Schwartz, and Frost (2008), Collins, von Unger, and Armbrister (2008), Bowleg (2008). On applications of intersectionality and intersectional research in the health sciences field in Canada, refer to Anderson (2004), Benoit et al. (2007), Hankivsky and Christoffersen (2008), Reid, Tom, and Frisby (2006), Varcoe and Dick (2008), Mulvihill, Mailloux, and Atkin (2001), Hulko (2009).

References

Anderson, J.M. 2004. Lessons from a postcolonial feminist perspective: Suffering and a path to healing. *Nursing Inquiry* 11(4): 238-46.

Bates, L.M., O. Hankivsky, and K.W. Springer. 2009. Gender and health inequities: A comment on the final report of the WHO Commission on the Social Determinants of Health. *Social Science and Medicine* 69(7): 1002-4.

Benoit, C., L. Shumka, B. McCarthy, M. Jansson, R. Phillips, and H. Hallgrimsdottir. 2007. Laborers, managers and counselors: A comparative analysis of intimate work in the sex industry. Paper presented at "Intimate Labors Conference," University of California, Santa Barbara, 4-6 October.

Bowleg, L. 2008. When black + lesbian + woman ≠ black lesbian woman: The methodological challenges of qualitative and quantitative intersectionality research. *Sex Roles* 59(3): 312-25.

Bredström, A. 2006. Intersectionality: A challenge for feminist HIV/AIDS research? *European Journal of Women's Studies* 13: 229-43.

Burman, E. 2004. From difference to intersectionality: Challenges and resources. *European Journal of Psychotherapy, Counselling and Health* 6(4): 293-308.

Carter, P., S. Sellers, and C. Squires. 2002. Reflections on race/ethnicity, class and gender inclusive research. *African American Research Perspectives* 8(1): 111-24.

Chuback, J., J.M. Embil, E. Sellers, E. Trepman, M. Cheang, and H. Dean. 2007. Foot abnormalities in Canadian Aboriginal adolescents with type 2 diabetes. *Diabetic Medicine* 24: 747-52.

Collins, P.Y., H. von Unger, and A. Armbrister. 2008. Church ladies, good girls, and locas: Stigma and the intersection of gender, ethnicity, mental illness, and sexuality in relation to HIV risk. *Social Science and Medicine* 67(3): 389-97.

Cummings, J., and P.B. Jackson. 2008. Race, gender and SES disparities in self-assessed health, 1974-2004. *Research on Aging* 30(2): 137-67.

Deeb-Sossa, N. 2007. Helping the "neediest of the needy": An intersectional analysis of moral-identity construction at a community health clinic. *Gender and Society* 21(5): 749-72.

Doyal, Lesley. 2009. Challenges in researching life with HIV/AIDS: An intersectional analysis of black African migrants in London. *Culture, Health and Sexuality* 11(2): 173-88.

Giddens, A. 1984. *The constitution of society: Outline of the theory of structuration.* Berkeley: University of California Press.

Greenwood, R.M., and A. Christian. 2008. What happens when we unpack the invisible knapsack? Intersectional political consciousness and inter-group appraisals. *Sex Roles* 59(3): 404-17.

Hankivsky, O. 2007. More than age and biology: Overhauling lifespan approaches to women's health. In *Women's health in Canada: Critical perspectives on theory and policy,* ed. M. Morrow, O. Hankivsky, and C. Varcoe, 64-93. Toronto: University of Toronto Press.

Hankivsky, O., and A. Christoffersen. 2008. Intersectionality and the determinants of health: A Canadian perspective. *Critical Public Health* 18(3): 271-83.

Hankivsky, O., and R. Cormier. 2009. *Intersectionality: Moving women's health research and policy forward.* Vancouver: Women's Health Research Network.

Hulko, W. 2009. The time- and context-contingent nature of intersectionality and inter-locking oppressions. *Affilia: Journal of Women and Social Work* 24(1): 44-55.

Kelly, U.A. 2009. Integrating intersectionality and biomedicine in health disparities research. *Advances in Nursing Science* 32(2): E42-E56.

Lorber, J. 1994. *Paradoxes of gender.* New Haven: Yale University Press.

–. 1997. *Gender and the social construction of illness.* Thousand Oaks, CA: Sage.

McCall, L. 2005. The complexity of intersectionality. *Signs* 30(3): 1771-1800.

Meyer, I.H., S. Schwartz, and D.M. Frost. 2008. Social patterning of stress and coping: Does disadvantaged social status confer more stress and fewer coping resources? *Social Science and Medicine* 67(3): 368-79.

Mulvihill, M.A., L. Mailloux, and W. Atkin. 2001. Advancing policy and research responses to immigrant and refugee women's health in Canada. Prepared for the Centres of Excellence for Women's Health. http://www.cewh-cesf.ca/en/resources/im-ref_health/im_ref_health.pdf.

Pearlin, L.I. 1999. The stress process revisited: Reflections on concepts and their interrela-tionships. In *Handbook of the sociology of mental health,* ed. C.S. Aneshensel and J.C. Phelan, 395-416. New York: Plenum.

Reid, C., and C. Herbert. 2005. 'Welfare moms and welfare bums': Revisiting poverty as a social determinant of health. *Health Sociology Review* 14(2): 161-73.

Reid, C., A. Tom, and W. Frisby. 2006. Finding the 'action' in feminist participatory action research. *Action Research* 4(3): 313-30.

Rowland Hogue, C.J. 2000. Gender, race and class: From epidemiologic association to etiologic hypotheses. In *Women and health,* ed. M. Goldman and M. Hatch, 15-23. San Diego: Academic Press.

Schulz, A.J., and L. Mullings, eds. 2006. *Gender, race, class and health: Intersectional approaches.* San Francisco: Jossey-Bass.

Steinbugler, A.C., J.E. Press, and J. Johnson Dias. 2006. Gender, race and affirmative action: Operationalizing intersectionality in survey research. *Gender and Society* 20(6): 805-25.

Varcoe, C., and S. Dick. 2008. The intersecting risks of violence and HIV for rural Aboriginal women in a neo-colonial Canadian context. *Journal of Aboriginal Health* 4(1): 42-52.

Vinz, D., and M. Dören. 2007. Diversity policies and practices: A new perspective for health care. *Journal of Public Health* 15(5): 369-76.

Warner, L.R. 2008. A best practices guide to intersectional approaches in psychological research. *Sex Roles* 59(5-6): 454-63.

Weber, L. 2006. Reconstructing the landscape of health disparities research: Promoting dialogue and collaboration between feminist intersectional and biomedical paradigms. In Schulz and Mullings, 21-59.

Weber, L., and D. Parra-Medina. 2003. Intersectionality and women's health: Charting a path to eliminating health disparities. In *Advances in gender research.* Vol. 7, *Gender perspec-tives on health and medicine,* ed. M.T. Segal, V. Demos, and J.J. Kronenfeld, 181-230. Oxford: Elsevier.

1

Why the Theory and Practice of Intersectionality Matter to Health Research and Policy

Rita Kaur Dhamoon and Olena Hankivsky

There is a growing sense that current approaches to health inequities in Canada and elsewhere are insufficient for increasing the understanding of multifactoral and multi-level complexities of health disparities and for identifying the most effective strategies to reduce them (Hankivsky and Cormier 2009; Hankivsky and Christoffersen 2008; Varcoe, Hankivsky, and Morrow 2007).[1] Traditional frameworks often fragment vulnerabilities into distinct categories such as sex, gender, race/ethnicity, socio-economic, sexuality, geography, or disease status, prioritize one category over others or look at two or three common variables at a time, and fail to fully consider and analyze the context and influence of social power inequities. Fully understanding health inequities requires alternative research frameworks, such as those emerging from an intersectional perspective, which can investigate the interaction of numerous characteristics of vulnerable populations, not only at the individual level but also at structural levels so as to capture the multiple contexts that shape individual lives and health statuses.

Intersectionality is concerned with simultaneous intersections between aspects of social difference and identity (as related to meanings of race/ethnicity, indigeneity, gender, class, sexuality, geography, age, disability/ability, migration status, religion) and forms of systemic oppression (racism, classism, sexism, ableism, homophobia) at macro and micro levels in ways that are complex and interdependent (Hankivsky and Cormier 2009). Across disciplines, but especially in the social sciences, intersectionality is now recognized as an important normative and empirical paradigm (Hancock 2007a). In the words of Bates, Hankivsky, and Springer (2009, 1002), "the intersectionality perspective brings to the fore the complexity and contingency of social inequities." In the realm of health, scholarship is emerging that demonstrates the significance of intersectionality.

For example, it has been shown to make a concrete difference to the understanding and interrogation of a variety of health issues such as HIV/AIDs (Collins, von Unger, and Armbrister 2008; Doyal 2009), mental health

(Kohn and Hudson 2002; Collins, von Unger, and Armbrister 2008; Warner 2008), violence against women (Crenshaw 1994; El-Khoury, Dutton, and Goodman 2004), and access to and quality of health care services (Iyer, Sen, and Östlin 2008). Numerous arguments have been put forward for its potential to enhance biomedical approaches to health (Weber and Fore 2007; Kelly 2009), existing tools for analyzing health inequities such as sex- and gender-based analysis (Clow et al. 2009), and conceptualizations of health determinants (Hankivsky and Christoffersen 2008). Moreover, the promise of intersectionality to create new and broader frameworks for health disparities research has been widely acknowledged (Schulz and Mullings 2006; Weber 2006; Weber and Parra-Medina 2003). And significantly, the need for more Canadian work in the field of intersectionality and health has been emphasized (Zawilski and Levine-Rasky 2005; Hankivsky et al. 2010; Hankivsky and Cormier 2009).

However, a number of obstacles impede intersectionality's progress in the realm of health. First, health researchers, practitioners, and advocates have paid little attention to the breadth of theoretical developments and current debates and discussions in the field. In other words, intersectionality as research paradigm has a longer and more substantive history in the theoretical literature than it does in some fields of research and policy. Although a significant body of empirical work (much of it qualitative) draws on the experiences of marginalized individuals and social groups, and reflects that intersectionality theory emerged from living practices, this close link between theory and practice has not been adequately incorporated into some dominant research paradigms. Conventional streams of the social sciences and policy development, for example, have been critical of oral traditions, narratives, storytelling, biography, and personal testimony because they are not seen as positivist, objective, rigorous, theoretical, or scholarly enough. Yet, methods considered anti-positivist are traditional tools of existing intersectionality work because they centre situated and experiential knowledge. This centring fosters a close link between established and emerging theories and established and emerging practices; it also counters positivist approaches that are limited to the study of static, categorical, error-free variables. But, because researchers in the mainstream are often focused on the "applied" side of knowledge production (whether from choice or because of disciplinary and policy conventions and requirements), theory is seen as too complicated, too abstract, or simply as irrelevant to research and policy processes. Without doubt, moving between these two realms is an imperfect exercise; the complexity and nuances of theory are not always well suited to the clarity and expedience required for practical applications. However, fostering the link between theory and practice, and thereby drawing on one of the building blocks of intersectionality, can expand and deepen the set of tools available to deconstruct the work of power.

Second, intersectional frameworks remain underutilized because developing theoretically informed and methodologically sound approaches for their health research application is in its nascent stages. In fact, many scholars have argued that there is a lack of methods and tools that can be drawn on by intersectionality researchers and policy makers in their applied work (Nash 2008; Hancock 2007a, 2007b; Phoenix and Pattynama 2006). Moreover, only recently has there been an explicit recognition that intersectionality can be applied to every type of research method, including quantitative methodologies, and that it has currency, relevance, and transformational potential vis-à-vis biomedical research, which has dominated the field. In this way, it is not simply the domain of "social" determinants health scholars. That said, it is also true that applications of intersectionality in health research are in their early stages. As Olena Hankivsky el al. (2010, 12) have argued, "more methodological development is needed so that research design can reflect innovative thinking about identity, equity, and power."

Third, despite often good intentions to undertake an intersectionality framework, conventional exclusionary paradigms of knowledge-production remain intact, in both the theory and policy realm, with the effect of oversimplifying and/or depoliticizing issues of difference. Indeed, some research only symbolically notes the importance of differences and intersections, and continues to assume and foreground categorical essentialisms (such as a universalized category of "woman"). Even where there is recognition of intersecting differences, the overall acceptance of this approach is slow, in large part because it complicates established straightforward modes of research and policy making. As Patricia Hill Collins (2009, xii) says, "Seemingly inclusionary knowledge produced in exclusionary contexts remains suspect, no matter how well intentioned the practitioners might be."

With these three issues in mind, this book seeks ways to illuminate, better understand, and bridge some of the distance by linking the theory to mainstream health research and policy contexts. What becomes clear is that a dialectical relationship exists between theory and practice, one where theories of intersectionality are informed by and informing of practice. In this particular chapter, we contribute to the central goals of the collection by first identifying and exploring five considerations that the theoretical literature raises for the application of intersectionality:

- What are the discursive parameters of intersectionality as a concept?
- What should be studied – interacting/intersecting identities, categories, processes, or systems of difference?
- How can the complexities that are foregrounded by this research paradigm be analyzed?

- Which model(s) is currently available and ideally suited to describe intersectionality methods?
- How does the researcher/analyst decide which interactions to analyze?

Although the following analysis is by no means a comprehensive survey of all intersectionality work, we synthesize some of the tensions and debates raised in the theoretical literature, linking them to those highlighted in this book, so as to develop one possible "model" framework for the application of the theory. In the second part of the chapter, the value and concrete implications of an intersectionality analysis for health research and policy are illustrated through a case example of cardiovascular disease (CVD). The case study reveals the significant gaps in health studies between intersectional theorizing and one area of health research and policy. Despite these gaps, and specifically the confines of current health research and policy in terms of operationalizing the key features of intersectionality, this chapter, like the others in the collection, begins to demonstrate the real transformative potential of an intersectionality-based analysis for identifying and responding to the health needs of traditionally vulnerable and excluded populations.

Part 1: Theoretical Considerations

The Discursive and Conceptual Framework of Intersectionality

Although the intersectionality discourse has been popularized since the 1980s through the work of American critical race scholar Kimberlé Crenshaw (1989, 1994, 1997), the analytical framework for examining the relationship between various aspects of identification and modes of oppression has been a long-standing feature of anti-slavery and anti-colonial struggles against practices of gendered racism. In nineteenth- and twentieth-century America, for example, Anna Julia Cooper, who was born a slave and later became an educator and earned a PhD; Mary Church Terrell, who was the first president of the National Association of Colored Women; and Sojourner Truth, who advocated for women's rights and fought against slavery – all spoke in different ways to the struggles facing women, blacks, and black women (King 1988, 42-43). As well, anti-racist and post-colonial feminists such as Audre Lorde (1984), bell hooks (1981, 1984, 1989), T. Minh-ha Trinh (1989), and Gayatri Chakravorty Spivak (1995) all deployed an intersectionality framework before the term became widely used. Overall, it was non-white women who challenged the universalizations and essentialisms of many struggles dominated by white women (such as the Western feminisms of the 1960s and 1970s) and non-white men (such as the American black civil rights movement) that initially developed frameworks of intersectionality. Yet, as the chapters in this book testify, intersectionality is a bourgeoning idea

(Phoenix and Pattynama 2006). In the words of Collins (2009, vii), "Despite the widespread belief that intersectionality has arrived, I think it is important to stop and recognize that this way of looking at and living within the world constitutes a new area of inquiry that is still in its infancy." It is a new and developing area of inquiry insofar as original and innovative conceptual frameworks, theoretical approaches, methodologies (qualitative, quantitative, and mixed), and cases have emerged over the last ten years. Thus, against a backdrop of a rich history in social struggles and writings by feminists of colour that pushed against the norms of earlier versions of feminism, intersectionality is a discourse and body of work in flux.

This perhaps is most clearly evident in the contestability regarding the very language of intersectionality. The concept of intersectionality has increasingly been contested because it continues to suggest that aspects of oppression merely meet at the intersection rather than mutually constitute one another. This has led some feminists to use alternative terms, such as "interlocking oppressions" (Razack 1998), "multiple jeopardy" (King 1988), "discrimination-within-discrimination" (Kirkness 1986-88), "multiple consciousness" (King 1988; Matsuda 1992), "multiplicity" (Wing 1990-91), "multiplex epistemologies" (Phoenix and Pattynama 2006, 187), "translocational positionality" (Anthias 2001), and "complexifying" (see Chapter 18 this volume).

What Is Being Studied and How?

When one adopts an intersectionality framework, it is important to be clear about what precisely is being examined; this is because the substantive content of what is studied shapes research conclusions as well as normative and policy directions. In the current theoretical literature, at least four kinds of interactions are analyzed: the identities of an individual, set of individuals, or a social group that are marked as different (such as a non-white woman, non-white women as a group, or a specific group of non-white women), the categories of difference (race, gender), the processes of differentiation (racialization gendering), and the systems of domination (racism, colonialism, sexism, and patriarchy). Sometimes these four aspects of analysis are distinct; at other times they merge into one another, or a combination exists as is the case with the study of interacting social locations. Although all four are consistent with intersectionality forms of analysis, each emphasizes something different in our understanding of subject formation and power. Here, the distinctions are explored so as to identify what is brought into view and what is eclipsed in each instance.

Identities of Individuals and Social Groups

Much feminist intersectionality analysis focuses on the individual or social group marked as oppressed. As Leslie McCall (2005, 1780) notes, in these instances, "the primary subject of analysis is typically a social group at a neglected point of intersecting master categories, or a particular social setting or ideological construction, or both." This kind of analysis often occurs through case studies and/or narratives of various othered subjects, such as black women, Third World women, Muslim women, and indigenous women – either as individuals, as a general group, or a specific group. An intersectionality analysis of these specific individuals and social groups especially emphasizes lived experiences and situated knowledge, whereby narratives of lived experience provide knowledge about the social location embodied by that individual or group.

This kind of embodied knowledge has been significant on a number of levels. First, and perhaps most importantly, it has emphasized and celebrated the voices, experiences, perspectives, and agency of those who are traditionally marginalized and erased in mainstream academic literature and public policy. Indeed, many of the authors in this book take up the marginalization of indigenous women, religious minorities, non-white immigrant women, those with mental health considerations, young girls, those with precarious status, such as women refugees and temporary workers, and so on. Second, experiences located in a particular identity provide a way to belong to a social group and thus open up collective relationships, shared spaces for living, and a sense of home. In particular, intersectionality-based research that foregrounds lived experiences helps us to see that marginalized people occupy multiple locations to advance their own freedoms and agendas of justice. Third, as well as providing knowledge about Others, a more nuanced analysis of subjects marked by *privilege* can be developed, thus illustrating that an intersectionality framework is "applicable to any group of people, advantaged as well as disadvantaged" (Yuval-Davis 2006, 201). Fourth, specific and general assessments can be made, especially with regard to differential experiences of discrimination. Embodied knowledge of an identity serves to contextualize oppression, discrimination, subject formation, and forms of resistance, and also illuminates how social locations and identities are changeable and contingent according to a spatial, temporal, and relational context.

The focus on identity, however, can become overdetermined in ways that are essentializing even when multiple aspects of identity are analyzed together. This occurs when a form of difference of one individual or specific group is collapsed as being representative of an entire social collectivity, even though individuals marked as a member of a group may not necessarily celebrate a mode of identification in the same way. Identities are historically and legally shaped but do not necessarily reflect how a person or group understand themselves. For example, the identities of some migrant women in Canada are shaped by the Live-In Caregiver Program and the immigration point system, First Nations women's identities are shaped by the Indian

Act, and the legal identities of transgendered people are determined by vital statistics legislation and medical norms. When identities are overdetermined, narratives of identity politics become conflated with descriptions of positionality (ibid., 195). Although these externally imposed norms are relevant to the lives of subjects, they are not necessarily in tune with self-directed modes of identification.

Furthermore, claims about identity often require that some sense of boundedness and thus some interpretations of difference are privileged over others even though a singular dimension of identity can be interpreted in many ways, both by the self and others, and identities are not always self-evident (for example, a mixed-race person may look white but may not identify as such). Essentializing representations of identity can be especially troubling because they invite researchers to seek out "authentic" subjects with the effect of determining who is purely the Other, who is really worth saving, and who is truly different (Trinh 1989, 88-89; Smith 1999, 74). Furthermore, the focus on identity can falsely pit groups against one another (indigenous men versus indigenous women) without recognition of how these groups may have much in common, even when identities are conceptualized in complex ways.

Certainly, feminists who use an intersectionality method are not unaware of this essentializing risk. As Leslie McCall (2005) says, feminists have developed anti-categorical approaches that deconstruct existing systems of categorization (for example, not just women, but many kinds of women), intracategorical approaches in which the experiences of a single social group (such as women of colour) are defined by an intersection of multiple dimensions, and intercategorical approaches in which there are complex relations among multiple groups within and across identities and analytic categories (such as black women in relation to other non-white women and to different groups of men). These are important techniques for countering hegemonic ways of seeing identity, but the risk of essentialism is unavoidable because claims of identity necessarily lead to some sense of boundedness. As a way to deal with this problem, many feminists do provide caveats regarding specificity, context, and the contingency of social group identity and experience, but these nuances can get lost in translation.

Categories of Difference

In feminist theory, identities and categories of difference are often conflated with one another (Yuval-Davis 2006, 203-5), whereby the identity of a subject at the intersections is synonymously described in terms of categories. In this regard, the issues raised above regarding identity are tied up with issues concerning categories (such as race, class, gender, sexuality, nationality, religion). Accordingly, whereas an analysis of categories is a useful starting point because it punctuates points of connection and disjuncture, this second area of study provides many of the same benefits and pitfalls as above. Rather than rehearsing the limitations mentioned above, we will focus on two additional problems raised within feminist theory as they relate to the study of categories.

The first problem concerns what Patricia A. Monture (2007, 199) calls a "race-class-gender trinity," whereby "some forms of oppression are explained as more damaging than others." There are, of course, some good reasons for this privileged trinity: decision makers are directly unsettled by the gendered non-white subject, and therefore feminists must confront dominant ways of organizing race, class, and gender (ibid.). Also, non-white feminists have had to counter racism and class privilege within white feminism and have thereby emphasized the trinity. Yet the privileging of this trinity not only masks less traditional modes of difference such as religion, spirituality and faith, chronic pain, addictions, place, mental health, disability, literacy, employment status, transnationality, age, migrant status, indigeneity, whiteness, gender identity and expression, and marital status – all of which are taken up by the authors in this book – but it also creates what Elizabeth Martinez (1993) aptly calls the "Oppression Olympics." In the Oppression Olympics, "groups compete for the mantle of 'most oppressed' to gain the attention and political support of dominant groups as they pursue policy remedies, leaving the overall system of stratification unchanged" (Hancock 2007b, 68).

The mantra of race-class-gender categories, in other words, emphasizes some kinds of difference at the exclusion of others. As many of the chapters in this book illustrate, the study of categories does not, of course, have to be confined to this trinity. Indeed, research has shown that an intersectionality lens is applicable to the dynamics between systems of disability, sexuality, and gendering (D'aoust 1999; Garland-Thomson 2002; Shuttleworth 2001), disability, race, culture, and ethnicity (Jakubowicz and Meekosha 2003; Kliewer and Fitzgerald 2001; Titchkosky 2002; Vernon 1999), and race and sexuality (Harper et al. 1997; Hawley 2001). But when the emphasis is on race-class-gender, analysts need to specify why these categories are chosen in preference to others.

A second potential problem with the study of categories is that they are sometimes treated as if they were analogous to one another. In other words, categories such as race, ethnicity, class, gender, and sexual orientation are treated as if they were alike in content and form. In these instances, a claim, for example, about the oppression of a black woman becomes another way of saying either that she suffers from a "triple oppression" because she is black, a woman, and working class, or that to be black or a woman is another way of being a member of the working class (Yuval-Davis 2006, 195-200). Yet, as Floya Anthias and Nira Yuval-Davis argue in their joint and separate work, each category has a different ontological basis that is irreducible to other social divisions (Anthias 1998, 2001; Anthias and Yuval-Davis 1983, 1992; Yuval-Davis 2006). Although categories of division are intermeshed in one another, they are not the same. To treat them as if they were would be to conflate positions, identities, and values. Given this, when studying interactive categories, it is important to avoid the problem of analytic conflation.

Processes of Differentiation and Systems of Domination

As well as analyzing identities or categories through an intersectionality approach, some feminist theories focus on interactive processes of differentiation and interactive systems of domination. Processes of differentiation are self-directed, other-directed, and other-imposed so as to constitute, organize, and govern identities and categories. This includes such processes as racialization, gendering, sexualization, ethnicization, and disabling. Systems of domination are those that organize the privilege of some norms and, by extension, some subjects over others. These include such systems as racism, colonialism, patriarchy, sexism, capitalism, homophobia, transphobia, oralism, disableism, and so on. In both cases, the focus is not on the intersection/interaction itself but on what the intersection/interaction reveals about power. Importantly, an analysis of identities and categories is not erased; instead, the study of processes and systems requires an examination of how identities and/or categories are constituted, resisted, and governed in the first place. Although the study of processes and systems can also be overdetermined, these further an understanding of difference in two key ways.

First, this focus shifts from "different" identities and bodies per se to doing or making of difference – namely, to the contextual processes and socio-political conditions in which representations of identity and categories of difference are produced, governed, and socially organized. The shift is especially necessary because identities and categories are sometimes treated as real *even when it is stated that they are socially constructed.* Some have used quotation marks around categories to emphasize their socially constructed nature. But quotation marks are inconsistently used or overused and therefore are not a good substitute. As Sherene Razack (1998, 165) argues, all social concepts lack scientific validity, but it is often race that appears in quotation marks, as if it were somehow more socially constructed than categories such as gender and class. To counter this tendency, the focus on processes of differentiation and how these processes are constituted by and constitutive of systems of domination would provide a way to critically examine how norms are produced and how they function in and through representations of identity and the body at different levels of socio-political life. Thus, rather than presenting essentialist characterizations of social groups, such an analysis would attend to the many manifestations of otherness. This is because an intersectionality framework reveals that similar kinds of processes of differentiation and systems of domination are operationalized in distinct and specific historical and temporal ways. For example, although the social locations of indigenous women and black women are both constituted through processes of racialized gendering, the different histories of colonization, slavery, gendered imperialism, and white supremacy function in distinct ways so as to position various non-white women differently. This theme of variation runs through many of the following chapters.

Second, in foregrounding the relationship between processes of differentiation and systems of domination, an intersectionality framework can be directly applied to critiques of power – how it operates to produce something specific, how it is resisted, and how difference is governed on a discursive and structural level. To put it differently, the study of processes addresses systemic issues and avoids the tendency to reduce issues of difference to individuals. Accordingly, it is not that analysts examine either interacting discourses or interacting structures, but how these operate together. In Foucauldian terms, the focus of analysis would therefore not strictly be an individual, or group, or institution (although these are not absent either) but the techniques of power. Subjects or categories, in this regard, are not to be studied outside the mechanisms of subjection, subjectivity, domination, and exploitation (Foucault 1982, 212-13). That is, researchers and policy makers are never looking solely at the identities of individual/social group or intersecting categories; rather, they are looking at specific ways, specific moments, and specific contexts in which subjects come into being *relationally*, and, how these processes function, and are resisted, within systems of domination. These are the micro and macro conditions that give meaning to a specific identity or category in the first place. This kind of analysis is hence analytically significant because it shifts the gaze from the othered identity and/or category of otherness to the relational processes of othering and normalization, and their pertinent contexts of power.

The Complexity of Identity Formation and Power

The theoretical literature also points toward a third consideration – namely, how to conceptualize the complexity of difference formation and the work of power, and how to navigate this complexity. The complexity arises for three reasons. First, an intersectionality analysis expands the focus from one dimension to many dimensions, and it simultaneously enables an analysis of the relationship between different dimensions. Thus, what is germane is not simply the fact of plural differences but the relationship between these. In particular, an intersectionality framework starts from the premise that each system needs the others in order to function. Mary Louise Fellows and Sherene Razack (1998, 335)describe this relationship in the following way: "Systems of oppression (capitalism, imperialism, patriarchy) rely on one another in complex ways. The 'interlocking' effect means that the systems of oppression could not be accomplished without gender and racial hierarchies; imperialism could not function without class exploitation, sexism, heterosexism, and so on." The link between these systems has been interpreted in many different ways, but the main point is that it goes beyond a unidimensional analysis.

Second, an understanding of subject formation and power is further complicated by an intersectionality framework because it serves to capture everyday, subjective, structural, and social levels of differentiation. Collins (1990, 227) describes these as multiple levels of domination, which include "the level of personal biography; the group or community level of the cultural context created by race, class, and gender; and the systemic level of social institutions." Anthias and Yuval-Davis refer to these levels of analysis as different social divisions that take on organizational, intersubjective, experiential, and representational forms (Anthias 1998; Anthias and Yuval-Davis 1983, 1992; Yuval-Davis 2006). An analysis of these levels complicates an understanding of subject formation and power by illuminating that it is not simply that interactions occur but that they occur in particular and multiple ways.

Issues of subject formation and power are complicated by intersectionality in a third way because such a framework shifts the focus from a binary-based understanding of difference (e.g., male/female) to one in which binaries are examined in terms of how they interact with one another. This shift is important because it reveals that there are few pure victims or oppressors because each "individual derives varying amounts of penalty and privilege from the multiple systems of oppression which frame everyone's lives" (Collins 1990, 229). Attention to the ways in which "an individual may be an oppressor, a member of an oppressed group, or simultaneously oppressor and oppressed" (ibid., 225) is especially important because it reveals the relational differences not only between norm-Other but also between different kinds of Others (Dhamoon 2009). In attending to these varying degrees and forms, we can avoid what Fellows and Razack (1998, 335) refer to as "the race to innocence," whereby one subject marked by otherness claims that her own marginality is the worst one and fails to interrogate her complicity (however unevenly manifest) in the position of other Others.

To summarize, when an intersectionality paradigm is adopted, three aspects of complexity need to be considered: the multi-dimensional ways in which power operates and subjectivity, subjection, and social location are subsequently constructed; the different levels at which interactions occur; and the differing degrees and forms of penalty and privilege between social locations and subjects. An intersectionality analysis may or may not attend to all three aspects of complexity, but when it does not, it is important to consider and name what kinds of complex relations and contradictory dynamics are being foregrounded and which are missed or underexamined in the analysis and why.

This complexity may make the application of an intersectionality framework seem impossible, but it is useful to bear the following in mind: First, a comparative framework can help to navigate this complexity. In particular, as a way to maximize the analytic capacities of an intersectionality framework, it is necessary to go beyond the examination of one set of interactions and instead to compare multiple interactions, compare across many levels of social life, and compare interactions relationally. Such an approach would help to attend to the variation within and across social differences. Second, research and policy making are inevitably incomplete and partial endeavours. A singular project is simply inadequate to address all the complexities of difference. Thus, it is essential to undertake quantitative, qualitative, and mixed methods research, and to bring different intersectionality methodologies into dialogue with other methodologies that are grounded in social constructivism (rather than biomedical models in the case of health).

This book alone demonstrates the breadth of methodologies that are grounded in an intersectionality paradigm, from discourse analysis of policies, laws, and strategies adopted by governments and community organizations, to a social determinants approach, ethnography and auto-ethnography, regression modelling, narrative-based studies, participatory action and community-based research, photovoice, situated standpoint, statistical data analysis, interview and survey analysis, as well as analytic perspectives drawn from hybridity theory, post-colonial feminism, indigenous philosophies, and political economy approaches. Some of these methods are in tension with one another, all reveal the limits of knowing, and some have been narrowly defined (for example, as noted by some of the contributors, the social determinants approach has failed to adequately integrate indigenous philosophies and perspectives). However, the important point is that there is no single ideal way to undertake intersectionality work; in fact, different kinds of complementary research are essential.

Which Model?
A fourth issue raised in the theoretical literature regards the particular model that is used to describe and explain the relationship between multiple systems of power and multiple modes of identification. As noted, at the base of an intersectionality framework is the idea that a unitary approach or a multiple approach are insufficient. As Ange-Marie Hancock (2007b, 64) states, this means that more than one category is addressed, that categories matter equally and that the relationship between them is an open empirical question, that a dynamic interaction exists between individual and institutional

factors, that members within a category are diverse, that analysis of the individual or set of individuals is integrated with institutional analysis, and that empirical and theoretical claims are both possible and necessary.

On this basis, an intersectionality model does not view systems of power or modes of identification in isolation, precisely because these exist, perform, and function through one another. Nor are they outside the subject and therefore extractable as pure or contained and non-contradictory entities. They are not simply added to each other and overlapping, hierarchically structured whereby one mode of difference is assumed to be salient over others, or merely multi-dimensional. Instead, it is important to examine how specific interactions occur in specific contexts and how these function in relation to other interactions at different levels of life and across time and space.

Several intersectionality models have been developed over the years to capture this complexity. Some are presented in the context of specific case studies (see Chapter 14 this volume, for example) but have general applicability. One general model that serves to illustrate the paradigmatic shift in thinking that is constitutive of intersectionality is the image of a matrix. Although not entirely satisfactory, the matrix captures the complex webs of power that produce, organize, and govern difference. In particular, rather than seeing systems of domination as having independent effects, or conceptualizing systems as independent but overlapping, or perceiving one or more systems as more significant even though these mutually reinforce others (Weldon 2006, 240-44), the metaphor of a matrix is premised on the idea that systems of domination are mutually dependent but analytically distinct. The idea of a matrix has, of course, been developed by Collins in her first edition of *Black Feminist Thought* (1990, 225) and is taken up by numerous feminists (including some in this book). Collins deploys the notion of a "matrix of domination" to make the shift away from additive models of oppression, which, she rightly argues, "are firmly rooted in the either/or dichotomous thinking of Eurocentric, masculinist thought" (ibid.).

The matrix of domination, she states, refers to how intersecting oppressions, such as race and gender, are actually organized at structural, disciplinary, hegemonic, and interpersonal levels (Collins 2000, 18). More specifically, the matrix addresses the "overall social organization within which intersecting oppressions originate, develop and are contained" (ibid., 228-29). As one example, Collins cites case studies of black women who head households. She deploys the matrix idea so as to attend simultaneously to racially segmented local labour market and community patterns, changes in local political economies, and established racial and gender ideologies for a given location (Collins 1990, 224). By examining how these differing aspects function through one another, she argues that it becomes possible to "deconstruct Eurocentric, masculinist analyses that implicitly rely on controlling images of the matriarch or the welfare mother" and produce generalizations across national and international contexts (ibid.). In addition, the matrix model not only centres black women's experiences, but it also shows that subjects can revise constraining definitions of family and community, thereby revealing their agency.

The image of the matrix has three key interrelated advantages. First, since the matrix itself is structured at different levels, it does not conflate how interactive processes of differentiation and systems of domination function at various levels of social life (such as level of personal biography, cultural context, and institutionally). Nor does it separate these social levels but instead provides a way to make linkages between them. As such, the matrix model describes and explains the relationship between the micro and macro – namely, how specific processes of differentiation and systems of domination interactively operate in the context of the broader structure of power.

Second, this model shifts the focus from one set of interactive processes of differentiation and systems of domination to the *relationship* between multiple interactive processes and systems, and thus attends to the issues of complexity discussed above. In particular, the model concerns itself not only with a neglected intersection but with how various intersectional meanings and effects of power are relationally constituted and how they produce relational differences. Attention to these differences provides a way to be precise about a specific set of interactive processes and systems, to recognize that social locations vary even when the same kinds of interactive systems are at play (that is, interactions between racialization, disability and ability, and gendering have different manifestations), and to locate the pattern of interactive norms that is upheld through such representations of difference (such as, in this case, whiteness, ability, and masculinity).

Third, since the matrix model is predicated on the idea that processes of differentiation and systems of power rely on one another, it illustrates that it is not possible to critique and thus disrupt one process and system without simultaneously disrupting them all. Thus, racism cannot be disrupted without also disrupting sexism, capitalism, homophobia, transphobia, disableism, and so on. As Fellows and Razack (1998, 335-36) state, "systems of oppression (capitalism, imperialism, and patriarchy) rely on one another in complex ways. This 'interlocking' effect means that the systems of oppression come into existence in and through one another so that class exploitation could not be accomplished without gender and racial hierarchies, imperialism could not function without class exploitation, sexism, heterosexism, and so on. Because the systems rely on one another in these complex ways, it is ultimately futile to attempt to disrupt one system without simultaneously disrupting others." The matrix idea therefore keeps the overall conditions of difference formation and power front and centre, and in doing so, it directs attention to issues of social (in)justice.

Which Interactions?

The final issue raised in the theoretical literature that should be considered in the practical application of intersectionality concerns the problem of deciding which differences and interactions to examine. Of course, several factors shape this choice, including analytic intelligibility, data availability, an interest in the specific social identities and/or categories that are most directly affected, the findings of particular case studies, the emphasis of particular research subjects who draw from their own experiences, and topical political issues that gain the attention of the public or governments. In other words, there is no preset list for determining which differences and interactions are most salient; indeed, the choice is often made pragmatically by context, is shaped by what the analyst knows about the particular topic (for, as analysts we never come to a topic value-free), or arises from a sense of engaged subjectivity (what the analyst is passionate about or is directly or indirectly affected by). Regardless, it is necessary not to predetermine the scope of an intersectionality project in ways that close off unexpected findings. Indeed, only by keeping the selection of social interactions open can one perceive which are relevant, for sometimes the findings can reveal that some interactions are less relevant or more salient than expected, that more research is needed before establishing relevancy, or that the set of interactions must be expanded.

As well, it is important for researchers to be self-reflexive about their own positionality and their relationships of power to knowledge production and research subjects. Intersectionality should not be approached as an academic or community-based fad – ours is not a call to well-meaning scholars and policy makers to claim the domain of difference by appropriating studies about non-white women, non-white lesbians and queers, migrant trans-sexuals, or other marginalized people – but requires instead that the researcher situates herself in the social matrix of domination. This kind of situated framework has been especially successful through participatory and community-based research, which brings together academics and other stakeholders such as community partners and policy makers in order to actively define research questions and approaches, and to analyze and interpret data. This is a challenging process that demands a commitment to collaborative work, self-reflection about power dynamics, and a willingness to name uncomfortable relations of penalty and privilege. Therefore, it should not be idealized (Hankivsky et al. 2010). But, as many authors in this book argue, much evidence shows that the capacity of participatory and community-based research to illuminate the multiplicity of differences and key interacting systems is strengthened when individual experiences and perspectives are socially contextualized.

Moreover, though several factors may determine the choice of which interactions will be studied, the choice should be driven by the specific aspect of power that is to be critically analyzed, or, to put it differently, the site of struggle. This means that there is a need to step back and examine how specific interactive processes and systems function and how these affect social differences and people's lives in the context of a matrix of domination. Another way to put this is to say that what drives the research is a critique of how power operates and of its effects. Critiques of power have without doubt been the foundation of feminist intersectionality work: as a mode of critique, not only has intersectionality decentred woman as the normative subject (Brah and Phoenix 2004, 78), but it has also provided a way to critique everyday practices of othering, challenge modes of oppression and domination, render power visible, reconsider what we think we know and how, and challenge the separation of theory and practice. That is, an intersectionality framework provides a way to express, theorize, and act in social struggles. This praxis – the integral relationship between intersectionality theories and practices – can therefore generate agency and active citizenry: in exposing and challenging (established and emerging) dominant ways of organizing and responding to difference, intersectionality can further agendas of anti-oppression and social justice. This place-based oppositional ethos is intrinsic to this analytic framework.

To undertake intersectionality work is neither glamorous, nor without its challenges. Indeed, even in hegemonic feminist circles and other equality-seeking spaces, there is still much resistance to displacing the centrality of singular categories such as "woman" in favour of a more nuanced framework. But intersectionality work is "important work because people's lives depend on it" (Collins 2009, xi) and because, when social justice drives the research, it becomes possible to identify differentials in access and resources, what specific services are needed, what policy areas require institutional support and development, and how people are exercising their agency. In sum, for researchers, the choice of "which interactions" starts not with a particular set of interactions but with what an understanding of interactions reveals about how power functions, how to disrupt relations of domination, exploitation, powerlessness, violence, and how to foster agency and transformation.

A Theoretical Framework for Intersectionality Research

Drawing on the theoretical considerations identified above, we suggest that an ideal intersectionality framework includes the following considerations. First, whatever conceptual framework is employed, the historical foundations, contestability, and specificity of terms used in reference to it should be clearly laid out. Second, to be clear about what kinds of differences are to be analyzed and also to centre critiques of power, the emphasis needs to shift from a preoccupation with identities and categories of difference to an analysis of the interactive processes of differentiation that produce and govern subjects (and that subjects generate and resist), and how these processes work in relation to the systems of domination. Third, as a way to attend to the complexity underlying an intersectionality lens – namely, the multiplicity and relationality between systems that are distinct in character, content, and effect but that function and enable one another; the differing levels at which power operates and subject formation occurs; and the various degrees and forms of penalty and privilege that shape everyone's lives – there is enormous value in comparing the operation and effects of interactive processes of differentiation and systems of domination relationally, across one another, and at different levels. Such comparisons can be undertaken by deploying a range of quantitative, qualitative, and mixed methodologies. Fourth, in order to examine the relationships between interactions and how these function relationally and within a broader context, it is necessary to go beyond unidimensional, additive, and hierarchical models of analysis to deploy images such as the matrix, which better capture the complexity and the overall conditions in which difference is constituted and organized. Finally, though one must not predetermine which differences and inter-actions are significant to research and policy, it is nonetheless critical that the research and policy be directed by social justice agendas. Otherwise, they are inconsistent with intersectionality analysis.

Part 2: An Intersectionality Framework and Canadian Health Research and Policy

Despite significant theoretical developments, the potential of intersectional-ity frameworks has not been realized in the context of health research and policy (Carter, Sellers, and Squires 2002; Hankivsky et al. 2007; McCall 2005; Morrow and Hankivsky 2007). The challenges of applying theory have been well articulated and include the complexity and relevance of theory for ap-plied research and policy development and implementation. Some of the challenges also resonate with those highlighted in the theoretical section above. To begin, researchers in the mainstream health field find it difficult to interrogate their blind spots and are not clear about how to framework and design research in light of the variety and density of multiple differences (Davis 2008; Hankivsky et al. 2007; Lorber 2006). They remain uncertain as to how, when, and where an intersectionality method should be applied (Davis 2008, 78; Hankivsky and Cormier 2009), including how to determine whether all possible interactions might be relevant at all times or when some of them might be most salient (Bredström 2006; Verloo 2006). Thus, a dis-juncture remains between the theory and practice in health research and policy. Although this disjuncture can be difficult to reconcile, in this section, we aim to identify areas of consistency as well as existing gaps. We consider why these occur and provide some preliminary directions for applying the theory in the health research and policy fields, recognizing that the need to attend to issues of difference, as an intersectionality framework does, is urgent.

Although dual and multiple attachments have long been part of Canadian identity, and the most recent census data demonstrate that Canada is home to people of more than two hundred ethnic origins with increasing numbers identifying multiple ancestries (Statistics Canada 2008), most research emphasizes a single marker or small number of dominant expressions of difference. Although research is made easier by labelling people according to coherent and static categories, which are often treated as separate rather than overlapping (Morris and Bunjun 2007), this approach is inadequate for addressing "the complexity of social locations and experiences for understanding differences in health needs and outcomes" (Hankivsky and Cormier 2009, 6). In fact, it has great human and economic costs (Iyer, Sen, and Östlin 2008). However, Canadian health research and policy tend to lag behind intersectional theoretical developments in that they are still focused on identities and categories of difference, using an additive approach to understanding them and, to a lesser extent, examining select interactions between factors as frameworks of investigation.

Some explanation for this disconnection between theory and practice in conventional health research and policy may be found in the dominance of two existing approaches in the field, both of which attempt to deepen an understanding of difference but fail to attend to multiple processes of differentiation, systems of domination, and the complexities of difference, and also narrowly define social injustices and health inequities. The first approach to health disparities research in Canada and elsewhere often limits itself to considerations of socio-economic status and/or race/ethnicity, with little attention to sex and gender (Heymann et al. 2006; Weber 2006). In many instances, this research also fails to apply an analytic framework that understands disparities as occurring within the context of social power inequities. In other words, the focus on socio-economic status and race/ethnicity rather than the actual local, national, and global processes that produce economic inequity and racism has the effect of extracting the identity and category of difference from its context of power. As Lynn Weber and Deborah Parra-Medina (2003, 195) explain, "few health disparities researchers have addressed the conceptual distinction between distributional and relational conceptions of social inequalities or the measurement issues that accompany them." This is despite the established link between theory and practice in much intersectionality work that is based on lived social inequities and the basis of generating theories from the ground up.

The second approach – in part responding to the exclusion of sex and gender within health disparities research, gender-based analysis (GBA), and more recently, sex- and gender-based analyses (SGBA) – has privileged these dimensions of difference (sex and gender) over others: SGBA differs from GBA in its explicit emphasis on sex and on how sex interacts with gender to create health conditions, living conditions, and problems that are unique, more prevalent, and more serious, or for which there are distinct risk factors for women or men (Health Canada 2003a). GBA is supposed to *intersect with* a diversity analysis, and SGBA is meant to be applied *within the context of* a diversity framework, attending to the ways in which determinants such as ethnicity, socio-economic status, (dis)ability, sexual orientation, migration status, age, and geography interact with sex and gender to contribute to exposures to various risk factors, disease courses, and outcomes. The SGBA framework, however, maintains the primacy of sex and gender, resulting in a failure to accurately acknowledge and capture how sex and gender interact with or in fact may be less important than other factors (Hankivsky et al. 2007; Varcoe, Hankivsky, and Morrow 2007). This results in what an SGBA is intended to avoid – missing and misreading the experiences of a significant portion of the population (CIHR 2006).

In sum, even if the two approaches discussed in this section – that is, health disparities research that focuses on socio-economic status and/or race/ethnicity, and GBA/SGBA, which focuses on sex and gender – were to be combined, the problem of a race-class-gender trinity may remain. Moreover, the kind of relationships of difference/health disparities illuminated through the matrix model would be missed. To illustrate some of these concerns, and in particular, those related to GBA/SGBA, we draw on a research case study of cardiovascular disease, which appears in Health Canada's *Exploring Concepts of Gender and Health* (2003a).

A Case Study: Policy Research on Cardiovascular Disease

Exploring Concepts of Gender and Health is a key capacity-building tool for demonstrating to researchers, policy analysts, program managers, and decision makers how to include GBA in their work. The guide includes key concepts in GBA, how to integrate GBA within the research-policy-program development cycle, and case studies to exhibit in concrete terms how GBA can be a catalyst for change. Among its case studies is cardiovascular disease (CVD), which includes myocardial infarction, ischemic heart disease, valvular heart disease, peripheral vascular disease, arrhythmias, high blood pressure, and stroke. Even though CVD is the number-one killer of Canadians (Statistics Canada 2006), the privileging of sex and gender in *Exploring Concepts* demonstrates the exclusionary nature of GBA/SGBA.

According to *Exploring Concepts* (Health Canada 2003a, 20), CVD "has a history of being considered a men's disease," and the historical lack of attention to sex and gender differences "has had far reaching consequences for accurate diagnosis, effective treatment and prevention of cardiovascular disease (CVD) for women." In response, the document calls for more evidence-based research that focuses on both sex- and gender-based factors that combine to affect cardiovascular health. It explains that "we are learning that sex-based factors affect the presentation of symptoms of myocardial infarctions. Gender-related factors affect when women and men seek treatment as well as the responses of health practitioners to men and women presenting with cardiac symptoms" (ibid.). Although it is noted that "the combined effects of sex and gender, *in interaction with other health determinants,* affect health status, health system responses and eventual health outcomes" (ibid., emphasis added), with few exceptions – including references to Aboriginal women and diabetes, and the relationship between ethnicity, gender, socio-economic status, and stressors – the case study is limited to examples of sex and gender differences in CVD, specifically in the areas of risk factors, symptoms and patterns of disease, diagnosis and interventions, and outcomes of CVD.

Moreover, in making recommendations for the future, the guide emphasizes the need for CVD health promotion and disease prevention programs that take note of the differences in the social roles of women and men. It also calls for research on the underlying pathophysiology of heart disease and stroke, and how these differ for men and women, including research on the effectiveness of prevention interventions. Although it also advocates for "more research to investigate how other social determinants of health (e.g., income and poverty, culture and racism) have an impact on the development of CVD over a person's life cycle and how these determinants can be addressed to improve health outcomes for women and men" (Health Canada 2003a, 24), this point suggests an additive rather than an intersectionality framework, and it is not elaborated on or emphasized in any detail. This is further evidenced by the guide's conclusion: "This CVD case study illustrates the need to integrate an understanding of sex and gender into research methods and analyses" (ibid.). Although choosing these dimensions of difference in preference to others does illuminate some health disparities, the primacy assigned to the unitary categories of sex and gender not only occludes a more comprehensive understanding of the actual operations and effects of patriarchy and sexism as they relate to health, but it also masks difference among groups that are organized through processes of gendering, sometimes with the effect of erasing differences such as those related to transgender and transsexual identity (which also challenge the conventional relationship between sex and gender).

Stressing sex and gender in relation to CVD extends beyond Health Canada's *Exploring Concepts of Gender and Health.* For example, in 2004, the associate deputy minister of health stated that "we now know that the risk factors, symptoms and patterns of cardiovascular disease (CVD) are different for women and men. However CVD has not always been understood in terms of its sex and gender-based differences, and therefore has not been appropriately addressed by the health system. From studies on using aspirin as a preventative medicine, to doses of drugs for treatment, the exclusion of women in medical research on CVD has led to numerous potentially fatal pitfalls in both diagnosis and treatment for women" (CIHR 2004)."

Recently, Louise Pilote (2007, 789) and the Gender and Sex Determinants of Cardiovascular Disease: From Bench to Beyond team have asserted the "importance and contribution of sex and gender to the development, manifestation, management and outcomes of cardiovascular disease" and have identified key knowledge gaps that need to be addressed in order to "gain a better understanding of why cardiovascular disease affects women and men differently." In their review and identification of key knowledge gaps, they maintain the binary of women/men and marginalize factors beyond sex and gender in their assessment of CVD.

The lack of attention to how sex and gender interact with or are modified by other determinants of health or may be less relevant than other factors wrongly essentializes the experiences of women and men, reifies inequities among groups, and arguably leads to the production of faulty and incomplete knowledge (Hankivsky and Christoffersen 2008). The production of sex and gender differences is an important consideration. And yet, it cannot be assumed that these are the most important aspects of difference for conducting health research or for developing, implementing, or evaluating policy. If researchers continue to ignore the complexity of people's lives, the evidence base that is generated may reify rather than help to ameliorate a range of inequities (Hankivsky et al. 2007).

Specifically, a better understanding of difference-making is required, including how discourses and the materialities of sex and gender interact with and are affected by discourses of race/ethnicity, language, cultural background, disability, geography, and sexuality. And though it has been acknowledged that intersectionality theory has enormous potential to shape the future of SGBA (Clow et al. 2009), the position that we take here is that what is required is a framework that moves beyond GBA/SGBA that can evaluate and investigate the interaction of and relationship between numerous aspects of difference, not only at the individual level but also at structural levels. Recently, an important Canadian primer has emerged on applying an intersectionality perspective in the health field, providing new directions for research and policy development (Hankivsky and Cormier 2009). The framework outlined in this primer resonates with the tenets of the ideal theoretically informed intersectionality analysis presented here. Most importantly, both prioritize capturing the multiple interactive processes and systems that shape individual lives and health, and that structure social disparities, without producing overdetermined accounts of social groups and social categories. In practice, however, this is an ideal that researchers and policy makers can only strive to realize. Nevertheless, revisiting the case study of CVD clarifies the various ways in which an intersectionality-based analysis differs from that of GBA or SGBA.

CVD through an Intersectionality Framework

To ground this analysis, it is useful to begin by considering the implications of highlighting CVD mortality along male/female binaries. Narrowly reporting that CVD causes 31 percent of male deaths and 33 percent of female deaths (Statistics Canada 2006) obscures the rates of mortality among vulnerable subgroups. For example, compared to the general Canadian population, CVD is 1.5 times more prevalent among First Nations and Inuit populations (Health Canada 2007). Aboriginal women experience higher death rates than the general Canadian female population for both ischemic heart disease and stroke (Foundation 1999). Refugees have higher incidence and mortality rates for cardiovascular diseases than other immigrants (DesMeules et al. 2004). South Asians have the highest CVD mortality, compared with individuals of Chinese and European descent (Gupta, Singh, and Verma 2006; Sheth et al. 1999). Those with less than post-secondary education and women living in northern, remote, and rural communities are also less likely than their southern counterparts to die from CVD (WHI 2006). Similar conclusions are also evident outside the Canadian context. For instance, though CVD is recognized as the leading cause of death and disease in the United States, it is acknowledged that CVD is disproportionately experienced by racial/ethnic and low-income groups (USDHHS 2002). In the UK, it has been reported that the incidence and prevalence of coronary heart disease is higher in ethnic minority communities than in those of their white counterparts (Khunti and Samani 2003). Indigenous Australians have higher CVD mortality rates than the general population (AIHW 2002).

Although such differences focus on specific identity groups rather than processes of differentiation or systems of domination, they show the value of analyzing differences beyond the scope of sex and gender. Yet, despite such emerging evidence, it is also true that "most ... knowledge about prevention and treatment derives from studies conducted in developed countries and predominantly among white populations" (Yusuf et al. 2001b, 2862). Moreover, though it is also true that most traditional CVD research, including clinical trials, has excluded women, the current prioritization of sex and gender raises questions that are central to understanding power within an intersectionality framework: Who is being studied and why? Who is being compared to whom and why? (Hankivsky and Cormier 2009; Lorber 2006). And, of course, what are the real consequences for morbidity and mortality if researchers fail to undertake inclusive CVD research, including the uncovering of the fundamental causes and full range of experiences surrounding CVD?

It has been recognized that coronary heart disease is "a multifactorial disease, and a multiplicity of interacting factors are involved in its development" (Ockene and Ockene 1992). In fact, there are so many interrelationships between the complex levels of influence on CVD, which are so poorly understood that "no recent publication has attempted a comprehensive causal path diagram depicting them" (Frank et al. 2006, 18). Because of its unique defining features, an intersectionality framework can be instructive in starting the work of both identifying and better understanding the factors, relationships, and processes that are essential for advancing the evidence base around CVD so as to attend to the diversity of the Canadian population. It can answer questions that traditional methods of inquiry cannot address because it focuses on the relationship between multiple aspects of difference simultaneously; as a result, it promotes an understanding of, as Gita Sen (2008) argues, "better slices of reality."

First, intersectionality does not presume – a priori – the importance of one mode of difference over another. Instead, it encourages a contextual analysis that probes beneath single identities, experiences, and social locations to consider a range of axes of difference to better understand any situation of disadvantage (Yuval-Davis 2006, 194). There is some overlap between an intersectionality framework and the social determinants perspective, which provides evidence that "the greatest effect on whether people develop life-threatening diseases is usually from factors out of their personal control and fundamentally tied to culture and socioeconomic status" (Wharf Higgins et al. 2006, 222). Intersectionality, however, seeks to broaden the range of factors beyond socio-economic status and culture, which so often dominate determinants of health literature. And yet, this is in stark contrast to how CVD has been researched. Certain researchers such as Dennis Raphael (2002) have called for a lifespan approach for examining the links between determinants such as income and health, including CVD. But at this time, little research has even begun to examine any issues of difference in relation to CVD, let alone intersecting factors and their counterpart interacting processes. Indeed, the cultural influences and experiences of developing and having CVD are in their nascent stages of investigation (Daly et al. 2002; King et al. 2007; King et al. 2006; Wong and Wong 2003).

In response, Kathryn M. King et al. (2007, 806) have argued that "given the exceptional burden of CVD and the diversity of Canada's population – strategies for CVD risk reduction need to explicitly incorporate ethnocultural affiliation and gender." Importantly, King et al. signal the need to consider the relation between variables; her recommendation, however, is only one possible starting point for improving the breadth and depth of CVD research as it is necessary to go beyond an additive approach, expand the analysis even beyond ethnocultural affiliation and gender, avoid essentialist characterizations of difference that do not attend to relations of privilege and penalty, and contextualize health disparities within a matrix of domination.

Second, research framed under the umbrella of intersectionality often begins from the premise that individuals have subjective knowledge of their own lives and the context in which they live. For instance, the Native Women's Association of Canada (NWAC 2007, 14) recently asserted that "we Aboriginal women of Canada have a collective history and intimate knowledge of our health determinants and needs, and the relationship of these with those of Aboriginal men ... and our children, as well as our communities." Accordingly, it is important to consider whether research is being generated through genuine collaboration between researchers and researched. On this basis, with regard to CVD, the choice of which interactions to examine is, in part at least, shaped by the power of communities to define their own "health problems"; this requires critical reflection of the authority of researchers within that relationship. Although such analyses may include behavioural and physiological risk factors, response to these will follow actions on risk conditions or psychosocial risk factors in which community self-determination is respected (Raphael 2002). This type of involvement, which prioritizes experiences from those who are actually affected by research and policy decisions, may also ensure that representations of difference or systems of domination that influence health, like CVD, are not essentialized by researchers and are more fully examined and understood. And, this may lay the ground for bottom-up social justice analysis and collective action for change. At the same time, though there needs to be accountability to the communities served by a policy (because lived experiences inform policy and indicate whether it is successful), policy making needs to be self-reflexive, specifically so as to shift the gaze from the othered to the processes of othering and normalization.

Third, and simultaneously, an intersectionality framework would also ask whether research and policy are properly framed within current cultural, societal, and/or situational and institutional contexts, and thus attend to the differing levels of analysis that Collins and Yuval-Davis identify. This is especially important in terms of CVD. In the effort to reduce the incidence and costs of CVD, a significant amount of research and most heart health policies in Canada and elsewhere focus on CVD risk factors such as smoking, alcohol, physical inactivity, obesity, high blood pressure, high blood cholesterol, and on modifying behaviours that increase these risks, whereby the onus is on the individual. For example, until recently the Canadian Heart Health Initiative focused on risk factors and health behaviours. The new strategy does prioritize the cross-cutting theme of reducing the impact of cardiovascular outcomes that results from disparities, but it continues to prioritize as a key theme the prevention, detection, and management of major risk factors. Other examples of such foci include the 2005 Public Health Agency of Canada's (PHAC) Healthy Living Strategy, which targets three areas: healthy eating, physical activity, and healthy weight, hoping to improve all by 2015. A Healthy Heart Kit, made available on the PHAC website by Health Canada and the Heart and Stroke Foundation of Canada, also emphasizes "lifestyle factors" (PHAC 1999, 2003).

From an intersectional perspective, individual-level strategies, which focus on medical and lifestyle risk factors, may ignore the social processes of differentiation by which structural factors at both micro and macro levels shape the development, experiences, and outcomes of CVD as well as other diseases. As Alan Petersen and Deborah Lupton (1996, 29) argue, "risk is not a static, objective phenomenon, but is constantly constructed and negotiated as part of the network of social interaction and the formation of meaning." Similarly, attempts to implement prescriptive health information are "embedded within social relations of gender, class, ethnoracial group membership, and ability" (Angus 2008, 92) that are rarely acknowledged or understood. Not surprisingly, programs and interventions that are aimed at risk modification and self-care tend to have poor outcomes as they are useful to a limited number of people – namely, those who are wealthier and more educated (Wharf Higgins et al. 2006). Moreover, policies often "blame" individuals for their health problems while ignoring, for example, the effects of systemic discrimination within the health care system itself, which provides different care and treatment for vulnerable subgroups.

For instance, South Asian ethnicity is an independent predictor of poor outcomes after coronary bypass grafting (Brister et al. 2007). Racial/ethnic differences in cardiac care have been well documented (Halwani 2004; Lillie-Blanton et al. 2002; Mensah et al. 2003), whereby cardiac rehabilitation is available to a very small number of Canadian patients (Rachlis 2004, 298). In the US, research has demonstrated that African Americans and Latinos receive poorer treatment in the health care system than whites (Weber and Fore 2007, 197). African Americans are less likely than whites to undergo costly invasive cardiovascular procedures, and Hispanics are less likely than whites to receive catheterization and percutaneous transluminal coronary angioplasty (Ford, Newman, and Deosaransingh 2000). Though none of these studies adequately problematize identity categories (and thus tend to essentialize social differences), they are important insofar as they alert policy researchers/makers to the ways in which health is shaped by processes of racialization and systems of white privilege. Situating health disparities within a social context is a key step in moving toward an intersectionality framework.

Based on such research, a convincing body of evidence thus now exists to indicate that economic and social conditions, rather than medical treatments and lifestyle choices, are the major factors determining whether persons develop CVD (Raphael 2002; Tanuseputro et al. 2003; Wharf Higgins et al. 2006). For example, even after traditional risk factors are controlled, people living in lower-income areas are much more likely to be obese, to smoke, to be physically inactive, and to develop CVD when compared to those in well-off neighbourhoods (Diez Roux et al. 2001; HSF 2006). Rural populations, especially Aboriginal persons living in rural areas, have high risks of CVD (Monsalve et al. 2005). Julia Wong and Shirley Wong's study (2003) analyzing the dataset from the National Population Health Survey found that immigrant women tended to have worse CVD risk factors than non-immigrant women (regardless of race or birth country). Significant variation in CVD has been established along the lines of age, sex, ethnic group, and geographic areas (Anand et al. 2006; Franzini and Spears 2003; Tanuseputro et al. 2003). Overall, however, the available research is sparse in terms of understanding the differences in risk factors between groups, and little attention has been paid to the broader contexts that shape and influence the risk factors for heart disease or stroke. Here, an intersectionality framework would be invaluable, not only because it would provide a more nuanced and multi-faceted understanding of how various interacting social processes of differentiation affect the health of variously positioned social groups differently, but also because it would set an understanding of disparities within the overall conditions of domination – namely, Canada's matrix of domination.

One area where this kind of contextualization is apparent is in the evaluation of government policies. These have not gone unnoticed in the literature, but even well-intentioned analyses highlight the importance of making the links between policy, the reduction of CVD risk factors, and the improvement of personal health practices. This is reflected in the Health Canada (2003b, 67) statement that attention should be paid to public policies because they "can mediate the effect of inequities in risk for CVD by decreasing exposure to risk factors or facilitating the adoption of healthy behaviours." What is often missing from such interpretations is that government creates policies that shape political, economic, and social contexts, which in turn cause poverty, inequality, and social exclusion. This has led researchers such as Joan Wharf Higgins et al. (2006, 223) to conclude that "there is little North American research that is devoted to understanding how the social determinants of health relate to CVD."

Significantly, even if better attention were paid to socio-economic conditions *in addition* to risk factors, this would not necessary tell the whole story. Though not dealing specifically with CVD, Tony Blakely et al. (2006) have shown that smoking (a risk factor) contributes to approximately 10 percent of the difference in mortality rates between Maori and Pakeha (Europeans) in New Zealand, and that socio-economic disparities explain another third of the gap. The researchers highlight that this leaves an almost eight-to-nine-year difference in life expectancy unaccounted for and in need of further investigation. An intersectionality analysis may help to inform such explorations of knowledge gaps by directing researchers to pay explicit attention to issues of power, specifically so as to develop policies that address social inequities as they relate to health. In Canada, this means that it is important to examine the ways in which societal norms, typically characterized by the Eurocentric values of white, able-bodied, heterosexual, middle-class men, are shaped by those who have power (Hankivsky and Christoffersen 2008).

In a settler nation such as Canada, the effects of colonialism and the role of immigration are especially important to examine in the health context, but these remain obscured even by well-intentioned researchers. As Sonia S. Anand et al. (2001) concluded, since a significant proportion of Aboriginal people live in poverty, which is a risk factor for CVD, improvements to their socio-economic status may be key to reducing CVD within this population group. And yet, as is the case in many health studies, the authors do not explicitly link socio-economic status and colonialism. It is not possible to fully comprehend the current status of Aboriginal health and well-being – in its diversity – without acknowledging the legacies, ongoing treatment, and racism experienced by this population in Canada and elsewhere (Browne and Fiske 2001; Kirmayer, Brass, and Tait 2000; Stephens et al. 2006; Waldrum, Herring, and Young 2006). As Mohawk scholar/activist Taiaiake Alfred (2005, 163) has argued, though diversity exists among the Onkehonwe (original peoples), health problems are a main legacy of colonial dislocation and physical dispossession of the land: "The social and health problems besetting Onkehonwe are the logical result of a situation wherein people respond or adapt to unresolved colonial injustices." Such problems are evident in colonial psychologies of self-hating, repressed rage, drug and alcohol dependency, and an overall social climate of racism. As a response to these problems, Taiaiake Alfred and Jeff Corntassel (2005, 613) develop a framework for a resurgent indigenous movement, which includes a commitment to decolonize the diet. In this regard, they link the physical body to the ongoing conditions of colonialism and practices of reindigenization, and thereby contextualize the processes of differentiation in a way that is consistent with an intersectionality framework.

Immigration is also a significant site through which to operationalize an intersectionality framework, not only because just over one in five Canadians is a first-generation immigrant, but also because, since 2001, a growing body of literature has shown the differences between immigrant and non-immigrant health. The identity and category of "immigrant" needs to be problematized because it carries notions of a non-white person who is professionally challenged and has a particular labour market location (Folson 2004, 30).

Furthermore, we do not know enough about differences between and among immigrant populations. Claudio E. Pérez (2002) has demonstrated that, though immigrant men have a lower risk of heart disease than Canadian-born men, this difference disappears after ten years (Newbold and Danforth 2003). The reasons for this change are often linked to dietary factors associated with migrating to Western environments (Yusuf et al. 2001a). Significant gaps remain, however, in understanding the full effects of migration, dislocation, isolation, Canadian immigration policies, stress, and the loss of identity, language, culture, and meaningful employment as factors in CVD (Buzzelli and Newbold 2006; Oxman-Martinez and Hanley 2005; Sheth et al. 1999; Shookner and Chin-Yee 2003).

Furthermore, an understanding of CVD in Canada must also be linked to the global context, including global factors, processes, and the changes that have been occurring internationally. In their examination of CVD, Salim Yusuf et al. (2001b, 2862) observed that "social and economic transitions have resulted in major changes in population demography, industrial structure, income levels, expenditure patterns, education levels, family structures, eating habits and physical activity." Salim Yusuf et al. (2001a, 2751) reveal why space is an important intersection by explaining, "with urbanization ... there is a decrease in energy expenditure (through less physical activity) and a loss of the traditional social support mechanisms. In addition to increased migration of individuals from rural to urban areas, rural areas are themselves also being transformed. For example, increased mechanization in agriculture and increased use of automobile and bus transportation in rural areas are leading to a decrease in physical activity." And finally, as Roger S. Magnusson (2007, 3, emphasis in original) explains, "globalization creates ... new *process challenges* to an effective response to national health problems." That is, coordinated strategies including all relevant global actors are required to ensure that the appropriate groundwork for population-wide health improvements, including in CVD, can be realized. These national and global considerations can be more fully examined through an intersectionality framework because the emphasis is on different levels of socio-political life and the relational dynamics between interactive micro and macro processes of differentiation and systems of domination.

Overall, an intersectionality framework embraces rather than avoids the complexities that are essential to understanding social inequities, which in turn manifest in health inequities. From this perspective, social and health disparities, including those which shape and mediate experiences of illness, are seen as interactive and contextual. Intersectionality provides a lens through which to understand the cumulative, interlocking, and historically embedded influences on experiences, opportunities, and life chances, including risk factors for, experiences of, treatment, and outcomes of diseases, such as CVD. In opening new avenues of inquiry, it also points to how effective comparative research is at different levels of analysis for understanding the various experiences of CVD.

Conclusion

A key challenge for mainstream health research and policy, as noted above and as demonstrated by the CVD case study, is that the discourse lags far behind theoretical developments, many of which are rooted in existing oppressive practices and practices of resistance. At a practical level, an "ideal" intersectionality-based analysis requires the development of new approaches that cross health pillar and disciplinary boundaries, and that experiment with a range of existing methodologies (such as quantitative, qualitative, and mixed methods). As Weber and Parra-Medina (2003, 223) state, this requires "funding for research and practice into how to conduct interdisciplinary work that truly achieves an integration of ideas," which may be challenging in political contexts where funding cuts and other crises such as the 2008 global economic downturn make it difficult to advocate for resources necessary for such work. It also requires health information and data that best represent multiple groups and reflect significant variations within those groups across genders, socio-economic statuses, social classes, and sexual orientations (Weber 2006), so that comparisons can be made across interactions without essentialist conclusions, and inequities can be understood in terms of processes of differentiation and systems of domination. At present, there is a paucity of research and data, including linked databases and other surveys, that can provide the information necessary for a fully developed and robust intersectionality analysis. In sum, what is clear is that much more work is required to even begin to grasp what an ideal intersectional-type framework may look like in health research and policy.

Nevertheless, as we have attempted to illustrate, and as the following chapters will demonstrate, even at this point in health research and policy evolution, intersectionality, in all its assortments and stages of development, provides productive avenues for moving investigations of health disparities forward. Intersectionality demands that health policy researchers and policy makers begin to ask new and different questions. Using this framework will not, of course, lead to a complete understanding of any type of phenomenon, for – at any given point in time – it is possible to garner only a partial perspective on power. Indeed, partiality and contextual knowledge are intrinsic to intersectionality work. This does not take away from the fact that such work, as will be illustrated throughout this collection, has great potential for improving the existing evidence base. Indeed, one of the primary goals of an intersectionality framework is the inclusion of previously ignored and excluded populations. This has considerable implications for health research and policy because it requires analysts to be transparent about who has been the subject of inquiry and who has been excluded from the benefits of research that provides evidence for programs, services, and policies. Thus, it can drive research and policy to be more responsive to social justice agendas and in the process counter relations of privilege and penalty. This is when an intersectionality framework is at its best. Similarly, Hancock (2007b, 73) argues that it provides "the best chance for an effective diagnosis and ultimately an effective prescription" for social and health problems.

Note

1 Sections of this chapter appear also in "Considerations for Mainstreaming Intersectionality," *Political Research Quarterly* (forthcoming January 2011). The authors wish to acknowledge permission granted by the journal for the reprinting of these excerpts.

References

AIHW. 2002. *Australia's health 2002*. Canberra: Australian Institute for Health and Welfare.

Alfred, T. 2005. *Wasáse: Indigenous pathways of action and freedom*. Peterborough: Broadview Press.

Alfred, T., and J. Corntassel. 2005. Being indigenous: Resurgences against contemporary colonialism. *Government and Opposition* 40(4): 597-614.

Anand, S.S., F. Razak, A.D. Davis, R. Jacobs, V. Vuksan, K. Teol, and S. Yusuf. 2006. Social disadvantage and cardiovascular disease: Development of an index and analysis of age, sex, and ethnicity effects. *International Journal of Epidemiology* 35(5): 1239-45.

Anand, S.S., S. Yusuf, R. Jacobs, A.D. Davis, Q. Yi, H. Gerstein, P.A. Montague, and E. Lonn. 2001. Risk factors, atherosclerosis, and cardiovascular disease among Aboriginal people in Canada: The Study of Health Assessment and Risk Evaluation in Aboriginal Peoples (SHARE-AP). *Lancet* 358(9288): 1147-53.

Angus, J. 2008. Contesting coronary candidacy: Reframing risk modification in coronary heart disease. In *Contesting illness: Processes and practices*, ed. P. Moss and K. Teghtsoonian, 90-106. Toronto: University of Toronto Press.

Anthias, F. 1998. Rethinking social divisions: Some notes towards a theoretical framework. *Sociological Review* 46(3): 557-80.

–. 2001. Beyond feminism and multiculturalism: Locating difference and the politics of location. *Women's Studies International Forum* 25(3): 275-86.

Anthias, F., and N. Yuval-Davis. 1983. Contextualizing feminism: Gender, ethnic, and class divisions. *Feminist Review* 15: 62-75.

–. 1992. *Racialized boundaries: Race, nation, gender, colour and class and the anti-racist struggle*. London and New York: Routledge.

Bates, L.M., O. Hankivsky, and K.W. Springer. 2009. Gender and health inequities: A comment on the Final Report of the WHO Commission on the Social Determinants of Health. *Social Science and Medicine* 69(7): 1002-4.

Blakely, T., J. Fawcett, D. Hunt, and N. Wilson. 2006. What is the contribution of smoking and socioeconomic position to ethnic inequalities in mortality in New Zealand? *Lancet* 368(9529): 44-52.

Brah, A., and A. Phoenix. 2004. Ain't I a woman? Revisiting intersectionality. *Journal of International Women's Studies* 5(3): 75-86.

Bredström, A. 2006. Intersectionality: A challenge for feminist HIV/AIDS research? *European Journal of Women's Studies* 13(3): 245-58.

Brister, S.J., Z. Hamdulay, S. Verma, M. Maganti, and M.R. Buchanan. 2007. Ethnic diversity: South Asian ethnicity is associated with increased coronary artery bypass grafting mortality. *Journal of Thoracic and Cardiovascular Surgery* 133(1): 150-54.

Browne, A., and J. Fiske. 2001. First Nations women's encounters with mainstream health care services. *Western Journal of Nursing Research* 23(2): 126-47.

Buzzelli, M., and B. Newbold. 2006. *Immigrant rites of passage: Urban settlement, physical environment quality and health in Vancouver.* Paper 06-12. Vancouver: Centre for Research on Immigration and Integration in the Metropolis (RIIM), Vancouver Office of the Metropolis Project.

Carter, P., S.L. Sellers, and C. Squires. 2002. Reflections on race/ethnicity, class, and gender inclusive research. *African American Perspectives* 8(1): 111-24.

CIHR. 2004. What's sex and gender got to do with it? Integrating sex and gender into health research. Final Report prepared by the Canadian Institutes of Health Research. http://www.cihr-irsc.gc.ca/.

–. 2006. Gender and sex-based analysis in health research: A guide for CIHR researchers and reviewers. Canadian Institutes of Health Research. http://www.cihr-irsc.gc.ca/.

Clow, B., A. Pederson, M. Haworth-Brockman, and J. Bernier. 2009. *Rising to the challenge: Sex and gender-based analysis for health planning, policy and research in Canada.* Halifax: Atlantic Centre of Excellence for Women's Health.

Collins, P.H. 1990. *Black feminist thought: Knowledge, consciousness, and the politics of empowerment.* Boston: Unwin Hyman.

–. 2000. *Black feminist thought: Knowledge, consciousness and the politics of empowerment.* New York and London: Routledge.

–. 2009. Building knowledge and transforming institutions. In *Emerging intersections: Race, class and gender in theory, policy and practice,* ed. B.T. Dill and R.E. Zambrana, vii-xiv. Chapel Hill: Rutgers University Press.

Collins, P.Y., H. von Unger, and A. Armbrister. 2008. Church ladies, good girls, and locas: Stigma and the intersection of gender, ethnicity, mental illness, and sexuality in relation to HIV risk. *Social Science and Medicine* 7(3): 389-97.

Crenshaw, K. 1989. Demarginalizing the intersection of race and sex: A black feminist critique of antidiscrimination doctrine, feminist theory and antiracist politics. *University of Chicago Legal Forum:* 139-67.

–. 1994. Mapping the margins: Intersectionality, identity politics, and violence against women of colour. In *The public nature of private violence,* ed. M.A. Fineman and R. Mykitiul, 93-118. New York and London: Routledge.

–. 1997. Intersectionality and identity politics: Learning from violence against women of colour. In *Reconstructing political theory: Feminist perspectives,* ed. M.L. Shanley and U. Narayan, 178-93. University Park: Pennsylvania State University Press.

Daly, J., P. Davidson, E. Chang, K. Hancock, D. Rees, and D.R. Thompson. 2002. Cultural aspects of adjustment to coronary heart disease in Chinese-Australians: A review of the literature. *Journal of Advanced Nursing* 39(4): 391-99.

D'aoust, V. 1999. Complications: The deaf community, disability and being a lesbian mom – A conversation with myself. In *Restricted access: Lesbians on disability,* ed. S. Raffo, 115-23. Seattle: Seal Press.

Davis, K. 2008. Intersectionality as buzzword: A sociology of science on what makes a feminist theory successful. *Feminist Theory* 9(1): 67-85.

DesMeules, M., J. Gold, A. Kazanjian, D. Manuel, J. Payne, B. Vissandjée, S. McDermott, and Y. Mao. 2004. New frameworks to immigrant health assessment. *Canadian Journal of Public Health* 95(3): 22-26.

Dhamoon, R. 2009. *Identity/difference politics: How difference is produced, and why it matters.* Vancouver: UBC Press.

Diez Roux, A.V., S.S. Merkin, D. Arnett, L. Chambless, M. Massing, F.J. Nieto, P. Sorlie, M. Szklo, H.A. Tyroler, and R.L. Watson. 2001. Neighborhood of residence and incidence of coronary heart disease. *New England Journal of Medicine* 345(5): 99-106.

Doyal, L. 2009. Challenges in researching life with HIV/AIDS: An intersectional analysis of black African migrants in London. *Culture, Health and Sexuality* 11(2): 173-88.

El-Khoury, M.Y., M.A. Dutton, and L.A. Goodman. 2004. Ethnic differences in battered women's formal help-seeking strategies: A focus on health, mental health, and spirituality. *Cultural Diversity and Ethnic Minority Psychology* 10: 383–93.

Fellows, M.L., and S. Razack. 1998. The race to innocence: Confronting hierarchal relations among women. *Journal of Gender, Race and Justice* 1(2): 335-52.

Folson, R.B. 2004. Representation of the immigrant. In *Calculated kindness: Global restructuring, immigration and settlement in Canada,* ed. R.B. Folson, 21-32. Halifax: Fernwood.

Ford, E., J. Newman, and K. Deosaransingh. 2000. Racial and ethnic differences in the use of cardiovascular procedures: Findings from the California Cooperative Cardiovascular Project. *American Journal of Public Health* 90: 1128-34.

Foucault, M. 1982. Afterword: The subject and power. In *Michel Foucault: Beyond structuralism and hermeneutics with an afterword by Michel Foucault,* ed. H.L. Dreyfus and P. Rabinow, 208-26. Chicago: University of Chicago Press.

Foundation, H.S. 1999. The changing face of heart disease and stroke in Canada 2000. Public Agency of Canada. http://www.phac-aspc.gc.ca.

Frank, J., G. Lomax, P. Beard, and M. Locke. 2006. Interactive role of genes and the environment. In *In healthier societies: From analysis to action,* ed. J. Heymann, C. Hertzman, M.L. Barer, and R.G. Evans, 11-34. Oxford: Oxford University Press.

Franzini, L., and W. Spears. 2003. Contributions of social context to inequalities in years of life lost to heart disease in Texas, USA. *Social Science and Medicine* 57(10): 1847-61.

Garland-Thomson, R. 2002. Integrating disability, transforming feminist theory. *NWSA Journal* 14(3): 1-32.

Gupta, M., N. Singh, and S. Verma. 2006. South Asians and cardiovascular risk: What clinicians should know. *Circulation* 113: e924-e929.

Halwani, S. 2004. Racial inequality in access to health care services. Paper presented at "Race Policy Dialogue Conference," Ontario Human Rights Commission. http://www.ohrc.on.ca.

Hancock, A.-M. 2007a. Intersectionality as a normative and empirical paradigm. *Politics and Gender* 3(2): 248-54.

–. 2007b. When multiplication doesn't equal quick addition: Examining intersectionality as a research paradigm. *Perspectives on Politics* 5(1): 63-79.

Hankivsky, O., L. Blackwood, R. Hunt, S. Pigg, M. Morrow, C. Reid, and C. Patton. 2007. Gender, diversity and evidence-based decision making. *Health Law in Canada* 28(1): 1-15.

Hankivsky, O., and A. Christoffersen. 2008. Intersectionality and the determinants of health: A Canadian perspective. *Critical Public Health* 18(3): 271-83.

Hankivsky, O., and R. Cormier. 2009. *Intersectionality: Moving women's health research and policy forward.* Vancouver: Women's Health Research Network.

Hankivsky, O., C. Reid, R. Cormier, C. Varcoe, N. Clark, C. Benoit, and S. Brotman. 2010. Exploring the promises of intersectionality for advancing women's health research. *International Journal for Equity in Health* 9(5): 1-15.

Harper, P.B., A. McClintock, J.E. Munoz, and T. Rosen, eds. 1997. Queer transexions of race, nation and gender: An introduction. *Social Text* 52-53: 1-4.

Hawley, J.C., ed. 2001. *Post colonial, queer: Theoretical intersections.* New York: State University of New York Press.

Health Canada. 2003a. Exploring concepts of gender and health. Women's Health Bureau, Health Canada. http://www.hc-sc.gc.ca/hl-vs/alt_formats/hpb-dgps/pdf/exploring_concepts.pdf.

–. 2003b. The growing burden of heart disease and stroke in Canada: 2003. Heart and Stroke Foundation. http://www.cvdinfobase.ca.

–. 2007. First Nations, Inuit and Aboriginal health: Diseases and health conditions. Government of Canada. http://www.hc-sc.gc.ca.

Heymann, J., C. Hertzman, M.L. Barer, and R.G. Evans. 2006. *Healthier societies: From analysis to action.* Oxford: Oxford University Press.

hooks, b. 1981. *Ain't I a woman? Black women and feminism.* Boston: South End Press.

–. 1984. *Feminist theory: From margin to center.* New York: South End Press.

–. 1989. *Talking back: Thinking feminist, thinking black.* Boston: South End Press.

HSF. 2006. Tipping the scales of progress: Heart disease and stroke in Canada 2006. Heart and Stroke Foundation. http://www.heartandstroke.com/atf/cf/%7B99452D8B-E7F1-4BD6-A57D-B136CE6C95BF%7D/Tipping_the_Scales_new.pdf.

Iyer, A., G. Sen, and P. Östlin. 2008. The intersections of gender and class in health status and health care. *Global Public Health* 3(1): 13-24.

Jakubowicz, A., and H. Meekosha. 2003. Can multiculturalism encompass disability? In *Disability, culture and identity,* ed. N. Watson, 180-99. Harlow, UK: Pearson Education.

Kelly, U.A. 2009. Integrating Intersectionality and Biomedicine in Health Disparities Research. *Advances in Nursing Science* 32(2): E42–E56.

Khunti, K., and N.J. Samani. 2003. Improving the delivery of coronary care for ethnic minorities. *Heart* 89: 479-80.

Kohn, L.P., and K.M. Hudson. 2002. Gender, ethnicity and depression: Intersectionality and context in mental health research with African American women. *African American Research Perspectives* 8: 174–84.

King, D.K. 1988. Multiple jeopardy, multiple consciousness: The context of a black feminist ideology. *Signs: Journal of Women in Culture and Society* 14(1): 42-72.

King, K.M., P. LeBlanc, W. Carr, and H. Quan. 2007. Chinese immigrants' management of their cardiovascular disease risk. *Western Journal of Nursing Research* 29(7): 804-26.

King, K.M., P. LeBlanc, J. Sanguins, and C.M. Mather. 2006. Gender-based challenges faced by older Sikh women as immigrants: Re-organizing and acting on the risk of coronary artery disease. *Canadian Journal of Nursing Research* 38(1): 16-40.

Kirkness, V. 1986-88. Emerging Native women. *Canadian Journal of Women and Law* 2(2): 408-15.

Kirmayer, L.J., G.M. Brass, and C.L. Tait. 2000. The mental health of Aboriginal peoples: Transformations of identity and community. *Canadian Journal of Psychiatry* 45(7): 607-16.

Kliewer, C., and L.M. Fitzgerald. 2001. Disability, schooling and the artifacts of colonialism. *Teachers College Record* 103(3): 450-70.

Lillie-Blanton, M., O.E. Rushing, S. Ruiz, R. Mayberry, and L. Boone. 2002. Racial/ethnic differences in cardiac care: The weight of evidence. Prepared for the Henry J. Kaiser Family Foundation and Morehouse School of Medicine. http://www.kff.org.

Lorber, J. 2006. Shifting paradigms and challenging categories. *Social Problems* 53(4): 448-53.

Lorde, A. 1984. *Sister outsider.* New York: Crossing Press.

Magnusson, R.S. 2007. Non-communicable diseases and global health governance: Enhancing global processes to improve health development. *Global Health* 3(2): 1-16.

Martinez, E. 1993. Beyond black/white: The racisms of our time. *Social Justice* 20(1-2): 22-34.

Matsuda, M.J. 1992. When the first quail calls: Multiple consciousness as jurisprudential method. *Women's Rights Law Reporter* 14: 297-300.

McCall, L. 2005. The complexity of intersectionality. *Signs: Journal of Women in Culture and Society* 30(3): 1771-1800.

Mensah, G.A., A.H. Mokdad, E.S. Ford, K.J. Greenlund, and J.B. Croft. 2003. State of disparities in cardiovascular health in the United States. *Circulation* 111(10): 1233-41.

Monsalve, M.V., H.V. Thommasen, G. Pachev, and J. Frochlich. 2005. Differences in cardiovascular risks in the Aboriginal and Non-Aboriginal people living in Bella Coola, British Columbia. *Medical Science Monitor* 11(1): CR21-28.

Monture, P.A. 2007. Racing and erasing: Law and gender in white settler societies. In *Race and racism in 21st century Canada: Continuity, complexity, and change,* ed. S.P. Hier and B.S. Bolaria, 197-216. Peterborough: Broadview Press.

Morris, M., and B. Bunjun. 2007. Using intersectional frameworks in research: CRIAW. In *Women's health in Canada: Critical perspectives on theory and policy,* ed. M. Morrow, O. Hankivsky, and C. Varcoe. Toronto: University of Toronto Press.

Morrow, M., and O. Hankivsky. 2007. Feminist methodology and health research: Bridging trends and debates. In *Women's health in Canada: Critical perspectives on theory and policy,* ed. M. Morrow, O. Hankivsky, and C. Varcoe, 93-123. Toronto: University of Toronto Press.

Nash, J.C. 2008. Re-thinking intersectionality. *Feminist Review* 89(2): 1-15.

Newbold, K.B., and J. Danforth. 2003. Health status and Canada's immigration population. *Social Science Medicine* 57(10): 1881-1995.

NWAC. 2007. Social determinants of health and Canada's Aboriginal women: NWAC's submission to the World Health Organization's Commission on the Social Determinants of Health. Native Women's Association of Canada. http://www.nwac.ca/sites/default/files/reports/NWAC_WHO-CSDH_Submission2007-06-04.pdf.

Ockene, I., and J. Ockene. 1992. *Prevention of coronary heart disease.* Boston: Little, Brown.

Oxman-Martinez, J., and J. Hanley. 2005. Health and social services for Canada's multicultural population: Challenges for equity. Paper presented at the policy forum "Canada 2017 – Serving Canada's Multicultural Population for the Future," Multicultural Program, Department of Canadian Heritage, Gatineau, QC, July 13.

Pérez, C. F. 2002. Health status and health behaviours among immigrants. *Health Reports* (Statistics Canada Catalogue 82-003) 13: 1-12.

Petersen, A., and D. Lupton. 1996. *The new public health: Health and self in the age of risk.* St. Leonards, Australia: Allen and Unwin.

PHAC. 1999. The healthy heart kit. Public Health Agency of Canada.

–. 2003. Centre for Chronic Disease Prevention and Control: Cardiovascular disease. Public Health Agency of Canada. http://www/phac-aspc.gc.ca.

Phoenix, A., and P. Pattynama. 2006. Editorial. *European Journal of Women's Studies* 13(3): 187-92.

Pilote, L. 2007. Sex-specific issues related to cardiovascular disease: A synopsis of the 2007 supplement. *Canadian Medical Association Journal* 176(6): 789-91.

Rachlis, M. 2004. *Prescription for excellence: How innovation is saving Canada's health care system.* Toronto: HarperCollins.

Raphael, D. 2002. Social determinants of health: Why is there such a gap between our knowledge and its implementation? Powerpoint presentation at Ryerson Polytechnic University, Toronto, 4 October. http://www.medanthro.net.

Razack, S. 1998. *Looking white people in the eye: Gender, race, and culture in courtrooms and classrooms.* Toronto: University of Toronto Press.

Schulz, A.J., and L. Mullings, eds. 2006. *Gender, race, class and health: Intersectional approaches.* San Francisco: Jossey-Bass.

Sen, G. 2008. Intersectionality in health and health care: Review of research and policy. Paper presented at the "Intersectionality from Theory to Practice: An Interdisciplinary Dialogue" workshop, Simon Fraser University, Vancouver, 17 April.

Sheth, T., C. Nair, M. Nargundkar, S. Anand, and S. Yusuf. 1999. Cardiovascular and cancer mortality among Canadians of European, South Asian, and Chinese origin from 1979-1993: An analysis of 1.2 million deaths. *Canadian Medical Association Journal* 161(2): 132-38.

Shookner, M., and F. Chin-Yee. 2003. An inclusion lens: Looking at social and economic exclusion and inclusion. Canadian Social Welfare Policy Conference proceedings, University of Ottawa, Ottawa, 15-17 June. http://ccsd.ca.

Shuttleworth, R.P. 2001. Symbolic contexts, embodied sensitivities, and the lived experience of sexually relevant interpersonal encounters for a man with cerebral palsy. In *Semiotics and disability,* ed. B.B. Swadener, 75-96. Albany: State University of New York Press.

Smith, L.T. 1999. *Decolonizing methodologies: Research and indigenous peoples.* London: Zed Books.

Spivak, G.C. 1995. Can the subaltern speak? In *The post-colonial studies reader,* ed. B. Ashcroft, G. Griffiths, and H. Tiffin, 24-28. London and New York: Routledge.

Statistics Canada. 2006. Causes of death, 2004. Government of Canada Publications. http://www.publications.gc.ca.

–. 2008. Canada's ethnocultural mosaic, 2006 census. Government of Canada. http://www.statcan.ca.

Steinbugler, A.C., J.E. Press, and J. Johnson Dias. 2006. Gender, race, and affirmative action: Operationalizing intersectionality in survey research. *Gender and Society* 20(6): 805-25.

Stephens, C., J. Porter, C. Nettleton, and R. Willis. 2006. Disappearing, displaced, and undervalued: A call to action for indigenous health worldwide. *Lancet* 367: 2019-28.

Tanuseputro, P., D.G. Manuel, M. Leung, K. Nguyen, and J. Johansen. 2003. Risk factors for cardiovascular disease in Canada. *Canadian Journal of Cardiology* 19: 1249-59.

Titchkosky, T. 2002. Cultural maps: Which way to disability? In *Disability/postmodernity,* ed. T. Shakespeare, 101-11. London and New York: Continuum.

Trinh, T. Minh-ha. 1989. *Woman, Native, other.* Bloomington: Indiana University Press.
USDHHS. 2002. *Morbidity and mortality: 2002 chartbook on cardiovascular, lung, and blood diseases.* Washington: U.S. Department of Health and Human Services.
Varcoe, C., O. Hankivsky, and M. Morrow. 2007. Introduction: Beyond gender matters. In *Women's health in Canada: Critical perspectives on theory and policy,* ed. M. Morrow, O. Hankivsky, and C. Varcoe, 3-30. Toronto: University of Toronto Press.
Verloo, M. 2006. Multiple inequalities, intersectionality and the European Union. *European Journal of Women's Studies* 13(3): 211-28.
Vernon, A. 1999. The dialectics of multiple identities and the disabled people's movement. *Disability and Society* 14(3): 385-98.
Waldrum, J.B., D.A. Herring, and T.K. Young, eds. 2006. *Aboriginal health in Canada: Historical, cultural, and epidemiological perspectives.* 2nd ed. Toronto: University of Toronto Press.
Warner, L.R. 2008. A best practices guide to intersectional approaches in psychological research. *Sex Roles* 59(5-6): 454-63.
Weber, L. 2006. Reconstructing the landscape of health disparities research: Promoting dialogue and collaboration between feminist intersectional and biomedical paradigms. In Schulz and Mullings, 21-59.
Weber, L., and E. Fore. 2007. Race, ethnicity, and health: An intersectional framework. In *Handbook of the sociology of racial and ethnic relations,* ed. H. Vera and J.R. Feagin, 191-218. New York: Springer.
Weber, L., and D. Parra-Medina. 2003. Intersectionality and women's health: Charting a path to eliminating health disparities. In *Advances in gender research.* Vol. 7, *Gender perspectives on health and medicine,* ed. M.T. Segal, V. Demos, and J.J. Kronenfeld, 183-230. Oxford: Elsevier.
Weldon, L. 2006. The structure of intersectionality: A comparative politics of gender. *Politics and Gender* 2(2): 235-48.
Wharf Higgins, J., L. Young, S. Cunningham, and P. Naylor. 2006. Out of the mainstream: Low-income, lone mothers' life experiences and perspectives on heart health. *Health Promotion* 7(2): 221-33.
WHI. 2006. The diversity of women's voice in Ontario: A synopsis of selected literature. Women's Health Institute. http://www.womenshealthcouncil.on.ca.
Wing, A.K. 1990-91. Brief reflections towards a multiplicative theory and praxis of being. *Berkeley Women's Law Journal* 6: 181.
Wong, J., and S. Wong. 2003. Cardiovascular health of immigrant women: Implications for evidence-based practice. *Clinical Governance* 8(2): 112-22.
Yusuf, S., S. Reddy, S. Ôunpuu, and S. Anand. 2001a. Global burden of cardiovascular diseases. Part I: Variations in cardiovascular disease by specific ethnic groups and geographic regions and prevention strategies. *Circulation* 104: 2746-53.
–. 2001b. Global burden of cardiovascular diseases. Part II: Variations in cardiovascular disease by specific ethnic groups and geographic regions and prevention strategies. *Circulation* 104: 2855-64.
Yuval-Davis, N. 2006. Intersectionality and feminist politics. *European Journal of Women's Studies* 13(3): 193-209.
Zawilski, V., and C. Levine-Rasky, eds. 2005. *Inequality in Canada: A reader on the intersections of gender, race and class.* Don Mills: Oxford University Press.

Part 1
Theoretical and Methodological Innovations

Edited by Sarah de Leeuw and Olena Hankivsky

2

Beyond Borders and Boundaries: Addressing Indigenous Health Inequities in Canada through Theories of Social Determinants of Health and Intersectionality

Sarah de Leeuw and Margo Greenwood

> Some people think that to be Indian, you have to do certain things, but I'm just saying that you're Indian no matter what you do ... I'm always thinking about that.
>
> – Shelley Niro, quoted in Abbott (1995)

We have a friend whose life, in great part, has been shaped and ordered by a small, laminated, wallet-sized piece of blue paper.[1] When our friend speaks of that piece of paper, and it is often with tears choking her sentences, she tells a story of pain, isolation, and sadness. Although she is a strong and vibrant woman, a survivor if you will, she attributes to that piece of blue paper a life that includes the loss of all possessions in many house fires, struggles with addiction, a sustained poverty for herself and her children, and separation from and violence in her immediate family. The piece of paper is roughly the same size as a driver's licence or health care card. That small square of blue is an enfranchisement card, a materially small yet immensely powerful reminder of far-reaching and broadly impacting colonial policies that for generations governed the lives of indigenous peoples in Canada.

Present in policy documents circulated by the Government of Canada until the late nineteen hundreds, enfranchisement was a practice that stripped indigenous peoples of the few rights to which their indigenous identity entitled them.[2] To be enfranchised was, by decree of the federal government, to no longer be an Indian (as that category was defined, constructed, and enacted by Ottawa).[3] And to no longer be an Indian in Canada meant, and continues to mean, receiving services that differ vastly from those accorded non-enfranchised Indians, including non-enfranchised Indians in one's own family, community, or circle of close friends and loved ones. Enfranchisement is a clear example of colonial efforts to impose identities. To have an identity assigned to them, to be categorized and defined, had and has eminently embodied repercussions for indigenous peoples in Canada, particularly in the realms of health and well-being. Due to the imposition of an identity, indigenous people were territorially confined to Indian reserves or displaced to Indian residential schools, both of which had deleterious health outcomes. In many respects, indigenous peoples in Canada, and their historical and current health profiles, are perfect examples of how discursive practices come to form, and to be embodied by, the subjects they name (Foucault 1972). In this chapter, then, we specifically hope to redress a paucity of work that merges intersectionality theory with explorations about the social determinants of indigenous people's health in Canada. We argue that conceptualizing indigenous people's health through theories of intersectionality and social determinants of health may offer a means of addressing, and perhaps even ameliorating, the state of unhealthiness experienced today by many indigenous peoples.

This chapter explores the linkages between identity constructions and embodied, lived, realities. Our argument is somewhat speculative in nature, an outcome of thinking about a topic still in its infancy (indigenous people's health in Canada) through an array of relatively recent theories and research foci (intersectionality and the social determinants of health). We are interested in providing a historically and critically informed evaluation of indigenous peoples' current health status in Canada. Specifically, we explore how colonial construction of indigenous identity, principally for the purposes of "managing Indians," translated into significant divides between indigenous peoples and into differential abilities to access health care or support services that could contribute to better states of well-being. We thus begin the discussion on a historical note, looking at a few key policies, laws, and documents that sought to name and categorize indigenous peoples for the purposes of management and administration. Using a theoretical approach that recognizes the multiple and complex interplays of marginalized social otherness, which are often discursively produced but are also often embodied at individual levels, we then explore the health profiles of indigenous peoples today. From there, we explore possibilities for improving their health and well-being. Specifically, we are interested in burgeoning discussions concerning the social determinants of health and how this emerging way of conceptualizing health in turn links with theories of intersectionality. Such linkages, we posit, may provide a framework that is complex, sensitive, and nuanced enough to address the powerful legacy of colonialism that is lived and embodied, differentially, by so many indigenous people today.

To Produce Indians: Intersectionality, Identity, and Colonial History in Canada

> Identity, for my mother, was a complex issue ... What kind of name described her? You were Indian or white ... or you simply had no name for yourself.
>
> – Lawrence (2004)

Intersectionality is a relatively recent theory that has yet to be fully realized in reference to indigenous peoples. This is not surprising given both the newness of the theory and the general lack of critical decolonizing scholarly literature about indigenous peoples and indigeneity generally (Alfred and Corntassel 2005; Gilmartin and Berg 2007; Lawrence 2003; Smith 1999). Further, the relationship between feminist scholarship and critical indigenous studies is not well developed or without tension (for discussion and exception, see Laduke 1998; Cooper 2003; Jaimes 2003; Smith 1999). On the other hand, as intersectionality is increasingly developed and deployed across the social sciences, including the health sciences, its relevance to research concerning indigenous peoples becomes progressively more evident. Broadly speaking, intersectionality is a theory that wrestles with, and attempts to explain, how socio-culturally constructed categories (predominantly but not exclusively categories such as gender, ethnicity, and sexual orientation) interact with and affect one another to produce differentially lived social inequalities among people (Buitelaar 2006; Cole 2008; Collins 2000; Davis 2008; Hancock 2007). The theory of intersectionality arose as a means to examine, in an increasingly nuanced and complex approach, the ways in which varied forms of otherness interact to produce differently striated realities of social marginalization and social exclusion (Collins 2000). The theory arose in part as a response to abbreviated understandings of power relationships and inequalities developed within the context of first- and second-wave feminist movements, movements that predominantly focused on gendered otherness as opposed to other categories that result in marginalization.

Intersectionality, then, might best be broadly understood as a theory that accounts for the relationships between categories of otherness and the ensuing marginalization resulting from those relationships (McCall 2005). This is the way we understand and deploy the theory throughout this chapter. We are, more specifically, interested in the ways the theory can be set in dialogue with ever-broadening conceptualizations about health and the well-being of indigenous people and their communities in Canada. For us, theories of intersectionality offer the potential to understand otherness, including the othered social and health realities that indigenous people live, as an arrogate state of being. Intersectionality moves away from attempting to understand marginalization through a focus on individual strands of a person's (or any subject's) being. For us, in its realization of relationality, the intersectionality theory complements growing discussions about the complexity and multiplicities involved in being indigenous, in the category of indigeneity, and in indigenous people's health and well-being. In this chapter, then, we employ an approach to intersectionality that recognizes the socially constructed nature of many categories and characteristics that have come to define and delimit the lives of indigenous people in Canada. Concurrent to this recognition is our realization that indigenous people cross multiple boundaries and are shaped by various boundaries of distinction, each of which factor into their health statuses and the way that health services are delivered (or not delivered) to them. Finally, we are also interested in how social determinants shape and affect people's health and how those determinants manifest differently for indigenous peoples.

Health as socially determined is an idea garnering increased attention across many disciplines and geographies. Canada has proved to be a leader in the area, revealing that "there is robust evidence demonstrating that social determinants have far greater influence on health and the incidence of illness than conventional biomedical and behavioural risk factors" (Gleeson and Alperstein 2006, 266; see also Baum and Harris 2006; Raphael 2002; Lantz et al. 1998). Understanding people's health through a social determinants lens means thinking about the systems and structures in which people live as opposed to privileging inquires about individuals as separate from their social contexts (Marmot et al. 2008). It has been described as research that moves thinking from "the cell to the social" and as a practice of investigating "the causes of the causes." Social determinants foci shift from genetic or biomedical inquiries to examinations of why some people and communities are more prone to health deficits, or suffer more severely from their outcomes, as a function of their social contexts. The health and wellness of people is thus increasingly conceptualized in relation to the social contexts in which they work, play, love, and experience life, and to the social factors that affect them. This is a conceptualization that merges productively with theories of intersectionality, particularly when the latter has been employed to understand roles of (to name a few) gender, geography, class, sexual orientation, or racialization in the persistent health disparities in Canada (Hankivsky and Christoffersen 2008). Now recognized by the Public Health Agency of Canada and the United Nations' World Health Organization as powerful constituters of people's well-being (or lack thereof), social determinants of health include employment and working conditions, education and literacy, income and social status, social support networks, culture, gender, and child development (Anderson and Domosh 2002; Marmot 2005).

For indigenous people in Canada, these factors are, unto themselves, socially determined. In other words, colonization plays a significant role in determining how, for instance, education is accessed by indigenous people, how income is allocated, or even how a person can access social support networks and child development services. Colonialism is increasingly being realized – particularly by indigenous health scholars – as a determinant of the social determinants of health (Loppie and Wien 2008). This discussion rests on evidence that the health disparities experienced by indigenous peoples are profoundly linked to erosions of lineages, languages, cultures, and traditions, and to separations from family, land, and territory (Reading, Kmetic, and Giddion 2007; Smylie 2009). These, it is observed, all result from colonization, a practice to which non-indigenous peoples in Canada were not subject.

To "be indigenous" in Canada comes with a series of attendant challenges, many of which are best understood through intersectional analysis, particularly because of the differential and complex nature of marginalization experienced by different indigenous peoples. Conceptualized as a group inclusive of First Nations, Inuit, and Métis, and compared to broader, non-indigenous Canadians, indigenous peoples live with significant cultural, socio-economic, and health inequities: higher rates of youth suicide, lower levels of incomes and employment, loss of language and cultural traditions, higher rates of school incompletion, high rates of child apprehension, shorter life expectancy, higher rates of incarceration and interaction with the criminal justice system, and disproportionally high rates of both infectious and non-infectious diseases (Reading, Kmetic, and Giddion 2007; Richmond and Ross 2009). These social realties are lived, in various configurations and to varying degrees, as embodied and individualized realities: and they are lived differently depending on the "who's" and "how's" of the person experiencing them. Geography, gender, age, background, and class cannot be excluded from understandings of the socio-cultural and health inequities of indigenous peoples. Further, whatever the nature of disadvantage, it is often exacerbated due to twenty-first-century anti-indigenous racism (Larson et al. 2007), much of which has historical roots. As two (post) colonial feminist geographers have recently observed, national discourses are formulated within historical colonial relationships but are constantly re-enacted in contemporary politics (Anderson and Domosh 2002, 125)

The very act of naming indigenous peoples is a complex practice rife with assumptions locatable in Canada's colonial project. Once collectively referred to as Indians or Natives, those who occupied the lands now known as Canada are in actuality geographically, linguistically, and socio-culturally complex and heterogeneous peoples. The very act of inscribing on them one name (Indian/Native) was an act of colonial conceit predicated on assumptions that any person who was not a Eurocolonial settler was a member of a homogeneous and static "Other" group. Early in the country's history, then, nomenclature fashioned social categories that discursively produced a particular people by assigning them a series of constructions. Broadly speaking, to be named and thus understood as an Indian or a Native meant, usually without nuance and in a homogeneous manner, being categorized as savage and troublesome. This in turn necessitated non-indigenous people's stern transformative intervention in a dying race that was always requiring management. These colonial assumptions, particularly in the area of "management" concerns, translated into governance policies that reified the social categories and subjects to which they referred.

To be categorized as Indian has material consequences that are inseparable from other categorizations and classifications. For instance, indigenous women were named and managed differently from their male counterparts, often, as we will explore, in ways that actively accounted for governmental efforts to negate genealogical Indianness, at least in ways that compelled the state to commit resources to individuals (Browne and Fiske 2001; Lawrence 2003). Indigenous peoples were also managed differently depending on colonial assumptions about levels of civility, resulting, for instance, in different types of interactions with schooling systems – including residential schooling – that are now recognized as having profound health implications (Milloy 1999; Larson et al. 2007). Indigenous peoples were displaced and deterritorialized differentially across Canada; treaties were signed in some areas, whereas vast geographies were left untreatied, and reserves were allocated differentially depending, for instance, on the value attributed to the land by colonial settlers (Harris 2002). Early in Canada's colonial project, then, gender, social status, colonial concepts about indigeneity, and physical geography all intersected with one another to produce differently situated indigenous peoples. Although the nomenclature has shifted, erasing the echoes of these discourses from discussions about indigenous peoples remains impossible. The translation of lexiconic acts (naming) into policies, documents, laws, and strategies that became practices that bore down on bodies, thus arguably producing the often unhealthy indigenous peoples of the twenty-first century, is traceable in close readings of the Enfranchisement Act, the Indian Act, and their precursor, the Bagot Report. We thus offer a close reading of these colonial documents, arguing that the two acts played roles in directing and dictating indigenous people's identities, in allocating resources and reserve lands, in structuring Indian education, including residential schools, and in distributing resources associated with health. These all have contemporary implications. Indeed, the Indian Act continues to govern First Nations people across the country, with ongoing health implications.

The Indian Act of the twenty-first century (current until 16 January 2009 at the time of writing) is a continuation of previous policies and acts that, as we briefly discuss, were all preoccupied with managing Indians. The 1845 *Report on the Affairs of the Indians in Canada* (known as the Bagot Report) was one of the first documents to comprehensively address "the Indian question" in Canada. Presented to the Legislative Assembly of the Province of Canada, it was a summary of existing British imperial thought and practices about Indians. The report's authors were "interested in the welfare of this race ... [in] mass[ing] valuable information upon their present state, and [making] suggestions for improving it ... to form a judgment upon any scheme proposed for their future management" (Rawson, Davidson, and Hepburn 1845, 3). The report can thus be read as an archive of the discursivities on which were built subsequent colonial management schemes, including the Indian Act, concerned with indigenous people.

Reflecting perspectives of the time, the Bagot Report's concerns about managing Indians operated principally from the position that Indians were a dying race whose best interest was to be quickly absorbed into the Canadian state and associated states of modernity (ibid.). The report was primarily concerned with treaty negotiations, land and resource allotments, relationships between Indians and the Crown, and strategies related to the population's health and education. Informing all these concerns were questions about identity, about who and what constituted an Indian: in other words, "The Indian" had to be defined and categorized in order to be appropriately managed. Geographic location, proximity to Eurocolonial settlers, time spent in the presence of non-indigenous subjects, levels of educational attainment, and degree of Christianization were all understood as critical factors in what constituted the type of Indian the government was dealing with. The Bagot Report argued that, for policy considerations, there were "good" and "not-good" Indians. In doing so, the report produced, simultaneously, a homogeneous Indian-Other category positioned in antithesis to Eurocolonial settlers and a subcategory of otherness within that group. The federal government's fixation with nuanced distinctions of Indianness, as necessary for Indian management, did not end with the Bagot Report. It carried into the Act for the Gradual Enfranchisement of Indians (1869), an act – as we shall discuss momentarily – with direct implications for indigenous people's health and access to health care.

The Enfranchisement Act was focused on further reifying who was an Indian and who was not, by even more clearly defining it from Ottawa's perspective. It is widely understood that enfranchisement was a deeply gendered effort. A status Indian woman lost her status if she married a non-status man, "Indian" or not. However, non-status-Indian women in this latter configuration did not gain status. Categorization and identity had eminently material implications: according to the federal government, those who were enfranchised were "no longer ... deemed Indians within the meaning of the laws relating to Indians" (Government of Canada 1869, section 16). This abdicated the government's fiduciary responsibility to the enfranchised individual, to her offspring, and to all her subsequent descendents. Concern with reducing federal fiduciary responsibility had historical roots. As the Bagot Report rather bluntly stated, the government wanted to minimize costs associated with managing Indians and, to do so, argued for civilizing through assimilation: "It appears that the most effectual means of ameliorating the condition of the Indians, of promoting their religious improvement and education, and of eventually relieving His Majesty's Government from the expense of the Indian Department are: 1st, to collect the Indians in considerable numbers, and to settle them in villages, with a due portion of land for the cultivation and support. 2nd, to make such provision for their religious improvement, education, and instruction in husbandry as circumstances may from time to time require" (Kemp 1828, quoted in Rawson, Davidson, and Hepburn 1845, 7).

In many respects, then, the discourse of enfranchisement was a retooling of and a new construction of previous narratives about the need to civilize and assimilate Indians. Whatever else they may have been, the narratives were informed at least in part by Ottawa's interest in lessening costs associated with managing Indians.

Categorizing Indians, and the consequent ability of the government to deem some Indians no longer Indians as per the definitional categories assigned to them, was couched in a discourse of benevolent governmental recognition that some Indians, through hard work and effort, could morally surpass others and were thus "worthy" of no longer being categorized as Indians. This sentiment is abundantly clear in the 1876 Indian Act, an updated and newly rationalized iteration of the Enfranchisement Act, tabled because it was "expedient to amend and consolidate the laws respective to Indians" in order to control and manage the "reserves, lands, money, and property of Indians in Canada." The 1876 Indian Act stated that an Indian was enfranchisable depending on the degree of civilization he or she had attained, and the character for integrity, morality, and sobriety that he or she bore (Government of Canada 1876). Enfranchisement wording was not repealed from the Indian Act until 1985. By then, fewer than 350,000 people were recognized as status Indians in Canada, prompting some to suggest that, along with its historic antecedents, enfranchisement was tantamount to cultural genocide (Lawrence 2003; Holmes 1987). Indeed, despite the 1985 repeal of enfranchisement wording, and a subsequent reassignment of Indian status to nearly 100,000 people, multiple divides remain between those who held Indian status prior to 1985 and those who were granted it as a result of Bill C-31 (the bill that repealed enfranchisement for the Indian Act).

These divisions and ongoing classification of Indian(ness) result in what some call "Indian Act math" a set of equations that continues to play out in the lived realities of indigenous peoples today. The equations unfold as follows. First, despite self-identifying as Indian, First Nations, or Native, many indigenous people in Canada remain non-status Indians as per the dictates of the Indian Act. There are also, more clearly, non-indigenous non-status people across the country. Both of these groups, but particularly those who are indigenous, are non-status (NS) in relation to the Indian Act. But people who are status Indians are also subdivided. Those who held status under the Indian Act prior to 1985 are referred to as 6(1) Indians, whereas those who gained status through Bill C-31, or after April 1985, are categorized as 6(2) Indians (Barker 2008; Furi and Wherrett 2003). With reference to the Indian Act, and who will be recognized as having status (thus receiving particular government considerations as per the act), the three categories of NS, 6(1), and 6(2) extend to the classification of offspring. For example, children produced by a 6(1) and an NS union will be 6(2) – or, as Indian Act math puts it, $6(1) + NS = 6(2)$. Furthermore, $6(2) + NS = 6(2)$, $6(1) + 6(2) = 6(2)$, and $6(2) + 6(2) = NS$. In an almost magical operation, the Indian Act granted status to people once understood as enfranchised Indians: simultaneously, however, it produced another category by dictating that the children of two people who gained status post-1985 were not eligible for Indian status. The configurations of these three categorizations have embodied consequences. As we will explore, they result in an ongoing and particularized classification of people who are differentially able (or unable as the case may be) to access health care in Canada.

Even with the absence of enfranchisement language, the most current iteration of the Indian Act, inclusive of 6(1) and 6(2) wording, continues to reinforce the socially engineered categories on which it historically drew and rested. These categories in turn govern how, among many other things and as we will discuss below, indigenous people interact with the various systems of health care services in Canada. Arguably, differentiated abilities to access and interact with health care services produce further striations between indigenous people and within their communities (namely, based on healthiness versus unhealthiness). Because these extant striations appear to be so closely linked to historical discourse and practices of colonial social engineering, understanding the health status of indigenous people through intersectionality theory becomes all the more urgent. We believe it is imperative that the Indian Act, and other colonial forces such as the deterritorializing and reterritorializing of indigenous peoples onto reserves, be conceptualized as a determinant of the twenty-first-century health status experienced by indigenous peoples in Canada. Given its clear link to the policies, laws, and discourses discussed above, and given its increasingly realized link with the unhealthiness experienced by indigenous peoples in Canada, there is one further colonial force we believe worthy of some note before moving into the contemporary health profiles of indigenous peoples today. That force is residential schooling.

Residential schooling, which is now widely understood as a "national crime," has been described as an act of socio-cultural genocide perpetrated by ecumenical organizations and the Canadian government (Milloy 1999). It relied entirely on discursive foundations and policy imperatives, such as the ones explored above, that constructed indigenous peoples and indigeneity as fundamentally flawed and in need of transformation. Like most colonial practices, residential schooling was not a static or homogeneous undertaking (Pratt 1991; Thomas 1994). It was undertaken differently depending on the time and location of its unfolding, and it was executed according to shifting mandates dependent in part on the curricular ideologies of the churches overseeing it (Milloy 1999). Importantly, and with reference to theories of intersectionality, due to its shifting and somewhat amorphous nature, residential schooling had vastly different impacts on the wide array of children who experienced it. In British Columbia, the province we know best, former residential school students have received differing settlements for abuses suffered in the schools. They also speak about very different experiences, running the gamut from positive to horrendously torturous, and they identify staff and teachers treating them differently based on gender, racialization, and their genealogies and statuses within home communities. As a consequence, any meaningful healing for former students (and their children and children's children) must account for differently produced survivors, people who will live and experience the intergenerational effects of residential schooling in complex and intersecting ways and, as a consequence, will live quite different health outcomes associated with the spectrum of experiences related to the schools.

Embodied Inequalities: Indigeneity, Health, Social Determinants, and the Intersectional Legacies of Colonialism

> Jordan spent the last two years of his life in hospital. The reason
> he spent that time in hospital was because governments had to
> argue, wrangle and discuss who should pay for Jordan's care.
>
> – Crowder (2007)

It has been our contention thus far that Canada's colonial project, historically and with impacts into the present day, operated in significant part through a set of discursive practices (reports, laws, policies, legislations) that produced indigenous peoples as particular social subjects in need of management and transformation. It is also our suggestion that colonial discourses, which retain their power in the twenty-first century, are eminently tangible and material practices, particularly as they produced marginalized social subjects and, with specific reference to indigenous peoples in Canada, unhealthy or differentially healthy citizens. The differentiated natures of healthiness and unhealthiness, across varying geographies and between peoples and communities, are an outcome of intersecting and interconnecting factors: these factors are also lived differently based on the unique ways they collude and/or are embodied within individuals. Colonialism in Canada turned in part on categorizing, or socially engineering, groups of people for the purpose of management: the management project was further preoccupied with differentially subclassifying people based in part on location of residence, gender, level of civility, and age. It makes sense, then, that a lens of intersectionality has value when trying to understand indigenous peoples' states of being today.

With these premises in mind, it is important to reiterate what is well established with reference to indigenous people's health in Canada. As we and many others have documented elsewhere, indigenous peoples across Canada live what some call "Third World conditions of health" and what others refer to as the "embodiment of inequality" (Adelson 2005). Indeed, although Canada is ranked among the best places to live in the world, if the United Nations Human Development Index were applied to indigenous peoples living on-reserve, Canada would rank between sixty-eighth to eightieth in the world (Bennett, Blackstock, and De La Ronde, 2005; Silversides 2007; Webster 2006). Aboriginal people in Canada have higher rates of disease, die younger, and experience higher rates of mortality and morbidity than their non-Aboriginal counterparts (Allard, Wilkins, and Berthelot 2004). Their life expectancy, although increasing, still falls "well below" that of non-indigenous people (Adelson 2005). The potential years of life lost (PYLL) in areas with large indigenous populations was eighty-four, as opposed to fifty-six in regions with fewer indigenous people. Injuries, including suicide and accidents involving a motor vehicle, account for a significant number of PYLL in regions with large indigenous populations (thirty-two per one thousand persons at risk as opposed to twelve in areas with few indigenous people) (see also Statistics Canada 2008).

Indigenous people have higher rates of infectious disease, but chronic diseases such as type 2 diabetes and various cancers are also increasing within their communities. Rates of tuberculosis were eight to ten times higher in First Nations communities than in non-indigenous communities, and other infectious diseases such as hepatitis, chlamydia, and HIV/AIDS are all either more prevalent or increasing at higher rates in First Nations communities than in non-indigenous populations (Adelson 2005). In 2006, the homes of nearly one-fourth of all indigenous people in Canada needed major repairs, and indigenous people were almost four times more likely than their non-indigenous counterparts to live in a crowded dwelling (Statistics Canada 2008). Finally, results of the 2002-3 First Nations Regional Longitudinal Health Survey (RHS), a unique survey because First Nations communities implemented the research, and the data remain the property of the National Aboriginal Health Organization (NAHO), corroborates non-indigenous-driven demographic profiles about the poor state of indigenous people's health. According to the RHS, adult First Nations living on-reserve have less education, higher unemployment rates, and lower incomes than those living off-reserve. Both groups experience lower earnings than non–First Nations Canadians (NAHO 2002-3). Evidence from a wide variety of sources leaves little doubt that indigenous people do not have access to the same levels of healthy living that their non-indigenous counterparts enjoy. Given the linkages between poor mental health and community experience of health disparities and health inequities (particularly for indigenous people), it is perhaps not surprising that indigenous peoples in both Canada and other nations suffer disproportionately high rates of mental-health-related illnesses (Kirmayer, Brass, and Tait 2000; Kirmayer, Simpson, and Cargo 2003; Ypinazar et al. 2007).

In addition to living with increased rates of health inequities, indigenous people in Canada face specific and significant mental illnesses in greater abundance than their non-indigenous counterparts (Kirmayer, Brass, and Tait 2000). In indigenous communities, mental illnesses are commonly accompanied by high rates of suicide (particularly in youth), alcoholism, violence, and feelings of demoralization (NAHO 2002-3; Kirmayer, Brass, and Tait 2000; Loppie and Wien 2008). According to the Regional Health Survey, indigenous people aged fifteen and over who are living off-reserve are almost twice as likely as their non-indigenous counterparts to have suffered a major depressive episode in the past twelve months, and a high percentage of youth report feeling sad, blue, or depressed during two or more weeks in the previous year (females 37.1 percent and males 18.1 percent) (NAHO 2002-3). Compared with their non-indigenous counterparts, indigenous women and girls in Canada, as in other nations, continue to face disproportionally high rates of family violence in the home and sexual violence both inside and outside it (LaRocque n.d.; Browne and Fiske 2001). Although not much empirical research has examined the link between residential school survivors and mental illness, small psychiatrically intensive studies document that the vast majority of them suffer from a host of mental illnesses related directly to their time at school (Corrado and Cohen 2003). These illnesses included post-traumatic stress disorder, substance abuse disorders, and major depression (ibid.). Compared with non-indigenous

Canadians, indigenous people can somewhat problematically be essential-ized as universally experiencing health inequalities; there are, however, sig-nificant differences within and between various indigenous groups that are often lost in the stark comparisons between them and non-indigenous Canadians. Although the intradifferentiations of health within indigenous communities are receiving growing attention, the extant research is insuffi-cient. Much of the compelling research that does exist, and that warrants further attention, focuses on the resilience and capacities of some indigenous communities. It suggests that a community's defying of health (in)equality trends may be linked to cultural continuity, self-determination, and persistent attention to aspects of indigeneity (Chandler, Lalonde, and Sokol 2003).

Jurisdictional issues, arguably the result of social engineering, continue to hamper the well-being of many indigenous people in Canada, sometimes with tragic results. In an albeit extreme example, tensions between federal and provincial governments, particularly with reference to on- versus off-reserve health services, have even been implicated in the deaths of children (MacDonald and Attaran 2007). More generally, indigenous people's access, or lack thereof, to non-insured health benefits is an ongoing confusion for many, often the elderly and elders, for whom prescription medications, dental care, and ophthalmology services could improve standards of living. The confusion rests solely with categorizations of identity and the services various levels of government will or will not pay for. The striated access to non-insured health benefits is rooted in historical classification and categor-ization, the result being different "types" of indigenous people across Canada. Based on this typing (e.g., status versus non-status, on-reserve versus off-reserve), indigenous people are able to access (or not) different health services (Legal Services Society 2007). For a status First Nation living on-reserve, access to non-insured health benefits differs markedly from that of, for instance, even a member of his or her own family who lives off-reserve and does not hold a status card.[4] At the embodied level, this means that some individuals may be able to afford newer glasses or to access medications associated with diabetes. It even means, and this has important ramifications for the increas-ing number of people suffering the intergenerational effects of residential schooling, that some indigenous people are provided funds to access coun-selling and therapy services, whereas others are not. The disparities between people's ability to access non-insured health benefits are reasonably overt; the linkage of this access to historically produced categorizations of indigen-ous people is fairly clear. When, however, more distal or nuanced determin-ants of people's health and well-being are accounted for, the consequences of colonial practices for indigenous people become even starker.

These factors cannot be extricated from other social determinants of health, thus producing an "indigenized" version of the more universalized components often understood to comprise the social determinants of health. When this work is coupled with theories of intersectionality, what arises are new ways to understand the current health status of indigenous people in Canada. First, as alluded to earlier in the chapter, the colonial project cordoned off and contained many indigenous peoples within reserve spaces (Harris 2002). Today, in an increasingly urbanized landscape where services are ever-more centralized within cities, indigenous people face choices between accessing health services and living away from social networks and families, the latter of which is understood as a determinant of well-being. Location, which for indigenous people has deeply colonial roots, also dictates access to education and employment, both of which are determinants of health and well-being. As is consistent with theories of intersectionality, living with reduced levels of education or employment options and satisfaction plays out differently for men and women; strong evidence suggests that the levels of physical, sexual, and emotional violence faced by indigenous women can be correlated to income and education (LaRocque n.d.). Beyond the colonial geographies just discussed, which determine indigenous people's levels of education or access to educational options, the colonial classification and categorization of indigenous people also dictates access to education. As is the case for financial support for non-insured health benefits, one's Indian status (or non-status) also determines the federal government's level of fiduciary responsibility with reference to, for instance, funding for post-secondary education. Thus, if as established by the United Nations and the Public Health Agency of Canada, education and literacy are determinants of a person's health and well-being, the historical social engineering of Canada's colonial project must be understood to be negatively asserting itself in this realm as well.

The health and well-being of people, and by extension their communities and the populations they comprise, are complex phenomena. As we have illustrated, they are produced by matrices of power and domination (Collins 2000) of which colonialism is focal for indigenous peoples. It was the intent of this chapter to intervene into the paucity of literature considering the social determinants of indigenous people's health through a lens of intersectionality. We argued that to fully understand health or a lack thereof requires moving from the temporally immediate and the biomedical or behavioural into realms of the historic, the discursive, and the impositions of power; in the case of indigenous people in Canada, such an understanding cannot ignore colonialism, as it was enacted historically and as it continues to assert itself. We contend that understanding colonialism as a fundamental determinant, in conjunction with the other social determinants, can provide one means of explaining and understanding the state of indigenous people's health in Canada today. We added further to this, arguing that social determinants cannot be unhinged from characteristics such as gender, geography, age, and indigeneity (to name a few). By charting impositions of colonial power and the production of indigenous people's identities, followed by exploring their health as socially determined and deeply intersectional in nature, we hope we have added to a literature that seeks to illuminate and thus address the reasons behind persistent health disparities between indigenous and non-indigenous people in Canada.

Having said this, however, we return to our place of departure: our friend, who still holds the small blue piece of paper that was her enfranchisement card. Colonialism as a determinant of health was and is not lived homogeneously or evenly by indigenous people. It shifts, it is embodied differently, depending on the body concerned and where it is situated. Theories of intersectionality must be added to understandings about the social determinants of health and to understandings that the social determinants of health must be indigenized to account for colonialism. This complexifies the equation. But, we think, the solutions to the very complex problem of social and health inequities might rest in spaces of complexity – inequities lived and embodied in so many ways by indigenous people in Canada. We think our friend deserves this.

Notes

1 "We" are Sarah de Leeuw and Margo Greenwood, two women who live in northern British Columbia, who work as professors and researchers at the University of Northern British Columbia, and who have been writing, working, and researching together for over a decade.

2 Nomenclature continues to flummox many who develop policies referencing indigenous peoples in Canada. From a policy perspective, "indigenous" presents a difficult framework because only the categorization of "Indian" was originally recognized by the federal government in the Indian Act. The terms "Inuit" and "Métis" came later, culminating in the recognition of "Aboriginal" peoples in section 35 of the 1982 Constitution Act. Many "indigenous" policies were based on what was provided to "Indians" under the Indian Act and thus excluded Inuit and Métis people. These categorizations continue to make policies and legislations confusing.

3 Although the word "enfranchisement" was present in the Indian Act until the 1985 amendment, changes were enacted to its meaning after 1969 when the Trudeau Liberals introduced, but failed to pass, their White Paper. Also, it should be noted that "Indians" were allowed to vote after 1961 without having to enfranchise in Canada.

4 With reference to federal health programs dedicated to "Indians," only the Non-Insured Health Benefits (NIHB) program extends beyond the territorial "border" of the federal jurisdiction of the reserve. All other federal programs are based on the community and serve the residents of that community (technically, regardless of status). The NIHB program is available to individuals based on their status, according to the Indian Act, *regardless* of where they reside.

References

Abbott, L. 1995. A time of visions: Shelley Niro, Mohawk. http://www.britesites.com.
Adelson, N. 2005. The embodiment of inequalities: Health disparities in Aboriginal Canada. *Canadian Journal of Public Health* 96(Suppl. 2): 45-61.

Alfred, T., and J. Corntassel. 2005. Being indigenous: Resurgences against contemporary colonialism. *Government and Opposition* 40(4): 597-614.

Allard, Y.E., R. Wilkins, and J.M. Berthelot. 2004. Premature mortality in health regions with high Aboriginal populations. *Health Report* 15(1): 51-60.

Anderson, K., and M. Domosh. 2002. North American spaces, post colonial stories. *Cultural Geographies* 9: 125-28.

Barker, J. 2008. Gender, sovereignty, rights: Native women's activism against social inequality and violence in Canada. *American Quarterly* 60(2): 259-66.

Baum, F., and L. Harris. 2006. Equity and the social determinants of health. *Health Promotion Journal of Australia* 17: 163–165.

Bennett, M., C. Blackstock, and R. De La Ronde. 2005. *A literature review and annotated bibliography on aspects of Aboriginal child welfare in Canada.* 2nd ed. Ottawa: First Nations Research Site of the Centre of Excellence for Child Welfare and the First Nations Child and Family Caring Society of Canada.

Browne, A., and J. Fiske. 2001. First Nations women's encounters with mainstream health care services. *Western Journal of Nursing Research* 2: 126-47.

Buitelaar, M. 2006. "I am the ultimate challenge": Accounts of intersectionality in the life-story of a well-known daughter of Moroccan migrant workers in the Netherlands. *European Journal of Women's Studies* 13(3): 259-76.

Chandler, M.J., C.E. Lalonde, and B.W. Sokol. 2003. Personal persistence, identity development, and suicide: A study of Native and non-Native North American adolescents. *Monographs of the Society for Research in Child Development* 68(2): 1-128.

Cole, E.R. 2008. Coalitions as a model of intersectionality: From practice to theory. *Sex Roles* 59: 443-53.

Collins, P.H. 2000. *Black feminist thought: Knowledge, consciousness, and the politics of empowerment.* New York: Routledge.

Cooper, N. 2003. Arts and letters club: Two spirited women artists and social change. In *Strong women stories: Native vision and community survival,* ed. K. Anderson and B. Lawrence, 135-55. Toronto: Sumach Press.

Corrado, R.R., and I.M. Cohen. 2003. *Mental health profiles for a sample of British Columbia's Aboriginal survivors of the Canadian residential school system.* Ottawa: Aboriginal Healing Foundation.

Davis, K. 2008. Intersectionality as buzzword: A sociology of science perspective on what makes a feminist theory successful. *Feminist Theory* 9(1): 67-85.

Foucault, M. 1972. *The archaeology of knowledge.* New York: Pantheon Books.

Furi, M., and J. Wherrett. 2003. Indian status and band membership issues. Ottawa, Political and Social Affairs Division, Library of Parliament, Parliamentary Information and Research Service. http://www.2parl.gc.ca.

Gilmartin, M., and L. Berg. 2007. Locating postcolonialism: Commentary. *Area* 39(1): 120-24.

Gleeson, S., and G. Alperstein. 2006. The NSW Social Determinants of Health Action Group: Influencing the social determinants of health. *Health Promotion Journal of Australia* 17: 266-68.

Government of Canada. 1869. *An act for the gradual enfranchisement of Indians, the better management of Indian affairs, and to extend the provisions of the Act 31st Victoria, Chapter 42.* Ottawa: Government of Canada. http://www.ainc-inac.gc.ca/ai/arp/ls/pubs/a69c6/a69c6-eng.pdf.

–. 1876. *Indian Act.* Amendments to the Indian Act, 1910, 1911, 1927, 1951, 1970, 1981, and 1985. Kingston and Ottawa: Government of Canada. http://laws-lois.justice.gc.ca/PDF/Statute/I/I-5.pdf.

Hancock, A.-M. 2007. When multiplication doesn't equal quick addition: Examining intersectionality as a research paradigm. *Perspectives on Politics* 5(1): 63-79.

Hankivsky, O., and A. Christoffersen. 2008. Intersectionality and the determinants of health: A Canadian perspective. *Critical Public Health* 18(3): 271-83.

Harris, C. 2002. *Making Native space: Colonialism, resistance, and reserves in British Columbia.* Vancouver: UBC Press.

Holmes, J. 1987. *Bill C-31: Equality or disparity? The effects of the new Indian Act on Native women*. Background paper. Ottawa: Canadian Advisory Council on the Status of Women.

Jaimes, M.A. 2003. "Patriarchal colonialism" and indigenism: Implications for Native feminist spirituality and Native womanism. *Hypatia* 18(2): 58-69.

Kirmayer, L.J., G.M. Brass, and C.L. Tait. 2000. The mental health of Aboriginal peoples: Transformations of identity and community. *Canadian Journal of Psychiatry* 45: 607-16.

Kirmayer, L.J., C. Simpson, and M. Cargo. 2003. Healing traditions: Cultural, community and mental health promotion with Canadian Aboriginal peoples. *Australian Psychiatry* 11: 15-23.

Laduke, W. 1998. Power is in the earth. In *Talking about the earth,* ed. South End Press Collective, 67-79. Cambridge: South End Press.

Lantz, P.M., J.S. House, J.M. Lepkowski, D.R. Williams, R.P. Mero, and J.J. Chen. 1998. Socioeconomic factors, health behaviors, and mortality. *Journal of the American Medical Association* 279: 1703–8.

LaRocque, E. N.d. *Violence in Aboriginal communities*. Ottawa: Public Health Agency of Canada. http://dsp-psd.pwgsc.gc.ca/Collection/H72-21-100-1994E.pdf.

Larson, A., M. Gillies, P.J. Howard, and J. Coffin. 2007. It's enough to make you sick: The impacts of racism on the health of Aboriginal Australians. *Australian and New Zealand Journal of Public Health* 31: 322-29.

Lawrence, B. 2003. Gender, race, and the regulation of Native identity in Canada and the United States: An overview. *Hypatia* 18(2): 3-31.

–. 2004. *"Real" Indians and others: Mixed-blood urban Native peoples and indigenous nationhood*. Vancouver: UBC Press.

Legal Services Society – British Columbia. 2007. *Benefits, services, and resources for Aboriginal peoples*. Vancouver: Legal Services Society.

Loppie, C., and F. Wien. 2008. *Health inequalities and social determinants of Aboriginal peoples' health*. Prince George: National Collaborating Centre for Aboriginal Peoples' Health.

MacDonald, N., and A. Attaran. 2007. Jordan's principle, governments' paralysis. *Canadian Medical Association Journal* 177(4): 321.

Marmot, M. 2005. Social determinants of health inequalities. *Lancet* 365(9464): 1099-1104.

Marmot, M., S. Friel, R. Bell, T.A.J. Houweling, and S. Taylor. 2008. Closing the gap in a generation: Health equity through action on the social determinants of health. *Lancet* 372(9650): 1661-69.

McCall, L. 2005. The complexity of intersectionality. *Signs: Journal of Women in Culture and Society* 30(3): 1771-1800.

Milloy, J. 1999. *A national crime: The Canadian government and the residential schooling system, 1879-1986*. Winnipeg: University of Manitoba Press.

NAHO. 2002-3. *First Nations Regional Longitudinal Health Survey (RHS) 2002/2003: Results for adults, youth and children living in First Nations communities*. Ottawa: First Nations Centre.

Pratt, M.L. 1991. *Imperial eyes: Travel writing and transculturation*. New York: Routledge.

Raphael, D. 2002. *Social justice is good for our hearts: Why societal factors – not lifestyles – are major causes of heart disease in Canada and elsewhere*. Toronto: Centre for Social Justice Foundation for Research and Education.

Rawson, W.R., J. Davidson, and W. Hepburn. 1845. *Report on the affairs of the Indians in Canada*. Kingston, ON: Province of Canada, Report submitted by Charles Bagot to the Legislative Assembly, 20 March 1845.

Reading, J., A. Kmetic, and V. Giddion. 2007. *First Nations holistic policy and planning model: Discussion for the World Health Organization Commission on Social Determinants of Health*. Ottawa: Assembly of First Nations.

Richmond, C.A.M., and N.A. Ross. 2009. The determinants of First Nation and Inuit health: A critical population approach. *Health and Place* 15: 403-11.

Schulz, A.J., N. Freudenberg, and J. Daniels. 2005. Intersections of race, class, and gender in public health interventions. In *Gender, race, class and health: Intersectional approaches,* ed. A.J. Schulz and L. Mullings, 371-93. San Francisco: Jossey-Bass.

Silversides, A. 2007. The north "like Darfur." *Canadian Medical Association Journal* 177(9): 1013-14.

Smith, L.T. 1999. *Decolonizing methodologies: Research and indigenous peoples*. New York: Zed Books.

Smylie, J. 2009. The health of Aboriginal peoples. In *Social determinants of health: Canadian perspectives*. 2nd ed., ed. D. Raphael, 280-301. Toronto: Canadian Scholars' Press.

Statistics Canada. 2008. *Aboriginal peoples in Canada in 2006: Inuit, Métis and First Nations, 2006 census*. Ottawa: Minister of Industry.

Thomas, N. 1994. *Colonialism's culture: Anthropology, travel and the government*. Princeton, NJ: Princeton University Press.

Webster, P. 2006. Canadian Aboriginal people's health and the Kelowna deal. *The Lancet* 368 (9523): 275-76.

Ypinazar, V.A., S.A. Margolis, M. Haswell-Elkins, and K. Tsey. 2007. Indigenous Australians' understandings regarding mental health and disorders. *Australia and New Zealand Journal of Psychiatry* 41: 467-78.

3

A Cross-Cultural Quantitative Approach to Intersectionality and Health: Using Interactions between Gender, Race, Class, and Neighbourhood to Predict Self-Rated Health in Toronto and New York City

Jennifer Black and Gerry Veenstra

As noted throughout this volume, intersectionality-inspired research has made important theoretical and empirical contributions to the understanding of how intersections between axes of inequality such as gender, race, and class might shape important life outcomes such as health. This literature has, however, largely overlooked the role of "place" as a potentially relevant determinant of health, seldom considering how socio-political contexts might influence the intersections between gender, race, and class. Moreover, intersectionality researchers have seldom made use of the full repertoire of analytical tools – such as the inclusion of statistical interaction terms in regression models or the modelling of slopes in multi-level models – that are currently available for examining intersectionality from a quantitative perspective. In this chapter, we engage in a multi-level quantitative investigation of health disparities that considers statistical interactions between gender, race, and class and modelling of their slopes by neighbourhood of residence in Toronto and in New York City (NYC). We seek to provoke future discussions and to offer new questions about intersecting determinants of health and the role of innovative quantitative analyses for better understanding such health determinants. In so doing, we respond explicitly to three imperatives proffered by intersectionality scholars in recent years.

The first of these refers to the distinction between intracategorical and intercategorical intersectional analysis (McCall 2005; Siltanen and Doucet 2008). The *intracategorical* approach examines the experiences of people located at specific intersections of axes of inequality, illuminating the rich complexity of experiences that can accumulate at a given complex social location. A "thick" description of experiences accruing to a single social location can facilitate an understanding of how structural factors influence and are reinforced by personal identities, an understanding that can potentially encompass nearly the entirety of the structure/agency continuum. Because of the close attention paid to experiences at selected social locations, qualitative methods are especially useful here. The *intercategorical* approach examines experiences at multiple complex social locations, seeking to compare and contrast experiences across locations in order to determine which dimensions have a structuring effect on an outcome of interest and whether these effects are modified by their intersections with other dimensions (Siltanen and Doucet 2008). Comparisons of experiences across multiple social locations can provide insights into the characteristics of locations that are unique and identify those that are shared. Noting the plethora of intracategorical intersectional research and the relative paucity of intercategorical intersectionality research, Leslie McCall (2005) and others (such as Landry 2007) have called for more of the latter in order to supplement the many valuable insights provided by the former. This imperative applies especially to the health research domain where intercategorical intersectionality research is almost non-existent. In response, in this chapter we use statistical methods applied to two large survey datasets to investigate the degree to which health outcomes accrue to a host of complex social locations formed by intersections between four axes of inequality.

Second, there is growing agreement that intersectionality researchers need to move beyond the conceptual trinity of gender, race, and class to encompass other dimensions of inequality such as sexuality, disability, religion, nationality, or language (Siltanen and Doucet 2008). Although these have certainly been incorporated into a number of intersectionality research projects, the majority of research in the field continues to centre primarily on gender, race, and class. Our investigation of health predictors also focuses on gender, race, and class, each known to be associated with health and well-being in Canada and the United States, but we additionally consider a hitherto unexplored dimension of inequality: *residential neighbourhood location,* specially examining the aggregate wealth of neighbourhoods. We incorporate neighbourhood of residence into our study because we suspect that people's experiences of race, class, and gender differ across the varied settings that comprise a large urban city. For example, the experiences and social interactions that accompany personal wealth may differ by wealth of neighbourhood, and some of the interpersonal experiences that accompany race may differ by the degree of racial diversity in neighbourhoods. We also note that many studies have found that neighbourhood wealth is related to the health of residents beyond the health effect of the wealth of the individuals themselves (Diez Roux 2001; Kawachi and Subramanian 2007; Matheson, Moineddin and Glazier. 2008). In this chapter, we seek to determine whether this particular axis of inequality also interacts with the other axes and therefore deserves further attention from intersectionality-inspired health scholars.

Third, some scholars have suggested that certain key axes of inequality may be differently manifested across national contexts and that intersections between these axes may differ across these contexts as a result. Yasmin

Jiwani (2006) argues that the Canadian configuration of "race," for instance, surely differs from that of the United States. Direct comparison of the nature of inequality and intersections between axes of inequality across contexts, especially across national contexts, is another important line of investigation that deserves serious attention from intersectionality scholars. In this chapter, we replicate analyses conducted in Toronto with those undertaken in New York City. Although we use two different survey datasets and subtly different measures of key concepts, implementing the same analytical strategy in both cities means that we are able to provide some insight into how intersections between key axes of inequality might differ across urban or national contexts.

In the remainder of this introductory section, we describe our understanding of intersectionality theory and the assumptions and concepts that we believe can be meaningfully incorporated into our investigation of determinants of health disparities. We describe the neighbourhoods and survey datasets from Toronto and New York City used in our study and then briefly describe our multi-level regression modelling procedures. After describing our empirical results, we conclude the chapter by speculating about contributions that intersectionality theory can make to the health disparities literature.

Intersectionality Theory: Precepts and Suppositions

Large-scale systemic power relations apply when dominant groups in society can use power over subordinate groups to regularly secure material and social resources, and can exist simultaneously at the macro levels of structures and institutions and the micro level of interpersonal relationships (Collins 1993; Weber 2006). Many sociological traditions founded on analyses of systemic relations of power are "monist" in character (King 1988), intrinsically privileging one dimension of inequality over others. Nowadays, however, dimensions of inequality such as gender, race, and class are seldom treated in complete isolation from one another in sociological research. In the health determinants literature, for example, race and health researchers have long debated the degree to which class inequalities underlie racial/ethnic health differences. Thus, race could conceivably influence health indirectly via an effect on wealth; race could influence health after controlling for wealth and educational attainment; and wealth and education could have an effect on health after controlling for race. These would all represent *distinct additive* effects of race *and* class on health. Many investigations of these axes of inequality in sociological literatures have similarly treated gender, race, and class as additive processes with distinct – albeit often interconnected – effects on the lives of people. Intersectionality theory seeks to transcend the distinct additive approach to social inequality. The intersectionality principle of simultaneity maintains that all the axes and their corresponding identities should be considered in a given analysis (Landry 2007). Some axes and identities may be more relevant to a specific social context or outcome than others, but a social researcher should never discard or ignore an axis a priori. This is because intersections between axes are thought to create complex social locations that are possibly more central to the manifestation of social experiences and social outcomes than are any of the axes of inequality considered individually. Indeed, the most extreme expression of intersectionality theory would be to maintain that there are no distinct race, gender, class, or sexual orientation effects per se. *Multiplicativity* should supplant *additivity* (Zinn and Dill 1996). Racism + sexism + classism should be replaced by racism × sexism × classism (King 1988; Brewer 1993). Experiences of gender are racialized and classed; experiences of class are gendered and racialized, and so on.

From the principles of simultaneity and multiplicativity arise new versions of double jeopardy and triple jeopardy, renamed *multiple jeopardy* by Deborah King (1988), wherein disadvantaged identities experienced in tandem are seen to result in inordinate amounts of discrimination and disadvantage (even more disadvantage than one would predict from an additive perspective – an aggravating effect). That is, complex social locations comprising multiple disadvantaged identities are thought to lead to multiplicative disadvantage. And because of the relational nature of intersectional theories founded on notions of oppression and discrimination, some complex locations – such as the one inhabited by upper-class white men, for example – in turn are thought to experience multiplicative *advantage*.

From this theoretical perspective, by focusing on just one or two inequality identities, or by (mis)treating multiple axes of inequality as distinct rather than intersecting processes, a social researcher is in danger of profoundly misunderstanding the nature of structural processes, social experiences, and personal identities manifested in specific contexts and thus in danger of producing results and interpretations that are as misleading as they are incomplete. Yet despite the popularity of intersectionality theory and the growing body of applied intersectionality research containing numerous applications of both qualitative and quantitative methodologies, few researchers have explicitly applied intersectionality to health outcomes in quantitative studies. Some health researchers have unknowingly addressed some of the tenets of intersectionality theory by identifying statistically significant two-way interaction effects in multivariate regression models, partially addressing the principles of simultaneity and multiplicativity. In the United States, for example, Joan Ostrove, Pamela Feldman, and Nancy Adler (1999) investigated interactions between socio-economic status and race (white versus African American) as predictors of self-rated health and depression, and Kei Nomaguchi (2007) explored interactions between race (black versus white) and gender on the effect of marital dissolution on depression. In Canada, Zheng Wu et al. (2003) identified two-way interactions between race and socio-economic status for depression. But very few quantitative studies have investigated illness states associated with complex social positions arising from intersections between three axes of inequality (see Jackson and Williams 2006; Zambrana and Dill 2006). We think that this lack of attention to multiple combinations of inequality identities and the intersections between them represents an important gap in the health determinants literature that we seek to redress here.

Data and Methods
Both Toronto and NYC are extremely demographically and socio-economically diverse urban areas. Given that rich health and socio-demographic data are available for the residents and neighbourhoods of Toronto and NYC, they are ideal settings for investigating intersectionality and health within cities and among neighbourhoods.

Neighbourhoods
The City of Toronto created 140 neighbourhoods by aggregating abutting census tracts to establish meaningful boundaries used by government and community agencies for local planning. These neighbourhoods and the median household income reported by residents in the 2001 Canadian census (mean = $54,694, s.d. = $20,115) are depicted visually in Figure 3.1. Median neighbourhood income is shown in quintiles, with darker shades representing neighbourhoods with higher incomes. Median neighbourhood household income ranged from a low of $15,357 in No. 73 Moss Park to a high of $174,967 in No. 41 Bridle Path-Sunnybrook-York Mills. There is a clustering of high-income neighbourhoods in Toronto's central region in and around Bridle Path-Sunnybrook-York Mills. Two other pockets of high-income neighbourhoods include No. 131 Rouge, No. 134 Highland Creek, and No. 133 Centennial Scarborough in northeast Toronto, with area incomes over $72,000, and the part of southwest Toronto that includes No. 15 Kingsway South and No. 10 Princess-Rosethorn, with median incomes surpassing $100,000 per year. Toronto's three lowest-income neighbourhoods (No. 73 Moss Park, No. 72 Regent Park, and No. 74 North St. James Town) are located in the southern part of the city near the downtown core. Low-income neighbourhoods falling in the lowest quintile of income also cluster in the central parts of western Toronto and just east of central Toronto.

Thirty-four New York City neighbourhoods were defined by the NYC Department of Health and Mental Hygiene to identify residential location of survey respondents based on neighbourhood definitions constructed by the United Hospital Fund (UHF) to characterize areas with shared and distinct

Figure 3.1 Neighbourhood median household income in Toronto

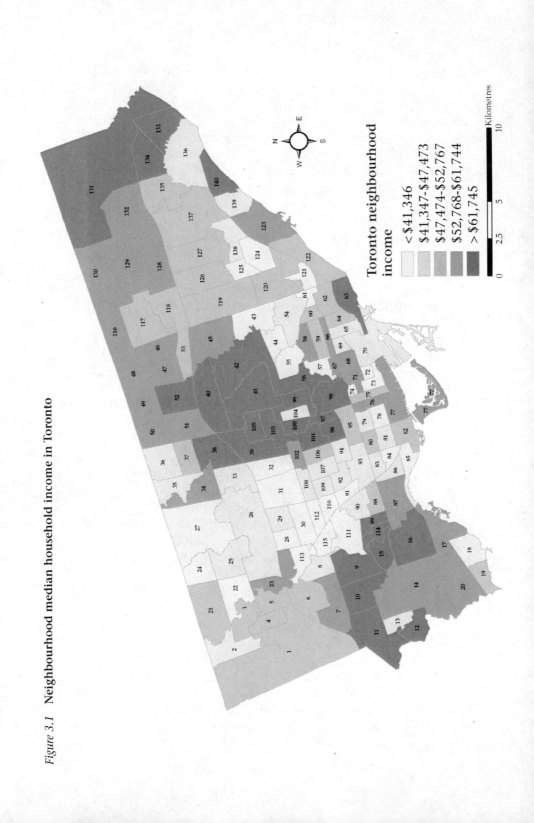

Toronto neighbourhood income

< $41,346
$41,347-$47,473
$47,474-$52,767
$52,768-$61,744
> $61,745

Kilometres
0   2.5   5   10

Toronto neighbourhood legend (neighbourhood number and name)

#	Name	#	Name	#	Name	#	Name
1	West Humber-Clairville	36	Newtonbrook West	71	Cabbagetown-South St. James Town	106	Humewood-Cedarvale
2	Mount Olive-Silverstone-Jamestown	37	Willowdale West	72	Regent Park	107	Oakwood-Vaughan
3	Thistletown-Beaumond Heights	38	Lansing-Westgate	73	Moss Park	108	Briar Hill-Belgravia
4	Rexdale-Kipling	39	Bedford Park-Nortown	74	North St. James Town	109	Caledonia-Fairbank
5	Elms-Old Rexdale	40	St.Andrew-Windfields	75	Church-Yonge Corridor	110	Keelesdale-Eglinton West
6	Kingsview Village-The Westway	41	Bridle Path-Sunnybrook-York Mills	76	Bay Street Corridor	111	Rockcliffe-Smythe
7	Willowridge-Martingrove-Richview	42	Banbury-Don Mills	77	Waterfront Communities-The Island	112	Beechborough-Greenbrook
8	Humber Heights-Westmount	43	Victoria Village	78	Kensington-Chinatown	113	Weston
9	Edenbridge-Humber Valley	44	Flemingdon Park	79	University	114	Lambton Baby Point
10	Princess-Rosethorn	45	Parkwoods-Donalda	80	Palmerston-Little Italy	115	Mount Dennis
11	Eringate-Centennial-West Deane	46	Pleasant View	81	Trinity-Bellwoods	116	Steeles
12	Markland Wood	47	Don Valley Village	82	Niagara	117	L'Amoreaux
13	Etobicoke West Mall	48	Hillcrest Village	83	Dufferin Grove	118	Tam O'Shanter-Sullivan
14	Islington-City Centre West	49	Bayview Woods-Steeles	84	Little Portugal	119	Wexford-Maryvale
15	Kingsway South	50	Newtonbrook East	85	South Parkdale	120	Clairlea-Birchmount
16	Stonegate-Queensway	51	Willowdale East	86	Roncesvalles	121	Oakridge
17	Mimico	52	Bayview Village	87	High Park-Swansea	122	Birchcliffe-Cliffside
18	New Toronto	53	Henry Farm	88	High Park North	123	Cliffcrest
19	Long Branch	54	O'Connor-Parkview	89	Runnymede-Bloor West Village	124	Kennedy Park
20	Alderwood	55	Thorncliffe Park	90	Junction Area	125	Ionview
21	Humber Summit	56	Leaside-Bennington	91	Weston-Pellam Park	126	Dorset Park
22	Humbermede	57	Broadview North	92	Corso Italia-Davenport	127	Bendale
23	Pelmo Park-Humberlea	58	Old East York	93	Dovercourt-Wallace Emerson-Junction	128	Agincourt South-Malvern West
24	Black Creek	59	Danforth Village-East York	94	Wychwood	129	Agincourt North
25	Glenfield-Jane Heights	60	Woodbine-Lumsden	95	Annex	130	Milliken
26	Downsview-Roding-CFB	61	Crescent Town	96	Casa Loma	131	Rouge
27	York University Heights	62	East End-Danforth	97	Yonge-St.Clair	132	Malvern
28	Rustic	63	The Beaches	98	Rosedale-Moore Park	133	Centennial Scarborough
29	Maple Leaf	64	Woodbine Corridor	99	Mount Pleasant East	134	Highland Creek
30	Brookhaven-Amesbury	65	Greenwood-Coxwell	100	Yonge-Eglinton	135	Morningside
31	Yorkdale-Glen Park	66	Danforth Village-Toronto	101	Forest Hill South	136	West Hill
32	Englemount-Lawrence	67	Playter Estates-Danforth	102	Forest Hill North	137	Woburn
33	Clanton Park	68	North Riverdale	103	Lawrence Park South	138	Eglinton East
34	Bathurst Manor	69	Blake-Jones	104	Mount Pleasant West	139	Scarborough Village
35	Westminster-Branson	70	South Riverdale	105	Lawrence Park North	140	Guildwood

Note: Toronto neighbourhood income represents median income for *n* = 140 Toronto neighbourhoods, categorized in quintiles based on Canadian dollars.
Source: Statistics Canada 2001; Canadian Census 2001.

Figure 3.2   **Neighbourhood median household income in New York City**

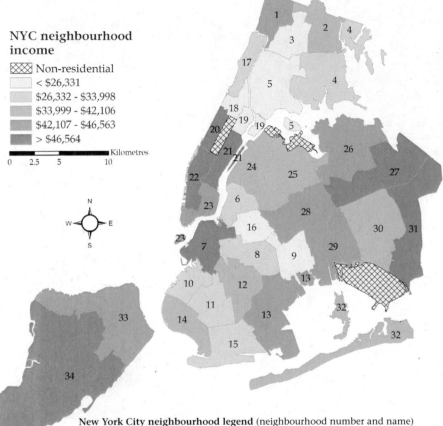

NYC neighbourhood income

- ⊠⊠⊠ Non-residential
- ☐ < $26,331
- ☐ $26,332 - $33,998
- ☐ $33,999 - $42,106
- ☐ $42,107 - $46,563
- ☐ > $46,564

Kilometres
0   2.5   5   10

New York City neighbourhood legend (neighbourhood number and name)

1	Kingsbridge-Riverdale	18	Central Harlem-Morningside
2	Northeast Bronx	19	East Harlem
3	Fordham-Bronx Park	20	Upper West Side
4	Pelhem-Throgs Neck	21	Upper East Side-Gramercy
5	South Bronx	22	Chelsea-Village
6	Greenpoint	23	Union Square, Lower Manhattan
7	Downtown-Heights-Slope	24	Long Island City-Astoria
8	Bedford Stuyvesant	25	West Queens
9	East New York	26	Flushing-Clearview
10	Sunset Park	27	Bayside-Meadows
11	Borough Park	28	Ridgewood-Forest Hills
12	East Flatbush-Flatbush	29	Southwest Queens
13	Canarsie-Flatlands	30	Jamaica
14	Bensonhurst-Bay Ridge	31	Southeast Queens
15	Coney Island-Sheepshead Bay	32	Rockaway
16	Williamsburg-Bushwick	33	Northern Staten Island
17	Washington Heights-Inwood	34	Southern Staten Island

Note: NYC neighbourhood income represents the weighted median income for *n* = 34 United Hospital Fund neighbourhoods weighted based on the median income of zip codes and their population that define each neighbourhood, categorized in quintiles based on US dollars. Non-residential areas include Central Park and airports.
Source: Bureau of the Census, 2000; US Census 2000.

identity. The neighbourhoods comprise adjoining zip codes. A composite measure of median neighbourhood income was created from 2000 US census data. Because the neighbourhood metric was an aggregate of zip codes, median zip code household income was multiplied by the number of households per zip code, summed to create an estimate of total UHF neighbourhood income, and then divided by the total number of households per neighbourhood. The final estimate represents a population-weighted measure of median neighbourhood-level household income and is depicted in Figure 3.2 (mean = US$39,241, s.d. = US$13,270). The median neighbourhood household income variable ranged from a low of $18,914 in No. 5 South Bronx to a high of $72,192 in No. 21 Upper East Side-Gramercy. Pockets of high-income areas occur in southern Manhattan and eastern Queens, and pockets of low-income neighbourhoods exist in Brooklyn, the Bronx, and northern Manhattan. Median income in No. 5 South Bronx, No. 19 East Harlem, No. 16 Williamsburg-Bushwick, and No. 18 Central Harlem-Morningside falls below the national poverty cut-off. (The federal poverty level for a family of five in 2005 was $22,610.)

Survey Samples

The individual-level Toronto data are from the Canadian Community Health Survey 2.1 dataset, which was collected by Statistics Canada in 2003. The target population for this cross-sectional survey was all persons twelve years of age and older residing in Canada, excluding individuals living on Indian reserves and Crown Lands, institutional residents, full-time members of the Canadian Armed Forces, and residents of some remote regions. A complex multipart sampling design was implemented to contact households, and one person was chosen randomly from each household to complete the survey. A total of 134,072 usable responses were obtained, representing a national response rate of 80.7 percent. We focus on the 10,898 survey respondents living in Toronto who were twenty-five and older at the time of the survey and who provided data for all the variables included in our analyses.

The New York City data come from 7,508 adults over twenty-five years of age who participated in the 2004 New York City Community Health Survey (NYCCHS) and who provided data for all the variables included in our analyses (NYCDOHMH 2005). The NYCCHS comprises computer-assisted telephone interviews conducted with non-institutionalized adults, with a landline telephone, who lived within the administrative boundaries of NYC. The survey used a stratified random sampling design with the United Hospital Fund neighbourhoods forming the sampling strata. The overall co-operation rate was 59 percent, based on the number of interviews completed divided by the total number of contacted households. Characteristics of the Toronto and NYC samples are described in Table 3.1.

Table 3.1

Sample characteristics

Variables	Toronto			New York City		
	Categories	Frequency	%	Categories	Frequency	%
Self-reported general health status	Excellent, very good, or good	9,160	84.1	Excellent, very good, or good	5,762	76.7
	Fair or poor	1,738	15.9	Fair or poor	1,746	23.3
Gender	Male	4,879	44.8	Male	3,044	40.5
	Female	6,019	55.2	Female	4,464	59.5
Educational attainment	Less than high school	2,203	20.2	Less than high school	1,145	15.3
	High school graduate	2,683	24.6	High school graduate	1,802	24.0
	Some college	3,621	33.2	Some college	1,561	20.8
	College graduate	2,391	21.9	College graduate	3,000	40.0
Household income	Lowest	380	3.5	Lowest	1,594	21.2
	Lower middle	852	7.8	Lower middle	1,596	21.3
	Middle	2,240	20.6	Middle	1,369	18.2
	Upper middle	3,823	35.1	Upper middle	1,468	19.6
	Highest	3,603	33.1	Highest	1,481	19.7
Racial/ethnic identity	White	9,482	87.0	White	3,099	41.3
	Black	208	1.9	Black	1,781	23.7
	South Asian	236	2.2	Hispanic	1,872	24.9
	Asian	320	2.9	Asian/Pacific Islander	522	7.0
	Other	652	6.0	Other	234	3.1
Age (years)	25-44	4,345	39.9	25-44	3,471	46.2
	45-64	3,708	34.0	45-64	2,647	35.3
	65+	2,845	26.1	65+	1,390	18.5
Nativity	Foreign-born	2,821	25.9	Foreign-born	3,240	43.2
	Canada-born	8,077	74.1	US-born	4,268	56.9
	Neighbourhood income (2001) n =140			*Neighbourhood income (2000) n = 34*		
	Mean	*S.D.*		*Mean*	*S.D.*	
	$54,694	$20,115		$39,241	$13,270	

Note: Instances in which percentages total other than 100 are due to rounding.

Survey Measures

To assess racial/cultural background in Toronto, survey respondents were asked "People living in Canada come from many different cultural and racial backgrounds. Are you: White? Chinese? South Asian (e.g., East Indian, Pakistani, Sri Lankan)? Black? Filipino? Latin American? Southeast Asian (e.g., Cambodian, Indonesian, Laotian, Vietnamese)? Arab? West Asian (e.g., Afghan, Iranian)? Japanese? Korean? Aboriginal (North American Indian, Métis or Inuit)? Other – specify." The interviewer was instructed to read all of the possible responses and record all of those that applied. This variable was recategorized for our purposes as follows: White, Asian (combining the Chinese, Korean, and Japanese categories), Black, South Asian, and "other" (combining all of the remaining categories). The NYCCHS classified racial and ethnic identity based on the following questions: "Please tell me which group best represents your Hispanic or Latino origin or ancestry" and "Which one or more of the following would you say is your race: White, Black or African American, Asian, Native Hawaiian or Other Pacific Islander, American Indian, Alaska Native, or something else?" The five-part mutually-exclusive race/ethnicity variable described in Table 3.1 was subsequently constructed by the NYC Department of Health. Respondents missing race/ethnicity data were assigned to a race/ethnicity group based on country of birth and the language of the survey. For the remaining observations with missing data, respondents were assigned to the majority race/ethnicity group in their neighbourhood. Only 13 percent of respondents in Toronto reported a racial/ cultural background other than White, whereas only 41.3 percent were coded as White in NYC.

Highest educational attainment and household income were used to assess class. Statistics Canada asked a series of survey questions pertaining to education to create the four-part education variable described in Table 3.1. To assess household income, respondents were asked "What is your best estimate of the total income, before taxes and deductions, of all household members from all sources in the past 12 months?" Statistics Canada subsequently calculated the "income adequacy" variable described in Table 3.1.[1] In NYC, level of education was based on the highest school grade completed. Household income was reported as a function of the US federal guidelines for poverty.[2] Although the income variables differ somewhat from one another, the proportional leaps in household income across the categories are quite similar. We note, however, that the NYC sample included proportionately more participants from the lowest two income categories than did the Toronto sample (42.5 percent versus 11.3 percent respectively).

The main outcome variable was self-reported general health status, assessed in NYC with the question "Would you say that in general your health is: Excellent, Very good, Good, Fair or Poor?" Toronto survey respondents were asked "In general, would you say your health is: Excellent? Very good? Good? Fair? Poor?" We distinguish between fair/poor and excellent/very good/good self-rated health in our analyses. The prevalence of fair/poor self-rated health was slightly higher in the NYC sample than in the Toronto one (23.3 percent versus 15.9 percent).

Statistical Methods

A series of multi-level binary regression models was implemented in STATA version 10 to predict fair/poor self-rated health in both cities.[3] All models controlled for age and for nativity (that is, born in Canada or elsewhere for Toronto residents and born in the US or elsewhere for NYC residents). In the first series of models, we investigated the additive effects of gender, race, class, and the wealth of neighbourhood of residence on health by calculating the main effects of each of these inequality variables on health before and after controlling for the others. These models reflect the standard additive approach to investigating health inequalities and represent the departure point for our investigation of intersectionality. By creating these models in a multi-level regression framework, we attempt to untangle the complex interconnectedness of contextual influences (characteristics of the neighbourhoods themselves, such as aggregate wealth) and compositional effects (the characteristics of the people who live there). If neighbourhood of residence persists as a health determinant after controlling for neighbourhood composition, residential neighbourhood location may be an axis of inequality that deserves further attention in intersectionality health research.

In the second set of models, to test the intersecting effects of gender, race, and class, a series of two-way interaction terms comprised all possible combinations of these three inequality axes was added to the final additive model derived in the previous stage of analysis for each city. These models, each of which examines the health outcomes associated with complex social locations derived from two intersecting axes of inequality, tell us whether the two-way interactions have a predictive effect on health above and beyond the additive approach, hence addressing the simultaneity and multiplicativity principles of intersectionality. Furthermore, the nature and direction of the interactions tell us whether or not a given multiplicative scenario displays multiple jeopardy as would be predicted by intersectionality theory. To facilitate these insights, we presented the odds ratios from two-way interactions in a table. Statistically significant two-way interactions tell us whether consideration of complex social locations provides better insights into the nature of disparities in self-rated health than using an additive approach. Finally, a third set of random slopes models allows us to determine whether relationships between self-rated health and each of gender, race, and class differ among neighbourhoods, which would represent another kind of two-way interaction between axes of inequality. Following convention, we consider results from these analyses as statistically significant if they exhibit *p*-values below 0.05.

Results

Additive Models

Tables 3.2 and 3.3 describe the additive models predicting fair/poor health for Toronto and NYC. These models depict the health effects of gender, race, class, and wealth of neighbourhood of residence while controlling for one another and for age and nativity. They provide a first indication of whether gender, race, class, and/or neighbourhood wealth have the potential to be relevant intersectionality axes of inequality in these contexts for predicting self-rated health and are the bases on which we build our investigation of intersectionality.

Table 3.2

Multi-level logistic models predicting fair/poor health in Toronto (2003)

	Odds ratio			
	Gender	Racial/ethnic identity	Class	Full additive model
Gender				
Female	1.152[a]	–	–	0.981
Male	1.000	–	–	1.000
Racial/ethnic identity				
Black		1.219	–	0.898
South Asian	–	0.965	–	0.822
Asian	–	1.120	–	1.060
Other	–	1.410[b]	–	1.118
White	–	1.000	–	1.000
Household income				
Lowest	–	–	5.089[c]	5.038[c]
Lower middle	–	–	3.797[c]	3.752[c]
Middle	–	–	2.514[c]	2.493[c]
Upper middle	–	–	1.570[c]	1.562[c]
Highest	–	–	1.000	1.000
Educational attainment				
Less than high school	–	–	2.574[c]	2.564[c]
High school graduate	–	–	1.813[c]	1.811[c]
Some college	–	–	1.530[c]	1.528[c]
College graduate	–	–	1.000	1.000
Neighbourhood income (in $10,000s)	–	–	–	0.971

$N = 10,898$ in all models; age and Canadian nativity controlled in all models; a $p < .05$, b $p < .01$, c $p < .001$.

Table 3.3

Multilevel logistic models predicting fair/poor health in New York City (2004)

		Odds ratio		
	Gender	Racial/ethnic identity	Class	Full additive model
Gender				
Female	1.239[b]	–	–	1.052
Male	1.000	–	–	1.000
Racial/ethnic identity				
Black	–	1.259[a]	–	0.785[a]
Hispanic	–	2.427[b]	–	1.269[a]
Asian/Pacific Islander	–	1.563[b]	–	1.071
Other	–	1.474[a]	–	1.094
White	–	1.000	–	1.000
Household income				
<100% poverty	–	–	7.173[b]	6.633[b]
100-200% poverty	–	–	4.340[b]	4.136[b]
200-400% poverty	–	–	2.274[b]	2.189[b]
400-600% poverty	–	–	1.712[b]	1.692[b]
>600% poverty	–	–	1.000	1.000
Educational attainment				
Less than high school	–	–	2.016[b]	1.849[b]
High school graduate	–	–	1.213[a]	1.168
Some college	–	–	1.213[a]	1.172
College graduate	–	–	1.000	1.000
Neighbourhood income				
(in $10,000s)	–	–	–	0.872[b]

$N = 7,508$ in all models; age and US nativity controlled in all models; a $p < .05$, b $p < .001$.

Regarding gender, in both Toronto and NYC women were more likely than men to report fair/poor health before, but not after, controlling for race and class. From an additive perspective, this suggests that the weak gender effect evident in both cities is probably explained by the mediating role played by class. With regard to racial/ethnic identity and health, no interpretable effects of note were identified in Toronto. However, Hispanics/Latinos, Asian/Pacific Islanders, and Blacks were all significantly more likely than Whites to report fair/poor health in NYC. After controlling for class and gender, these effects were attenuated for Asian/Pacific Islanders, reduced in magnitude for Hispanics, and reversed in direction for Blacks. These results suggest that class probably mediates the association between race/ethnicity and health in NYC.

Household income showed an extremely strong association with self-rated health in both Toronto and NYC. The magnitude of these associations was especially strong in the latter, where people living in the lowest income group had odds of fair/poor health that were approximately seven times as high as those in the highest income group, before and after controlling for the other axes of inequality. Educational attainment also manifested strong associations with health, the more so in Toronto where the least educated had odds of fair/poor health that were two and a half times as high as the best educated.

Finally, the multi-level models of Tables 3.2 and 3.3 tell us that significant variation occurs between neighbourhoods in both cities that is not explained by compositional differences in the age, nativity, gender, race, or class of residents within the neighbourhoods. Neighbourhood-level median household income explained much of this remaining variability in both contexts. In both cities, increased neighbourhood wealth was associated with a lesser likelihood of reporting fair/poor health: a $10,000 increase in neighbourhood median household income was associated with a 3 percent decrease in the odds of reporting fair/poor health in Toronto (OR = 0.971) and a 13 percent reduction in NYC (OR = 0.872), although in Toronto the neighbourhood wealth variable was not quite statistically significant ($p = 0.054$).

Interactions

First, we considered all two-way interactions between gender, race, and class. No statistically significant interactions were found between gender and income in either city. Gender and race interacted significantly in Toronto (but not in NYC), where South Asian women were much more likely than White women to report fair/poor health (OR = 3.280), whereas South Asian men were much less likely than White men to do so (OR = 0.414). (See Table 3.4.) A similar pattern, albeit less pronounced and non-significant, emerged for Black women and men. In addition, gender and education interacted in NYC (but not in Toronto) where the disadvantage for health of not completing high school versus completing a college degree was significantly larger for women (OR = 2.133) than for men (OR = 1.461). In Toronto, race and income interacted such that, among Asians, respondents with the lowest incomes were less likely than the highest-income earners to report fair/poor health (OR = 0.755). A similar pattern, but weaker and non-significant, emerged for Black Torontonians. Race and income did not interact significantly in NYC. Finally, race and education did not interact significantly in either urban context.

Next, we modelled the slope coefficients for gender, race, and class in each city to test whether the effects of these axes of inequality differed significantly among New York and Toronto neighbourhoods. The slope coefficients for

Table 3.4

Statistically significant interactions between axes of inequality

		Odds ratio	
		Toronto	New York City
Gender X race interactions			
Women	OR White (ref)	1.000	–
	OR Black	1.869	
	OR South Asian	3.280	
	OR Asian	1.010	
Men	OR White (ref)	1.000	
	OR Black	0.579	
	OR South Asian	0.414[a]	
	OR Asian	1.007	
Gender X education interactions			
Women	OR less than high school	–	2.133
	OR high school graduate		1.181
	OR some college		1.162
	OR college graduate (ref)		1.000
Men	OR less than high school		1.461[b]
	OR high school graduate		1.151
	OR some college		1.197
	OR college graduate (ref)		1.000
Race X income interactions[c]			
White (ref)	OR lowest income group	5.738	–
Black	OR lowest income group	0.979	
South Asian	OR lowest income group	3.001	
Asian	OR lowest income group	0.755[d]	
Gender X income interactions			
No significant interactions		–	–
Race X education interactions			
No significant interactions		–	–
Do the slope coefficients differ significantly among *neighbourhoods?*			
For gender?		–	–
For White versus non-White?		–	Yes
For lowest household income category versus the rest?		–	Yes
For having the lowest educational attainment versus having a high school diploma or higher?		–	–

$N = 7,508$ in all models; age and nativity controlled in all models.
a   The comparison with OR = 3.280 for South Asian women produced $p < 0.05$.
b   The comparison with OR = 2.133 for women produced $p < 0.05$.
c   All Race X income coefficients are interpreted relative to persons in the *highest* income group.
d   The comparison with OR = 5.738 for Whites produced $p < 0.05$.

gender on self-rated health did not vary significantly by neighbourhood in either city. After modelling the slope for a simple dichotomous variable distinguishing Whites from all others, we found that, where health was concerned, the effect of being White differed significantly by neighbourhood in NYC but not in Toronto. Slopes for income and education were also modelled by neighbourhood. The slope for a simple dichotomous variable, distinguishing respondents in the poorest category from all the other categories, varied significantly by neighbourhood in NYC but not in Toronto. Finally, modelling the slope for a dichotomous variable, distinguishing respondents in the least-educated category from all others, did not lead to significant variation by neighbourhood in either context.

In short, our multiplicative analyses provide evidence of interactions involving all of gender, race, class, and neighbourhood of residence for self-rated health outcomes, effects that seemingly played out very differently in the two urban areas.

Discussion

Our findings highlight the value of applying a multi-level intersectional approach to studying the complex, interrelated effects of gender, race, class, and place on health. Here we briefly discuss the meaning of these results in the context of current thinking about intersectionality theory and offer several suggestions for future health determinants research that also seeks to meaningfully incorporate intersectionality concepts.

Our greatest insight is that the additive approach is inadequate to the task of describing the health inequalities in Toronto and NYC. Knowing an individual's simple social location (such as female or poor) can provide insight about health outcomes, but understanding an individual's complex social location (female and poor) often provides additional information that helps to untangle the complex determinants of health outcomes. Multiplicativity was clearly relevant to inequality in self-reported health in both Toronto and New York City. A second important finding pertains to the principle of simultaneity. All four axes of inequality addressed in this study participated significantly in at least one two-way statistical interaction of note in at least one of the urban contexts. It is clear from our analysis of the intersecting roles of place, race, gender, and class that, had we not tested interaction terms and neighbourhood-level effects, a number of important insights would have been missed.

We were surprised by the nature of the actual manifestations of multiplicativity, few of which represented examples of multiplicative advantage or disadvantage. First, although the additive models for Toronto showed little association between gender and health, and little association between race and health, on examining the interaction between race and gender, we found that South Asian women tended to report poorer health than expected and that South Asian men tended to report better health than expected. Follow-up qualitative study is needed to identify social mechanisms that could work to produce such gendered health outcomes among South Asian Torontonians. Another surprising finding pertained to Asians and income in Toronto, with wealthier Asians more likely to report fair/poor health than those with lower incomes. Additional study is needed here as well to confirm and explain how income might be detrimental for the health of Asian Torontonians. Only one instance of multiple jeopardy emerged in our analyses, the case of the interaction between gender and education in NYC: our analyses indicate that a significant health penalty exists for women in NYC who possess few educational credentials.

Implications for Research and Practice

This chapter builds on a growing theoretical tradition of intersectionality research by describing the intersecting roles of place, race, gender, and class as determinants of health in Toronto and New York City. Here we make several suggestions for future research in this vein.

First, quantitative analyses offer useful tools for evaluating the intersecting determinants of health that have been largely overlooked to date. Databases containing rich health and demographic data about Canadians are publicly available and inexpensive, and intersectionality health researchers would benefit from using them. Acquiring the complex methodological and statistical prowess needed to take advantage of these datasets may not be feasible (or desirable) for many, but intersectionality scholars would certainly benefit by collaborating with quantitatively trained colleagues from the social sciences, as well as scholars from public health, epidemiology, and the health sciences who share an interest in understanding the determinants of health and who can contribute sophisticated analytical tools. Public health researchers also serve to gain from the theoretical and methodological contributions of intersectionality researchers. As of February 2009, only nine articles were identified by PubMed (the primary search engine used to access peer-reviewed biomedical research studies) with "intersectionality" as the search term. There remains a large gap in knowledge transfer from the social sciences literature to applied health researchers and practitioners who are positioned to translate lessons learned from intersectionality research into viable "real world" solutions geared toward reducing health disparities.

Second, although the neighbourhoods-and-health literature is growing, inspired by a rich tradition within geography on the significance of space and place for health and well-being (Gatrell 2002), intersectionality theorists have largely overlooked how geographic context shapes the intersections of inequality. Our analyses pointed out the important role of neighbourhoods in their own right. Questions remain about how and why neighbourhood residential context shapes access to health resources, health information and knowledge, social norms, transportation, experiences of discrimination, and expectations about health. Gender, race, and health scholars are well positioned to explore how these factors differ between places and spaces, and act to mediate other important dimensions of inequality. Our rationale for comparing Toronto to NYC was to examine whether intersecting relations between gender, race, and class vary between two large ethnically diverse urban centres in two countries. Clearly, these two places do not represent all Canadian and American cities, but given that several important differences were found in the significance, magnitude, and even direction of associations between interactions and self-rated health, we have opened the door for important discussions about the role of place and space for effects of inequalities on health.

In Toronto, we found significant interactions in the effects of race and gender and of race and income that were not observed in NYC; in NYC but not in Toronto we found significant interactions between gender and low educational attainment as well as neighbourhood differences in the effects of race and poverty. Further research is needed in order to identify underlying mechanisms that explain these between-city differences.

Our final thoughts relate to the usefulness of intersectionality theory for explicating disparities in health in general. We are pleased to have been pushed by this theoretical orientation to investigate a myriad of interactions that we would not have otherwise considered – many of them bore fruit empirically in these two cross-national urban contexts. Yet we found that only one of the interactions was in the directions predicted by the multiple jeopardy idea of intersectionality – that is, only one of them manifested a reinforcing or mutually constituting quality. This may be because the determinants of good and poor health are many and varied, and not all of them are intricately tied up in social and economic inequalities in society. To the degree that they are interconnected with such inequalities, then, intersectionality theory is well poised to help us better understand the nature of the social experiences that lead to lower levels of well-being; to the degree that they are not, intersectionality theory probably has little to tell us about why health outcomes vary.

In our analyses, we found several interactions that might benefit from further empirical investigation, such as the negative effect of income on health among Asians in Toronto (perhaps pertaining to the experiences of discrimination that may accompany fuller entry into North American society writ large) and the sharp divide between the health of South Asian men and women in Toronto (perhaps pertaining to a marked gender divide in power and authority in this particular cultural community). We encourage other scholars, possessing finer methodological tools than we can employ for understanding the lived experiences of Asians or South Asians in Canada, to further pursue the findings we have described here.

Notes

1 The income adequacy variable considers both household income and household size. Survey respondents placed in the lowest category had household incomes of less than $10,000 for households of one to four people and under $15,000 for households of five or more. Respondents placed in the lower middle category had household incomes of between $10,000 and $14,999 for households of one or two people, $10,000-$19,999 for households of three or four, and $15,000-$29,999 for households of five or more. Respondents placed in the middle category had household incomes between $15,000 and $29,999 for one or two people, $20,000-$39,999 for households of three or four, and $30,000-$59,999 for households of five or more. Respondents placed in the upper middle category had household incomes between $30,000 and $59,999 for one or two people, $40,000-$79,999 for households of three or four, and $60,000-$79,999 for households of five or more. Finally, respondents placed in the highest category had household incomes greater than $60,000 for one or two people and greater than $80,000 for households of three or more.
2 The lowest income category included respondents with household incomes below a poverty threshold. For families with one member the threshold was $9,310, for families with two members the threshold was $12,490, and so on. For families of eight the threshold was $31,570, and $3,180 was added to this value for every family member above eight.
3 For more information on multi-level regression modelling, see Raudenbush and Bryk (2002) and Diez Roux (2002).

References

Brewer, R.M. 1993. Theorizing race, class and gender: The new scholarship of black feminist intellectuals and black women's labor. In *Theorizing black feminisms: The visionary pragmatism of black women,* ed. S.M. James and A.P.A. Busia, 13-30. London: Routledge.

Collins, P.H. 1993. Toward a new vision: Race, class, and gender as categories of analysis and connection. *Race, Sex, and Class* 1(1): 25-45.

Diez Roux, A.V. 2001. Investigating neighborhood and area effects on health. *American Journal of Public Health* 91(11): 1783-89.

–. 2002. A glossary for multilevel analysis. *Journal of Epidemiology and Community Health* 56: 588-94.

Gatrell, A. 2002. *Geographies of health: An introduction.* Malden, MA: Blackwell.

Jackson, P.B., and D.R. Williams. 2006. The intersection of race, gender, and SES: Health paradoxes. In *Gender, race, class and health: Intersectional approaches,* ed. A.J. Schulz and L. Mullings, 131-62. San Francisco: Jossey-Bass.

Jiwani, Y. 2006. *Discourses of denial: Mediations of race, gender, and violence.* Vancouver: UBC Press.

Kawachi, I., and S.V. Subramanian. 2007. Neighbourhood influences on health. *Journal of Epidemiology and Community Health* 61(1): 3-4.

King, D.K. 1988. Multiple jeopardy, multiple consciousness. *Signs: Journal of Women in Culture and Society* 14(1): 42-72.

Landry, B., ed. 2007. *Race, gender and class: Theory and methods of analysis.* Upper Saddle River, NJ: Pearson Education.

Matheson, F.I., R. Moineddin, and R.H. Glazier. 2008. The weight of place: A multilevel analysis of gender, neighborhood material deprivation, and body mass index among Canadian adults. *Social Science and Medicine* 66(3): 675-90.

McCall, L. 2005. The complexity of intersectionality. *Signs: Journal of Women in Culture and Society* 30(3): 1771-1800.

Nomaguchi, K.M. 2007. Are there race and gender differences in the effect of marital dissolution on depression? In Landry 2007, 394-410.

NYCDOHMH. 2005. New York City community health survey. New York City Department of Health and Mental Hygiene. http://www.nyc.gov.

Ostrove, J., P. Feldman, and N. Adler. 1999. Relations among socioeconomic status indicators and health for African-Americans and whites. *Journal of Health Psychology* 4(4): 451-63.

Raudenbush, S.W. and A.S. Bryk. 2002. *Hierarchical linear models: Application and data analysis methods*. 2nd ed. Thousand Oaks: Sage.

Siltanen, J., and A. Doucet. 2008. *Gender relations in Canada: Intersectionality and beyond*. Don Mills: Oxford University Press.

Weber, L. 2006. Reconstructing the landscape of health disparities research: Promoting dialogue and collaboration between intersectional and biomedical paradigms. In *Gender, race, class and health: Intersectional approaches*, ed. A.J. Schulz and L. Mullings, 21-59. San Francisco: Jossey-Bass.

Wu, Z., S. Noh, V. Kaspar, and C.M. Schimmele. 2003. Race, ethnicity, and depression in Canadian society. *Journal of Health and Social Behavior* 44(3): 426-41.

Zambrana, R.E., and B.T. Dill. 2006. Disparities in Latina health: An intersectional analysis. In *Gender, race, class and health: Intersectional approaches*, ed. A.J. Schulz and L. Mullings, 192-227. San Francisco: Jossey-Bass.

Zinn, M.B. and B.T. Dill. 1996. Theorizing difference from multiracial feminism. *Feminist Studies* 22(2): 321-31.

4

Performing Intersectionality: The Mutuality of Intersectional Analysis and Feminist Participatory Action Health Research

Colleen Reid, Pamela Ponic, Louise Hara,

Connie Kaweesi, and Robin LeDrew

Feminist theorists and researchers have long claimed the need to pay attention to women's diversities. For over four decades, and more specifically in the last twenty years, feminist researchers have "grappled with questions around who is privileged epistemologically and how this affects the representation of voices and the interpretations of findings" (Reid and Frisby 2007, 96). As co-researchers with a five-year working relationship on the Women's Employability and Health Research Project (WEHP), we have been grappling with what it means to examine and embody women's diversity, and the implications this has for women's health.[1] We have collaborated on a feminist participatory action research (FPAR) project, engaged deeply with intersectional theory and analysis, and recently identified ourselves as an intersectional health research team (Clark 2009). Our process for working and writing together has been complex and rewarding, with constructive lessons along the way. Although our work is far from complete, we are pausing here to present our insights on how FPAR and intersectionality mutually inform one another and help illuminate the fluidity of our subject identities and the power relations that arose in our research relationships.

Through promoting participatory approaches to democratizing research, FPAR aims to bring diverse voices and perspectives into the research process with overt attention paid to what comes from the research and how women's health can be improved as a result. As a theoretical approach, intersectionality forces researchers to deeply consider the diverse identities and subjectivities that exist within and among women, and how these complexities inform research processes (Varcoe, Hankivsky, and Morrow 2007); it also "initiates a process of discovery, alerting us to the fact that the world around us is always more complicated and contradictory than we ever could have anticipated. It compels us to grapple with this complexity in our scholarship" (Davis 2008, 79). In this chapter, we describe our experiences conducting an intersectional analysis as a province-wide FPAR team located in British

Columbia. The intention of the project was to examine women's employability and health in relation to women-unfriendly shifts in provincial social policy and practices. The following research question guided our approach: How does an intersectional analysis illuminate aspects of an FPAR process?

This combination of theory and methodology requires feminist researchers to "grapple with this complexity" in their scholarship; it provides the tools and insights necessary to fully understand each person's individual intersections and how they shape the research process itself. Whereas intersectionality and FPAR offer the opportunity to facilitate deeper understanding of the complexities of women's lives, the potential they hold for understanding working relationships among diverse research teams has been relatively unexamined. Gaby Weiner (2004, 634) argues that although feminist action research is concerned with issues that matter to women, valuing women's lived realities and taking political action, it has been slow to take recent advances in feminist theory into account. On the other hand, intersectional researchers have rarely employed overtly participatory methods choosing to favour approaches that lead to enhanced theoretical sophistication. Using intersectionality as a theoretical approach within an FPAR project can provide greater insights into the analysis of women's health and diversities as well as the working relationships among research team members. In this chapter, we argue that despite the tensions that can arise in integrating an intersectional analysis into FPAR, in particular in terms of the impact on the research team members' health and well-being, bringing intersectional analysis and FPAR together has the capacity to illuminate the multiple and fluid identities of all members of a research team.

Feminist Participatory Action Research (FPAR)

Over the last three decades, there has been a rise in action research identified explicitly as feminist. This body of work explores how feminist perspectives on gender, as it intersects with other axes of oppression, are fundamental for engaging in action research that is representative, meaningful, and liberating in the context of women's lives (Reid and Frisby 2007). FPAR is a conceptual and methodological framework that enables a critical understanding of women's multiple perspectives and works toward inclusion, participation, action, and social change while confronting the underlying assumptions the researcher brings into the research process (Reid 2004). FPAR has made significant strides and contributions, especially in terms of encouraging subaltern voices to be heard and acted on through participatory methodologies (see, for example, Brydon-Miller, Maguire, and McIntyre 2004; McIntyre and Lykes 2004; Wang, Burris, and Ping 1996). Through advocating democratic practices at all stages of research (in terms of the questions that are asked, the research design, how and by whom data are collected, analyzed, and disseminated), it seeks to uncover and redress inequitable power relations that manifest in the everyday lives and experiences of historically marginalized women (Lykes and Coquillon 2006).

Increasingly, feminist participatory action researchers are uncovering the inevitable tensions and messiness of partnering with community members for social change and interrupting established research practices and paradigms (Lykes, Blanche, and Hamber 2003; Maguire 2001; Ponic 2007; Reid 2004). The tensions and messiness that arise during FPAR projects are a necessary component of social change and an indication that power relations are in fact shifting. This is especially true given the complex social and power differences among academic researchers, community-based researchers, and diverse participants that are typical in FPAR projects (Ponic 2007). What is needed, however, are tools and frameworks for both understanding and managing these complexities. Reflexivity is one such tool that requires all involved to critically examine the assumptions and beliefs brought to the research process as a tool for individual and mutual learning (Mauthner and Doucet 2003; Pillow 2003; Varcoe 2006).

Ideally, in FPAR, community members are actively involved in all stages of knowledge production, including identifying the research problem, data collection and analysis, and knowledge translation (Frisby et al. 2005). Conducting FPAR requires academic researchers to share some of their power within the research process and to promote community control. Doing so explicitly positions FPAR within a feminist social justice agenda, but it also makes the work more complex because of the necessity to interrogate, redefine, and transform traditional power relations both within broader social relations and the research process itself.

At times there has been an uneasy fit between overt feminist social justice agendas, as exemplified in FPAR approaches, and the development and refinement of feminist theory. This may partly result from claims that some feminist theories have become so esoteric and elitist that they are no longer pertinent to community-based or social change initiatives (Hemmings 2007). Certainly, it is not always clear how or which specific feminist perspectives ground FPAR projects (Frisby, Maguire, and Reid 2009). Weiner (2004) argues that although FPAR is concerned with understanding, valuing, and addressing issues that matter to women, it has been slow to take account of recent advances in feminist theory. Historically, however, researchers' willingness to continually engage in theory and critique has led to the rapid advancement in feminist knowledge and change. Bridging the gap between theory and practice is an important task for feminist participatory action researchers in order to make feminist theories relevant and avoid conducting research in colonizing and patronizing ways (McEwan 2001; Williams and Lykes 2003).

Intersectionality

Intersectionality theory is the study of multiple categories of identity and social relations that intersect with one another to produce systems of power, oppression, and privilege (McCall 2005). It has grown out of critical feminist concerns about the limits of privileging one category of analysis (gender) over others (race, class, sexual orientation, ability, and/or place), and it seeks to understand the fluid and contested ways in which they intersect to systematically shape the reality of women's lives (Collins 2000). It goes beyond the analytic approach of "adding" one social category to another, asking researchers to deeply consider the complex fluidity of social locations, identities, and processes (Hulko 2009). The core purpose of intersectionality is to facilitate profound analyses of social justice issues by interrogating the social and power relations that lie at their root (Hankivsky and Cormier 2009; Shields 2008).

Intersectionality theory can help illuminate the connections between individual subjectivities and broader social structures, as well as local and global experiences (Shields 2008). Intersectionality forces researchers to grapple in that uncomfortable territory of challenging assumptions, honestly considering alternative and at times oppositional world views and disrupting traditional power relations. Intersectionality can also inspire creative feminist inquiry that expands the potential for empirical and methodological advancements (Davis 2008). Indeed, it is an important and innovative advancement in feminist theory.

Yet a common critique of intersectionality is that it lacks specific methodological applications (McCall 2005; Simien 2007), making its usefulness to feminist goals of action and change uncertain. How to utilize intersectionality in interdisciplinary health research has also been unclear (Squier 2007). Kathy Davis (2008) points out that identifying the challenges in a theory is the necessary first step in improving it. In this light, specific methodologies for intersectional research have slowly begun to emerge (Hancock 2007); for example, a primer written by Olena Hankivsky and Renee Cormier (2009) offers a step-by-step illustration of how an intersectional lens can inform and deepen critical analysis throughout research and policy-making processes.

FPAR offers exciting potential for further operationalizing intersectionality, both in the analyses of findings and the relationships it produces. Given the community and participatory orientations of FPAR, its projects typically include a range of academic researchers, community-based researchers, community practitioners and service providers, and participants. The diversity and fluidity of social locations and subject identities that the various players bring to an FPAR process provide an opportunity to experience and document the dimensions and layers of intersectionality that would not necessarily arise in non-participatory, or more linear, approaches to research. Although this engagement can deepen understandings, it can also create complicated power relations. An FPAR approach is similar to an intersectional approach in its underlying principle regarding the pursuit of social justice as the primary goal of research (ibid.). Implicit within FPAR is the role of power and in particular the power a "community" has as a whole in influencing policy makers who make decisions that affect their lives directly. Further, FPAR recognizes that there are hierarchies of power within communities and differences in status among community members (Morris and Bunjun 2007). Yet, although feminist participatory action researchers have suggested intersectionality as a promising theoretical stance for advancing FPAR (Frisby, Maguire, and Reid 2009), and intersectional researchers have identified an epistemological coherence with more participatory approaches, there are no examples to date of analyses that aim to explicitly bridge them. What they do share is a commitment to reflexive practices. It is through this shared commitment that we, as a research team, explored how to bring intersectionality into our research practices and relationships.

WEHP Communities, Structure, and Methods

The Women's Employability and Health Research Project (WEHP) was a three-year FPAR venture that examined women's employability and how their efforts to survive affect their health and well-being. Employability was defined as women's relationship to the formal and informal economies. The four British Columbian communities involved in the project were characterized as rural-farming, northern-resource, remote-reserve, and urban-South Asian. They were selected because they represented the social, geographic, demographic, and economic diversities in BC in terms of the gap between women's and men's incomes, the local economy of the community, and socio-demographic factors such as ethnicity and migration status.

The WEHP was managed by Colleen as the principal investigator and Louise as the project coordinator. Pamela contributed research support and training, whereas the Coalition for Women's Economic Advancement provided intellectual guidance and administrative assistance. Local researchers were hired in each community, in one instance as an individual and in three others as teams of two to four women. Robin and Connie were members of two community teams. Figure 4.1 captures the structure and relationships in WEHP.

The community researchers were drawn to the project because it focused on the social determinants of women's health. In all cases, they felt a strong commitment to better understand the relationship between women's social status and health, and to taking action to improve women's health in their communities. The community researchers conducted one-on-one interviews and focus groups. In total, seventy women were involved as research

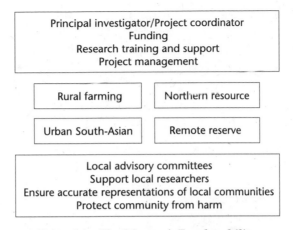

Figure 4.1   **The Women's Employability and Health Research Project (WEHP)**

participants, and sixty primary documents were generated for analysis. The community researchers wrote a report that detailed social, demographic, and economic characteristics of their community in relation to the research findings on women's health. These reports are now in circulation and have been used as the basis for many community actions.

In this chapter, we analyze our individual and collective reflexive processes as an intersectional research team. Our commitment to reflexivity meant that we were able to gather chunks of data from varying sources that were collected over the three-year project – email correspondence, meeting minutes, journal entries, and individual and shared reflections on questions around power, process, and intersectionality. In the early stages of the project, reflexive fieldnotes were used to better understand the working relationships among researchers within the four communities. Shortly into the project, our commitment to reflexivity expanded to include reflections on the broader project itself. Indeed, the excerpts included in this analysis resulted from our self-identified positionality as it emerged and shifted over the course of our project together. This chapter is a product not only of these threads of data but also of a collaborative writing process we engaged in together.

The FPAR Team: Multiple and Overlapping Relationships and Perspectives

Integrating an intersectional analysis into an FPAR process has the capacity to illuminate the multiple and fluid identities of all members of a research team (Hulko 2009). Davis (2008, 72) argues that intersectionality can be "employed by any feminist scholar willing to use her own social location, whatever it may be, as an analytic resource rather than just an identity marker." In order to harness our own social locations as analytic resources for our work together, we have been guided individually and collectively by a commitment to reflexivity. Throughout the project, we systematically recorded reflexive journal entries to document our work together, our evolving group process, and our emergent reflections and analyses. As a team, we kept notes of all discussions and meetings. Reflexivity is a tool that is central to both intersectionality theory and FPAR. We have also come to understand that intersectionality provides an appropriate theoretical approach for understanding our processes, as it is for thinking about others' lived realities; in other words, we embody and internalize intersectionality. In this regard, we use the term "intersection" as a way to capture the space between and across our various social locations and subject identities. On a collective level, consciously and reflexively engaging with each other has enabled us to uncover the depths and dimensions imbricated in our work together. In the spirit of reflexivity, we continually attempt to situate ourselves in the unique places from which we operate, all the while understanding the important connections that we share.

Colleen is an academically trained researcher who completed her doctoral studies in 2002 and, as a post-doctoral fellow, was the principal investigator for the WEHP. Louise facilitates capacity building within groups and organizations that wish to strengthen their ability to reach their goals, working from a feminist/anti-oppression/community economic development perspective. Working together since 2001, Colleen and Louise have enjoyed a tremendous synergy in ideas and passions around women's rights, social justice issues, and advocating for social change. Though their life trajectories have been very different, and they are at different stages of their lives personally and professionally, they have come together on key social issues that broadly relate to women's "place" in society. The Coalition for Women's Economic Advancement and the WEHP were born from this shared energy, enthusiasm, and passion. Pam is also an academically trained researcher who completed her doctoral studies in 2007. She was involved in the WEHP project as a research consultant, stepping in to support the team's research processes when Colleen was on maternity leave. Pam conducts FPAR in the social determinants of women's health, and like Colleen, has worked within and between academic and community-based research settings. Pam has long-standing working relationships with Colleen and Louise that were initiated via another FPAR project and sustained through mutual enthusiasm for the potential of FPAR to spark social justice efforts. Connie is a registered clinical social worker. She has extensive experience working in the social and health field and has lived in northern British Columbia since 1985. Finally, Robin graduated as a mature student from the University of Victoria. She practises social work in a small farming community where she has lived since the early 1970s. In the WEHP, Connie and Robin were the community researchers for the northern-resource and rural-farming communities, respectively.

Experiences of an Intersectional FPAR Research Team

The structure of the WEHP was intended to draw out women's "intersections" in relation to the research questions around employability and health. Adopting an intersectional analysis strengthened our understanding of women's diverse realities, all the while bringing attention to the remarkably similar ways in which women's paid and unpaid work affected health across and between diversities such as rural/urban/remote, north/south/interior and Aboriginal/South Asian/white. From the outset, we were clear that our theoretical goals required us to use intersectionality theory. Without doubt, adopting an intersectional analysis was the most meaningful and representative way to understand our research findings. It also had the unexpected impact of forcing us to more fully examine how our shared and unique intersections played out in our group dynamics and approaches to analysis and social action.

Navigating Place and Race

Control and Making Decisions for "Others"
Ideally, FPAR creates the space for community members to be involved in all aspects of the research process in an atmosphere of mutual respect (Frisby et al. 2005; Macaulay et al. 1999). Given the diversity of perspectives that are included, disagreements and conflicts should be anticipated by having mechanisms in place to address changes of research design, of personnel, and of mind (Macaulay et al. 1999; Ponic 2007). It is also important to ensure that all relevant partners are as involved as they want to be and in roles that are appropriate to their positions in the project (Gibson, Gibson, and Macaulay 2001). On a number of levels, these ideals were not our reality. The WEHP was not conceptualized by all the researchers who were ultimately involved, which meant that our processes for working together unfolded over time. Our group process was also shaped by changes in personnel (in two communities) that interrupted team building, by the fact that community researchers lived throughout the province with little direct access to each other, and by funding structures that circumscribed all our roles and potential involvement.

Throughout our work, there were key sources of tension that paradoxically created opportunities for better understanding our intersections while simultaneously complicating productive explorations of how our intersections were beneficial and instructive to the research process and findings. These sources of tension included access and control of funds, legitimacy and authority, jurisdiction and accountability, local gate keeping and support, and finally, education and skills.

Colleen, Louise, and Pam, as the team members primarily responsible for managing the project provincially and answering to the funders, often discussed these sources of tension while acknowledging the need to make unilateral decisions at the expense of coherence and mutuality. We faced the realities of insufficient funding, having three years to conduct the research, and being accountable to four funders and two research ethics boards (REBs). In our minds, handing down some decisions was the surest way to achieve what was promised and required. Yet one research team member of the rural-farming community wrote, "[I felt] frustration dealing with 3 other people [on the local team] plus Vancouver people and ethics committee. It has been resolved somewhat with a go-ahead but there are too many other distractions with us all on a personal basis for the project to feel cohesive." Robin reflected, "[We've faced] challenges feeling heard and valued, and difficulties confronting discussions about power. Although there is an overall buy-in to dissemination processes (writing for journals and books, conference presentations, etc), at times our roles are inequitable. And, we are dealing with these dynamics at a distance (over the phone) and via email – lots is lost in translation and in time and space."

In the northern-resource site, the community researchers had hoped that they would be able to control daily decisions that affected the research process. However, because grants were approved based on certain budgetary allocations and were administered by non-profit organizations in Metro Vancouver, making even small decisions was sometimes not possible. Connie commented,

> My values of community empowerment were challenged and I felt frustrated. I have lived in the North for 21 years and find myself always dealing with agencies in the South making decisions for the North. These decision-makers do not understand how the North works, how we are flexible, resourceful and need autonomy. Northern people have a pride in making their own way, taking control of their decisions and working cooperatively with each other. Dependence on set policies from external agents is difficult. In future, I will definitely ask more questions and have a clearer understanding of the expectations of the project.

Feelings of disillusionment were also fuelled by the sense that the imposed structures and decisions were changed occasionally and without notice: "It's hard to keep up the enthusiasm when the plans and rules keep changing from the ethics committee" (research team member, rural-farming). Whereas Colleen and Louise made some decisions as a way to expedite the research process, other decisions, such as the research ethics board's criterion of maintaining community confidentiality, were imposed "from above" on the entire team (see Reid et al. forthcoming 2011).

It is overly simplistic to portray the local researchers as sharing a singular perspective in contrast to Colleen, Louise, and Pam as the managers and key decision makers. All of us experienced moments of doubt, uncertainty, and discomfort, not only as a result of being forced to negotiate an imposed decision or structure but also because we did not know if the project would succeed at all. All of us negotiated these tensions throughout the project, at times feeling empowered and certain, and at other times disempowered and unclear. For instance, when the community researchers felt that decisions were being imposed, the sense of difference between local experience and project "headquarters" was strongest. This sense of difference was also amplified when project headquarters experienced resistance or "push-back" from the local researchers. For example, Louise said that "our ability to share all we think and believe is hampered by our [lack of] trust that what we share is valued by others on an equal basis with all members of the group."

When we did not feel the safety or trust within the group, we encountered stalemate and misunderstanding. On the other hand, when our individual autonomy, commitment, and effort were recognized and encouraged, team members felt a greater sense of coherence, shared goals, and mutuality. In some ways, when our relationships were rocky we "othered" each other. Othering involves privileging dominant social practices and experiences, and minimizing those from the margin (Young 1990). In our situation, when dominant practices were imposed by project headquarters in response to funder and REB requirements, the perspectives of community researchers and the needs for local control were minimized. Because othering is bred by a fear and intolerance of differences, it limited the degree to which we could exercise our capacities "in a context of recognition and interaction" (ibid., 55). We were left with the following questions: Can we foster enough trust across our intersections and within constraining structures to allow us all the freedom and cohesion to take our communal thinking and actions to the next level? Is it possible to do that given the complexities at play?

Only in our more recent work together, writing and presenting, have we identified how deadlines, external structures and expectations, and the imposition of decisions undermine the safety of our process and intensify the othering within our team. When this occurs, team members become more easily triggered and reactive, with a tendency to view each other's input as a set of fixed intersections rather than as the result of external pressures and difficulties with communication and control. Through our shared commitment to FPAR, we have learned that our ability to extend our thinking beyond our a priori social categories was most inhibited when we were not engaging collaboratively, mutually, and respectfully with one another.

In contrast, our commitment to creating a democratic working relationship, and our attention to developing these processes, has had a positive impact on our ability to do an intersectional analysis.

As an intersectional research team, our goal is to feel the safety and confidence to allow our individual "intersections" the fluidity necessary to generate a healthy and productive collective working environment. When individual needs are not met, our intersections become firmer, more entrenched, rigid, and static – leaving little possibility for intellectual or personal growth within the FPAR process. When we are not pressed with multiple demands and have the space and recognition for the work we are doing, our intersections become far more expansive, dynamic, and accommodating. This is not to say that we lose our individual perspectives: rather, it means that we are better able to truly engage in an intersectional analysis of our own and the research participants' lives.

When Good Intentions Mask White Privilege

As the project unfolded, Colleen and Louise realized that their original plan for it was logistically complicated, theoretically sophisticated, and methodologically difficult. Integrating an intersectional analysis into the structure of an FPAR project, through intentionally choosing Aboriginal and South Asian communities, led us into uncharted territory. In terms of the process itself, these two ethnically distinct communities showed striking similarities: in both, we had to hire new local researchers, we encountered challenges with regular communications, and fewer than expected actions resulted from the project. In both communities, we had to find additional resources from other aspects of the project to continue the work due to replacing the local researchers and the additional training and support required by newly hired researchers. And, as we are now engaged in co-writing and co-presenting our findings, the racialized women's voices, through the absence of the researchers as co-authors of this and other outputs, are lost.

The structure of the project, managing it from afar, and possibly the overt participatory and action orientation created a dynamic that positioned these communities as problematic and non-conforming. Despite our collective interest in better understanding racialized women's experiences, we did not uncover a way to do so collaboratively or meaningfully. What we are left to wrestle with is the possibility that, despite our good intentions, practices and assumptions of white privilege underpinned the project itself. What we fell prey to, which has been soundly argued in the literature, was the "invisibility" of whiteness in our FPAR project. When whiteness is invisible, it becomes a non-colour against which the non-white are measured as deviant (Ahmed 2004; Frankenberg 1993; Smith 1999).

An example comes from an examination of the report-writing process. Working closely with the researchers in the Aboriginal and South Asian communities, Colleen and Louise pushed and pulled at them to delve more deeply, produce "stronger" data, and to more firmly articulate outcomes and recommendations. Only after several months of these tensions did we fully examine what we were experiencing and how we viewed the work in these communities. Through ongoing conversations, we articulated how our understandings and imposition of what "good research" looks like were bound within our own culture and world view. Engaging reflexively with each other in the safety of our long-term relationship allowed us to see more truly and honestly what was at play. We realized that culture operates on all levels; it is not simply something to "ask" about. Rather, it permeates the ways that questions are asked and interpreted, the possibility for generating "outcomes" and "recommendations," and the inherent value of doing research in the first place. Only after this realization did we see the true value of the research and reports from these two communities. In the urban-South Asian community, a diverse group of South Asian women were asked questions and shared their experiences of immigration, work, family, and culture. Most of them had never explored their own experiences in the context of research, and through their involvement in this project, many were just learning about the possibilities for action-oriented research such as FPAR. In the remote-reserve community, women were asked about their experiences with employment, making ends meet, and supporting their often extended families. For the first time, gender issues, in terms of women's subordination and experiences of violence and abuse, were voiced in that community. They were also encouraged to share stories about the difficult legacy of the residential school system and how, as a community, they were wounded yet surviving. All of these actions are important indicators of "success" not typically valued in traditional research settings (Varcoe 2006).

Through our FPAR process, Colleen and Louise were able to shift how they judged and valued the research, and to become aware of the ways that their own social locations and intersections as white, Western, middle-class, and socially critical and aware women affected the work. We learned that our good intentions and social awareness did not prevent us from being blinded by our own privilege or from structuring a project that did not adequately embrace these communities and racialized women's voices. The researchers from these communities, through our prodding and questioning, began to learn that they held implicit taken-for-granted understandings of their own cultures that needed to be exposed and questioned. Indeed, our mutual commitments to intersectionality, FPAR, and reflexivity allowed these conversations to happen – we opened the possibility for discussing potentially explosive questions of racism and privilege. We learned that it is up to everyone to engage reflexively with each other, that it is necessary for all involved to understand and engage with the complex and shifting power relations at play (ibid.).

Yet the preceding analysis is by no means sufficient in addressing how we framed and struggled with concept and experience of ethnicity. In the first place, clustering the "racialized women's experiences" together is problematic in that it assumes that racialized women share a common experience of "race" while also suggesting that these concepts were not at play in the "white" communities. Ruth Frankenberg's (1993) seminal work in this area reminds us that whiteness is socially constructed. Mari Matsuda (1991, 1189) writes of "asking the other question": "When I see something that looks racist, I ask 'Where is the patriarchy in this?' When I see something that looks sexist, I ask, 'Where is the heterosexism in this?'" When the rural-farming research team asserted that "race isn't relevant here" (because most women in that community were white and of European descent), asking the other question demanded precisely that we ask about racism. Conversely, involving South Asian and Aboriginal women in the research requires research strategies and an analytic sharpness that prevent us from seeing these women's experiences as the product of their ethnicity alone. When we fail to ask the other question, what assumptions are being made, and what is lost?

By its very definition, intersectional analysis demands that we ask the other question. Of FPAR, it requires research structures, processes, and resources to support the research team in thinking across categories while simultaneously focusing on sites where multiple identities are performed. Not only does this necessitate a significant commitment from all members of the team in challenging and possibly abandoning preconceived ideas about social categories, but it also requires substantial resources (such as time and money) to engage meaningfully and deeply with one another (Varcoe 2006). Such processes can be time consuming and uncomfortable for research team members and require a significant commitment to unpacking and supporting group process work.

Negotiating the Power to Represent
Our research team was interested in analyzing the impact of systems of domination and oppression such as racism, sexism, and colonialism. In her notes, Louise described how she envisioned our feminist research: "Using a feminist lens meant that we would structure the research according to feminist understanding of the ethics and power relationships between researchers, research participants, and the community. We would also have some assumptions to start with, coming from accepted feminist theory and peer reviewed research. These would frame our understanding of the context for the research, including women's relative lack of control over their bodies, the product of their work, sexism and gender inequality and how it plays out in intimate relationships, the workforce, government, and policy development."

Yet developing approaches to weave these broader critiques into our analysis created uncertainty for some of the local researchers, specifically those from the rural-farming community. They felt that their research participants would not see their individual stories embedded in more structural analyses. For example, rather than criticizing the neo-conservative agenda of the past ten years as responsible for their conditions, the rural-farming research participants focused on the social worth of their unpaid work. They valued alternative health care and the grey economy, which consisted of barter and exchange. Paul Cloke and Jo Little (1997) describe the challenges faced by policy discourse in their rural research. Because the rural voices were granted authorship, the resulting narratives did not conform to accepted policy analyses and thus did not offer easily identifiable policy responses. In the rural-farming community, the participants' analyses reflected conservative values, and they rejected the language of feminism. Robin, one of the local rural-farming researchers who identified herself as a "radical feminist social worker," described how she negotiated her context vis-à-vis local politics and sensibilities: "I have had very radical ideas for much of my life. However, I have grown to respect the local conservative analysis even when I can't agree with it, and I continue to look for ways to help conservative women become more conscienticized."

The following quotation demonstrates how Robin made strategic decisions in order to engage women locally in the WEHP: "I remember deciding on the graphic for our poster. I was quite taken with the Rosy Riveter image and found it on the Internet. However, after passing it around the office for a reaction and getting not a very positive one, I settled for a much less political image of a woman in a business suit juggling items that reflect the multitude of women's work." What is revealing is that Robin consciously straddled her own political analysis and the opposing ones common in her community. Although she attempted to respect them, she also felt she had a role in conscienticizing conservative women. Robin occupies a unique intersection that is a combination of her age, her history, and her experiences living in this community. This history and set of experiences can be difficult to negotiate in the explicitly political approach of an intersectional FPAR team. An intersectional analysis can shed light on the varying dimensions at play in shaping the conservative ethos of this small rural community. Yet within the intersectionality literature, little attention is paid to who conducts the analysis and how decisions are made. How does engaging in an intersectional analysis put the local researcher at risk, especially within the community she is meant to represent?

Importantly, our commitment to FPAR helped to expose this tension while aiding us to untangle it. Although the feminist researcher's "job" is to conduct a socio-political analysis (Fine and Weiss 1996), in the context of FPAR there is a fine line between using power to privilege one analysis and questioning the validity of one's own analysis out of respect for, or in deference to, the research participants. As a team, we had to examine the power and impact of research as well as the reasons for engaging in the project in the first place. What helped us in this process, and in examining our respective answers to these questions, was our shared commitment to the ideals of FPAR, and in particular, our active engagement in reflexive work.

How Intersections Manifest in Research Relationships

As a research team, we were unprepared to deal with the complexity of engaging in intersectionality as "process," particularly in terms of the challenges that arise in trying to work between, through, and around multiple social locations. These challenges resulted in many difficult conversations concerning ethical questions and processes, decision making and control, and ownership of the research. As we applied intersectionality to our working relationships and came to identify as an intersectional research team, we were forced to wrestle with the discomforts exposed in challenging assumptions, honestly considering alternative opposed world views, and disrupting traditional power relations (Shields 2008). The process of exposing our assumptions and world views required us to examine our commitment to diversity, the differences and similarities among us, and the fluidity within our intersections (Hulko 2009). We realized that the broad analytic categories that we assigned to our research – gender, ethnicity, race, culture, place, and the economy – did not hold much meaning for us in our relationships and ability to work together. Rather, our various social locations, or intersections, manifested in the project itself in terms of confidence, safety and trust, embeddedness in the local community, political persuasion, access to resources, and experience with FPAR.

Through our individual and collective reflexive processes, we uncovered the machinations of our own internalized oppressions and privileges. Engaging in deep reflexivity is challenging work, and each of us struggled with the ways we have internalized our historical experiences of oppression and privilege. Internalization refers to the process whereby individuals incorporate and accept certain world views and experiences as truth (Pheterson 1990; Ponic 2007). This process occurs over time and contributes to the assumptions we make about others and ourselves, such as tendencies to mark those who perceive themselves to be different from us as "other" and therefore fearful (Lorde 1984). The psychosocial impact of internalizing oppression can manifest in feelings of shame, helplessness, and inferiority, whereas that of privilege can manifest in feelings of entitlement, superiority, and in some cases, guilt (Prilleltensky 2003). Importantly, how we internalize oppressions and privileges relates to the fluidity of our intersections. This means that most of us will have experienced, resisted, and internalized oppression and privilege at different times and realms of our lives.

This is not to say that we abandoned the a priori analytic categories that we originally identified. McCall (2005) articulates "anticategorical complexity" – the rejection of categories – as a viable approach to intersectional analysis, but we found that beginning with social categories in mind provided a useful analytic entry-point for establishing important connections and diversities among the research participants in the study and ourselves as co-researchers. Indeed, "it is equally a mistake to ban categories a priori – to deprive ourselves, in advance of inquiry, of access to conceptual frameworks and ideas that might be fruitful" (Martin 1994, 638). In this instance, FPAR has something to offer intersectionality: a deeper embodied approach to understanding analytic categories through the fluid expressions of research team members' internalized oppressions and privileges. Herein lies an opportunity for bringing together FPAR and intersectionality in such a way that more sophisticated analyses can be produced. The ways that we name these expanded social categories must not only speak to the individuals' realities but must also capture the more difficult terrain of how one engages with others and perceives and experiences difference within personal and professional relationships.

Confronting the Shadow in Women's Health Research

Our commitments to FPAR and intersectionality raised tensions and challenges that we continue to face. The ongoing complexities of our work have extended our collaboration far beyond the grant for the project. From an FPAR perspective, this level of commitment is often considered a success: a sustained academic-community partnership signals that the research processes were highly "democratized," that the questions asked were relevant and locally important, and that meaningful actions continue to unfold. However, the underbelly of our ongoing commitment to this research was our unpaid labour, volunteerism, and stress. For over two years, all of us have worked for no pay, attending conferences, writing manuscripts, participating in a visioning retreat, and communicating via email and teleconference. Working off the sides of our desk is partly a result of the composition of our research team itself – none of us are paid academic researchers in tenured positions, and all of us have "other jobs" and family obligations that require much of our time and attention.

In a study on the relationship between women's employability and health, it is deeply and disturbingly ironic that the research team members' own determinants of health are worsened due to their involvement. While we coalesced around our shared commitment to improving women's health, the protracted research process had a negative health impact on us all. This legacy leaves us concerned about our future work. Is it possible to engage in women's health research in such a way that all women's health is promoted?

From epistemological and methodological perspectives, bringing FPAR and intersectionality together is a necessary step forward. From our personal experience, however, it needs to be treated more cautiously. We remain committed to investigating the connections between FPAR and intersectionality, yet we are equally committed to promoting the health of diverse women's health researchers. Advocating for multiple, diverse perspectives in an intersectional health research team requires ongoing attention to how the health of team members is supported through the research process. Are members able to fully participate, or are they working off the sides of their desk? Are they drawn to the project because of their commitment to women's health, and do they feel able to withdraw when they are personally overwhelmed and overburdened? These are some initial questions that need to be raised when considering the possibilities for FPAR and intersectionality.

Moving Forward

Intersectionality promises an almost universal applicability,
useful for understanding and analyzing any social practice, any
individual or group experience, any structural arrangement, and
any cultural configuration ... It can ... be employed by any scholar
willing to use her own social location, whatever it may be, as an
analytic resource rather than just an identity marker.

– Davis (2008)

Intersectionality offered us an analytic approach to better understanding our practice as an FPAR team. It also provided us with greater insights into the richness of using our own fluid intersections as an analytic resource. Intersectionality encourages feminist participatory action researchers and research teams to engage reflexively with each other with the long-range goal of challenging world views and assumptions in order to generate analyses that cross-cut, intersect, and expand thinking around social categories. Intersectionality forces FPAR to delve into the depths of its process from the inside out, to explode expected categorizations, and to develop new and more meaningful ways to work together. It also forces FPAR to put difference and discomfort squarely on the table to be examined by all, to become accountable for the uses of power to control and silence.

In this project, we set out to answer how an intersectional analysis illuminates aspects of an FPAR process, yet we are left believing in the mutuality of intersectionality and FPAR. Despite the significant common ground in the philosophical underpinnings and social justice goals of intersectionality and FPAR, these two perspectives have rarely been combined in an explicit manner. Although intersectionality is poised to inspire creative feminist inquiry that expands the potential for empirical and methodological advancements (Davis 2008), it has also been soundly criticized for contributing few methodological strategies. FPAR offers a well-developed framework for intersectional researchers. By definition, FPAR brings multiple people, with their fluid intersections, to the table. With this comes the depth and richness of embodied experiences and what can be revealed in confronting assumptions and world views through reflexive practices. Through FPAR's well-developed methodological frameworks, all players involved in an FPAR project can be encouraged to think across and through their own multiple identities toward revealing additional intersections. In sum, FPAR offers intersectionality the possibility for unearthing more intersections.

Davis (2008, 77) writes, "with each new intersection, new connections emerge and previously hidden exclusions come to light. The feminist researcher merely needs to 'ask (an)other question' and her research will take on a new and often surprising turn. She can begin to tease out the linkages between additional categories, explore the consequences for relations of power, and decide when another question is needed or when it is time to stop and why." Certainly, FPAR is not the only solution to the critique of intersectionality as having few methodological strategies, but it does offer a promising approach for tackling and deepening what can be produced from an intersectional analysis. In our case, a commitment to intersectional analyses and FPAR, and the reflexive processes encouraged by both approaches, enabled us to grow from the challenges we raise here and to find ways to continue to do research together.

Acknowledgments
We are grateful to the Vancouver Foundation, Status of Women Canada, Canadian Institutes of Health Research, and Coast Capital Savings for funding support to the Women's Employability and Health Research Project. Colleen Reid thanks the Social Sciences and Humanities Research Council and the Michael Smith Foundation of Health Research for post-doctoral fellowship funding.

Note

1 As a team, we have principles that guide our co-writing and authorship. In publications, team members who do the substantive writing are credited first and second (in this case, Reid and Ponic). Team members who contribute reflections and edit the manuscript are listed alphabetically after those who do the majority of the writing (Hara, Kaweesi, and Ledrew).

References
Ahmed, S. 2004. Declarations of whiteness: The non-performativity of anti-racism. *Border-lands* 3(2). http://www.borderlands.net.au.
Brydon-Miller, M., P. Maguire, and A. McIntyre, eds. 2004. *Traveling companions: Feminism, teaching, and action research.* Westport, CT: Praeger.
Clark, N. 2009. Who are you and why do you care? Intersections of identity within the university. In Inside out: Reflections on personal and professional intersections, ed. E. Grise-Owens and K. Lay. Special issue, *Reflections: Narratives of Professional Helping* 15(2): 5-14.

Cloke, P.J., and J. Little. 1997. *Contested countryside cultures: Otherness, marginalisation, and rurality.* London: Routledge.

Collins, P.H. 2000. *Black feminist thought: Knowledge, consciousness, and the politics of empowerment.* 2nd ed. New York: Routledge.

Davis, K. 2008. Intersectionality as buzzword: A social science perspective on what makes a feminist theory successful. *Feminist Theory* 9(1): 67-86.

Fine, M., and L. Weiss. 1996. Writing the "wrongs" of fieldwork: Confronting our own research/writing dilemmas in urban ethnographies. *Qualitative Inquiry* 2(3): 251-74.

Frankenberg, R. 1993. *White women, race matters: The social construction of whiteness.* Minneapolis: University of Minnesota Press.

Frisby, W., P. Maguire, and C. Reid. 2009. The "f" word has everything to do with it: How feminist theories inform action research. *Action Research* 7(1): 13-29.

Frisby, W., C. Reid, S. Miller, and L. Hoeber. 2005. Putting "participatory" into participatory forms of action research. *Journal of Sport Management* 19(4): 367-86.

Gibson, N., G. Gibson, and A.C. Macaulay. 2001. Community-based research: Negotiating agendas and evaluating outcomes. In *The nature of qualitative evidence,* ed. J. Morse, J. Swanson, and A.J. Kuzel, 160-82. Thousand Oaks, CA: Sage.

Hancock, A.-M. 2007. When multiplication doesn't equal quick addition: Examining intersectionality as a research paradigm. *Perspectives on Politics* 5(1): 63-78.

Hankivsky, O., and R. Cormier. 2009. *Intersectionality: Moving women's health research and policy forward.* Vancouver: Women's Health Research Network.

Hemmings, C. 2007. What is a feminist theorist responsible for? *Feminist Theory* 8(1): 69-76.

Hulko, W. 2009. The time- and context-contingent nature of intersectionality and interlocking oppressions. *Affilia: Journal of Women and Social Work* 24(1): 44-55.

Lorde, A. 1984. *Sister outsider: Essays and speeches.* Feminist series. New York: Crossing Press.

Lykes, B., and E. Coquillon. 2006. Participatory and action research and feminisms: Towards transformative praxis. In *Handbook of feminist research: Theory and praxis,* ed. S. Hesse-Biber, 297–326. Thousand Oaks, CA: Sage.

Lykes, M.B., M.T. Blanche, and B. Hamber. 2003. Narrating survival and change in Guatemala and South Africa: The politics of representation and a liberatory community psychology. *American Journal of Community Psychology* 31(1-2): 79-90.

Macaulay, A.C., L.E. Commanda, W.L. Freeman, N. Gibson, M.L. McCabe, C.M. Robbins, and P.L. Twohig. 1999. Participatory research maximizes community and lay involvement. *British Medical Journal* 319: 774-78.

Maguire, P. 2001. Uneven ground: Feminisms and action research. In *Handbook of action research: Participative inquiry and practice,* ed. P. Reason and H. Bradbury, 59-69. London: Sage.

Martin, J.R. 1994. Methodological essentialism, false difference, and other dangerous traps. *Signs: Journal of Women in Culture and Society* 19(3): 630-57.

Matsuda, M.J. 1991. Beside my sister, facing the enemy: Legal theory out of coalition. *Stanford Law Review* 43(6): 1183-92.

Mauthner, N.S., and A. Doucet. 2003. Reflexive accounts and accounts of reflexivity in qualitative data analysis. *Sociology* 37(3): 413-31.

McCall, L. 2005. The complexity of intersectionality. *Signs: Journal of Women in Culture and Society* 30(3): 1771-1800.

McEwan, C. 2001. Postcolonialism, feminism and development: Intersections and dilemmas. *Progress in Development Studies* 1(2): 93-111.

McIntyre, A., and M.B. Lykes. 2004. Weaving words and pictures in/through feminist participatory action research. In Brydon-Miller, Maguire, and McIntyre 2004, 57-78.

Morris, M., and B. Bunjun. 2007. *Using intersectional frameworks in research.* Ottawa: Canadian Research Institute for the Advancement of Women.

Pheterson, G. 1990. Alliances between women: Overcoming internalized oppression and internalized domination. In *Bridges of power: Women's multicultural alliances,* ed. L. Albrecht and R.M. Brewer, 34-47. Gabriola Island, BC: New Society.

Pillow, W.S. 2003. Confession, catharsis, or cure? Rethinking the uses of reflexivity as methodological power in qualitative research. *Qualitative Studies in Education* 16(2): 175-96.

Ponic, P. 2007. Embracing complexity in community-based health promotion: Inclusion, power and women's health. PhD diss., University of British Columbia.

Prilleltensky, I. 2003. Understanding, resisting, and overcoming oppression: Toward psycho-political validity. *American Journal of Community Psychology* 31(1-2): 195-201.

Reid, C. 2004. *The wounds of exclusion: Poverty, women's health, and social justice.* Walnut Creek, CA. Left Coast Press.

Reid, C., and W. Frisby. 2007. Continuing the journey: Articulating dimensions of feminist participatory action research. In *Handbook of action research: Participative inquiry and practice.* 2nd ed., ed. P. Reason and H. Bradbury, 93-105. London: Sage.

Reid, C., P. Ponic, L. Hara, R. Ledrew, C. Kaweesi, and K. Besla. Forthcoming 2011. Living an ethical agreement: Negotiating confidentiality and harm in a feminist participatory action research project. In *Feminist methodologies in community research,* ed. G. Creese and W. Frisby. Vancouver: UBC Press.

Shields, S. 2008. Gender: An intersectionality perspective. *Sex Roles* 59: 301-11.

Simien, E.M. 2007. Doing intersectionality research: From conceptual issues to practical examples. *Politics and Gender* 3(2): 264-71.

Smith, L.T. 1999. *Decolonizing methodologies: Research and indigenous peoples.* London: Zed Books.

Squier, S.M. 2007. Beyond nescience: The intersectional insights of health humanities. *Perspectives in Biology and Medicine* 50(3): 334-47.

Varcoe, C. 2006. Doing participatory action research in a racist world. *Western Journal of Nursing Research* 28(5): 525-40.

Varcoe, C., O. Hankivsky, and M. Morrow. 2007. Introduction: Beyond gender matters. In *Women's health in Canada: Critical perspectives on theory and policy,* ed. M. Morrow, O. Hankivsky, and C. Varcoe, 3-32. Toronto: University of Toronto Press.

Wang, C., M.A. Burris, and X.Y. Ping. 1996. Chinese village women as visual anthropologists: A participatory approach to reaching policymakers. *Social Science and Medicine* 42(10): 1391-1400.

Weiner, G. 2004. Critical action research and third wave feminism: A meeting of paradigms. *Educational Action Research* 12(4): 631-44.

Williams, J., and B. Lykes. 2003. Bridging theory and practice: Using reflexive cycles in feminist participatory action research. *Feminism and Psychology* 13(3): 287-94.

Young, I.M. 1990. *Justice and the politics of difference.* Princeton: Princeton University Press.

5
Adding Religion to Gender, Race, and Class: Seeking New Insights on Intersectionality in Health Care Contexts

Sheryl Reimer-Kirkham and Sonya Sharma

On 29 October 2008, Monia Mazigh, wife of Maher Arar who was arrested in Syria on suspicion of terrorist activities, gave an interview to the Canadian Broadcasting Corporation's national show *The Current* (Tremonti 2008). While her husband was being held, she said that she attempted to find work but was turned down due to her husband's status and her traditional Islamic dress, despite having a PhD and having lived in Canada for many years. Her experience is just one example of the interlocking oppressions of race, religion, class, and gender, and more poignantly, the stark racialization of religion since 9/11.

The racialization of visible minority religious Canadians is not new. In 1914 the *Komagata Maru* arrived in Vancouver, BC, carrying 376 Indian Sikh and Hindu passengers (Ricketts 2008). The boat, chartered by Gurdit Singh, sailed to Canada to challenge the law recently passed by the Canadian government to limit immigration. The BC press prepared for its arrival with such headlines as "Hindu Invasion of Canada." After spending many days in the harbour, the passengers were refused entry and forced to return to India.

With such historical and current experiences of racialized religious oppression, we explore in this chapter what might be added when religion is brought into intersectional analysis and – conversely – what is overlooked when religion is left out. The context of health care services provides fruitful ground for our exploration. Beginning with a brief overview of key aspects of intersectionality as currently theorized, we define religion and spirituality, and consider their relationship to culture, ethnicity, and race. We explore the place of religion in public life, which has been largely informed by the processes of secularization, and more recently, the trends of the "subjective turn" (Heelas and Woodhead 2005), with its sacralization and "new" spiritualities, and globalization, with its increase in religious pluralism (Thomas 2005). We then draw examples from a study of religious and spiritual plurality in health care to illustrate the significance of religion and spirituality to the theorizing of intersectionality and to health-related practices and health care provision.[1] Intersectional analyses that incorporate the lens of religion and spirituality in health studies, we suggest, provide new insights into identity as a site for connection, and marginalizing practices through racialized, gendered, and classed religion.

Theorizing Intersectionality, Adding Religion

Although intersectional analysis is a relatively new form of social study, women's everyday lives over the centuries have born constant witness to the reality of intersectional oppressions. At different points of the women's movement, various compounding factors have been strongly named as exacerbating women's conditions. Indeed, the paradox of intersectional theory is that it is perhaps most clearly understood when it is lived and yet remains difficult to operationalize as a method of analysis or as policy.

Anastasia Vakulenko (2007) traces the historical development of intersectional analysis, beginning in the 1970s and '80s with the critique voiced by black feminists regarding their omission from what was presented as a homogeneous shared experience of "woman," which imposed the essentialist standard of the white, middle-class, heterosexual woman. Whereas early intersectional analysis tended to focus on overlapping categories of identity, Vakulenko notes that a more current development conceptualizes gender, race, sexuality, and so on in terms of systemic forces that shape societies, rather than as individual traits. Intersectional analysis pays attention to macro-institutional and micro-interpersonal power relations that create and sustain social hierarchies (Weber and Parra-Medina 2003). Contemporary uses, and the approach we take here, reflect current understandings of the indivisible relationship between the self and the social, where "structural influences are always subsumed and internalized in the individual" (Vakulenko 2007, 186).

The work of intersectional analysis has been carried out in various ways. Analyses of large data sets have shown how patterns of gender, race, and class inequality vary with the composition of economic activity in various locales (McCall 2005), emphasizing systematic forces that shape societies. Other analyses focus on local lived experience of intersectionality at the level of the individual. What becomes important, Nira Yuval-Davis (2006, 199) emphasizes, is differentiation between various kinds of difference, which can help "to avoid conflating positionings, identities and values." Yuval-Davis argues that divisions between people, such as class, gender, race, and sexuality, are grounded in autonomous processes and discourses that are not static but vary in meaning and importance, depending on time and place and the ways these are interrogated.

Theories of intersectionality have traditionally examined the interactions of gender, race, and class. Since Kimberlé Crenshaw's (1991) article first proposed a theory of intersectionality, other structures and cultures of difference have been theorized such as (dis)ability, sexuality, and age. Religion has been less considered. Feminist scholars and academic theorists have been wary of conservative religion that has sought to colonize political and social organizations (Fernandes 2003) and perpetuate patriarchy (Klassen 2003). And yet, religion and spirituality are an intricate part of many people's lives, complicating intersections of gender, race, and class. As revealed by the experiences of Monia Mazigh in the opening example, religion and spirituality cannot be dismissed as a separate categorization of difference and individual choice but are, in reality, integrated into the lived experiences of many.

This brings us to how religion and spirituality are defined and how they are conceptualized in relation to culture, ethnicity, and race. Interestingly, the very attempts at defining religion and spirituality have been described as originating from Western thought and growing "out of a Christian-informed imperialistic view" (Anderson and Dickey Young 2004, ix). Traditionally, religion has been understood as carrying transcendent (sacred) and social dimensions, with its practice typically occurring through relatively formal social institutions. In contrast, spirituality has been viewed as a more personal expression of values and beliefs. Modernity, urbanization, and migration have caused many scholars to re-evaluate how these occurrences have affected the phenomena of religion and spirituality. We locate our definitions of religion and spirituality in a time characterized by the crossover of cultures, races, and faith traditions, where forms of spirituality and religiosity are consistently challenged, negotiated, and generated. From this stance, defining the many ways that people live out their relationship to the divine or to the sacred is particularly difficult. Church or temple attendance does not define people's religiosity. Likewise, one's spirituality is not defined by attendance at an ashram, healing touch, or astrological sessions. Linda Woodhead's (2008, 55) explanation of religion aligns with how we are considering religion in this chapter: "[It is] a name we give to a complex set of social practices which structure individual agency, and are in turn recursively structured by it. At the heart of these practices there is a collective articulation and celebration of the sacred, which is experienced as transcending the everyday world. Religions seek to embody the sacred-transcendent not only by way of sacred objects, buildings and spaces, but in their collective lives."

Spirituality, on the other hand, is "understood as personal, unique, self-validating, authentic, and authoritative ... emphasizing individual experience" (Anderson and Dickey Young 2004, 219). A first place to acknowledge intersectionality, then, is in the languaging of religion and spirituality. With a history of dichotomous relationship between these two terms in both everyday and academic discourse – as reflected in the common social disclosure of "I'm spiritual but not religious" – we suggest that these two classifications rarely operate in isolation from each other but rather inform one another and have various meanings depending on the context in which they are lived out (Pesut et al. 2008), intersecting in interesting historical, political, economic, and social ways. Moreover, dichotomous constructions of religion and spirituality tend to be applied to categorize everyone within either of these positions, yet some individuals (such as atheists) may opt out of both.

The relationship of religion to culture, ethnicity, and race is conceptualized in various ways, often with considerable ambiguity. Race, culture, and ethnicity are frequently used, sometimes interchangeably, to denote "difference" (and often inferiority), with little consistency in how these terms are applied. A point put forward in this chapter is that, increasingly, religion is also used as a metonym for difference and, when imbricated with culture, ethnicity, and race, implicitly infers colonial images of the racialized Other, so as to position those who are not white Christians on the margins and thus reinscribe long-standing patterns of exclusion and inclusion. Spirituality, though regularly presented as inclusive and diverse, has also been criticized as complementing dominant social relations. Neil Henery (2003) observes that rather than redressing Western racism, the spirituality literature, by its disregard of religion, essentially marginalizes and dismisses ethnic minorities who adhere to religion over spirituality, resulting in what Yuk-Lin Renita Wong and Jana Vinsky (2009, 1343) refer to as "invisible Euro-Christian ethnocentrism and individualism." Thus, any intersectional theorizing must accommodate variations in the influence of religion and spirituality, the blurring between culture, ethnicity, race, and religion, and the power dynamics at play.

The Marginalization – and Presence – of Religion in Public Life

Many scholars have argued that religion in the West has lost its clout to modernity, losing its influence in "the operation of non-religious institutions" such as the "state and the economy," but also in the "social standing of religious roles and institutions" and "the extent to which people engage in religious practices" and beliefs (Bruce 2002, 3). Secularity has undoubtedly taken root in the context of health care where empiricism has been embraced and the sacred sidelined by agendas of cure, technology, and medical advancement. As secularization joined with Enlightenment rationalism have played out in the academy, theological and religious thought has been nearly erased from this venue of public discourse, sometimes in dismissive, pejorative fashion, resulting in references to "secular fundamentalism" (Berger 1997).

Despite such predictions of the irrelevance of religion to Canadian society, the religiosity of newcomers and the individual (re)turn to sacralization challenge the notion of Canada as a secularizing nation. Increasingly, scholars argue that, amid secularization, there is and has been a flourishing of religious and spiritual plurality, as evidenced in what is referred to as the "global resurgence of religion" (Thomas 2005). Globally, the proportion of people attached to the world's four biggest religions – Christianity, Islam, Buddhism, and Hinduism – rose from 67 percent in 1900 to 73 percent in 2005 and is speculated to reach 80 percent by 2050 (Micklethwait 2007). With global migration has come increased diversity in religious affiliations and spiritual practices in countries such as Canada. Increased immigration from Asia, the Middle East, and Africa has created ever-growing Muslim, Buddhist, Sikh, and Hindu communities. Diasporic communities in the context of globalization tend to retain strong religious identities. Whereas a decline has been noted in mainline Protestant and Catholic churches, other churches, particularly those of evangelical and charismatic Christianity, have grown.

Also coexisting with, and challenging, secularization is the (re)sacralization of day-to-day life in Western societies that relocates the sacred in a new individual and holistic manner (Vincett, Sharma, and Aune 2008, 3). In part, such transformation finds its roots in the women's movement in which the conventional gendered constructions of religious traditions were challenged, particularly in relation to female leadership. Many women responded by forming collectives that affirmed their voices and roles, offering an alternative to those who felt marginalized by or peripheral to traditional religion(s). Since the 1960s, these collectives have been among the fastest-growing religions in terms of adherents and distinct groups – from Wicca, ecofeminists, goddess feminists and neo-pagan groups, to various healing practices, astrological, herbs, and tarot work, transpersonal psychology, theosophy, and channelling (Anderson and Dickey Young 2004, 218-19). There are many who may not view themselves as belonging to these new religious or spiritual movements per se but nonetheless carry out spiritual practices indirectly linked to them.

Included in our consideration is atheism, a movement that has had a resurgence of its own. Atheism gives people a space to inhabit, highlighting the growth and complexity of the pluralism of belief. In the public realm, the recent UK Atheist Bus Campaign arose in "an effort to disseminate a godless message to the greater public" (Lyall 2009). Similar campaigns have been initiated in Canada, the US, Brazil, and Spain, demonstrating an effort to capture all sides of the discussion. For some, this message has given them a voice, whereas for others, it has meant an opening to a discussion on god versus a refusal of divine possibility.

Increasing societal plurality, represented by the concurrent social flows of the (re)sacralization of society, the resurgence of religion, growth in atheism, and continued secularity, suggests the need for a more intentional incorporation of religion and spirituality into our intersectional theorizing. Several factors can account for the near absence of religion and spirituality from intersectional analysis, beginning with a distaste for religion's complicity with patriarchy, colonialism, and historical dominance whereby "the church" or "the mosque" had/has remarkable control over domestic and public aspects of people's lives (Daly 1968; Ruether 2000). The complexity of Canada's religious landscape also makes religiosity and spirituality difficult to assess and measure (Beaman 2006). The strong influence of secularism in the academy, largely argued by white European male academics and focused primarily on Christianity and traditional church attendance (Vincett, Sharma, and Aune 2008, 2), has also inferred the study of religion and spirituality as irrelevant. The consequence of dismissing, excluding, and/or attacking religious and spiritual difference, Woodhead (2008, 57) argues, is that secularity becomes "'neutral,' detached from 'culture,' and has no sacred commitments of its own. It is then that 'religion' becomes a marker of the subjugated other, whilst the privileged become the possessors of pure truth, transparent rationality, and the engines of progress."

With recognition of religion's continued influence has come a proliferation of empirical research that has begun to examine the diversity, multiplicity, and complexity of spiritual and religious life (Heelas and Woodhead 2005; Sharma and Young 2007; Beyer and Beaman 2007; Aune, Sharma, and Vincett 2008). Notably, the study of "lived religion" has gained ground: "The study of lived religion situates all religious creativity within culture and approaches all religion as lived experience ... Religion approached this way is situated amid the ordinary concerns of life, at the junctures of self and culture, family and social world ... Religion is always religion-in-action, religion-in-relationships between people, between the ways the world is and the way people imagine or want it to be" (Orsi 2003, 172).

Religious and spiritual practices are where public and private blur, where race, culture, and gender intersect, producing a more complex living out of religion and spirituality than is presumed by secularization theories that fit white Western Christian contexts. The complexities of lived religion/spirituality, intersected by other social classifications such as race, class, and gender, come into focus in health care.

Studying Intersectionality in the Context of Health Care

Religious communities have long been involved in caring for the sick and dying. Likewise, beliefs with reference to supernatural and metaphysical worlds have historically been relied on to bring health and healing, and they represent a fairly universal phenomenon (Spector 2008). To sideline religion and spirituality from health care services is a relatively recent move, one that can be tied to the advent of Western biomedicine, with its preference for medical science, technologies, and rational empiricism. Biomedicine has been characterized by its separation of mind and body, mechanistic metaphors, aggressive interventions, and distancing style that detaches patients from their social relationships and culture (Gaines and Davis-Floyd 2003). It has been massively exported through the nineteenth and twentieth centuries to discredit and supplant what became known as "traditional medicine" or "folk medicine," those healing practices typically deeply rooted in religious beliefs (Dole 2004; Gaines and Davis-Floyd 2003).

Importantly, biomedicine, though still the pre-eminent model, has been influenced by humanist and holistic movements, both of which figure largely in nursing discourse and both of which open up some space for the reintroduction of religion and spirituality into health care services. For the most part, scholarship has focused on this one category (religion/spirituality) as it relates to health and health care in isolation from other social categories, with the side effect of obscuring and oversimplifying other interpenetrating realities. The context of health care, then, with its long-standing yet uneasy relationship with religion and spirituality, proves a fascinating ground for the exploration of religion as addition to intersectional analysis. In the discussion that follows, we centre on two themes brought into focus in a current ethnographic study through the lens of intersectionality: how intersecting subject positions are negotiated for connection, and how marginalizing practices are mobilized – and resisted – through intersecting constructions of racialized, classed, and gendered religion.

By way of brief background, the study, which examined the negotiation of religious and spiritual plurality in health care, focused on the following research objectives:

- to describe how religious and spiritual plurality are negotiated in health care provider/recipient encounters
- to examine ways in which health care contexts shape the negotiation of religious and spiritual plurality
- to critically analyze ways in which societal contexts shape the negotiation of religious and spiritual plurality in health care
- and to facilitate knowledge translation into practice, health policy, and education.

Interviews and participant observation were conducted with twenty health care professionals, twenty-one spiritual care providers, sixteen patients/family members, and twelve administrators and decision makers in various acute care settings, for a total of sixty-nine participants. Regarding religion, thirty-five participants self-identified as Christian, ten as Sikh, two as Muslim, two as Jewish, two as Native spiritualities, two as atheist, one as alternative spirituality, one as Hindu, and nine as none specified. Underlining the heterogeneity of those who self-identified as Christian were many participants best described as "fusers" (Vincett 2008), who represent new forms of spiritualized Christianity that bring together traditional Christianity with neo-pagan practices.

Informed by post-colonial feminist perspectives (Reimer-Kirkham and Anderson 2002), we accounted for intersectionality in several ways in this project: we recruited a diverse sample to give insight into the interplay of various social identities and structuring forces; we designed interview questions to elicit data regarding lived intersectionality (such as how difference is negotiated in health care encounters); and we analyzed data through the theoretical lens of intersectionality (with early memos and codes for intersectionality). Yuval-Davis (2006) suggests examining data from the differing levels in which social divisions operate (such as institutionally and inter-subjectively) and comprehending how social representations, constructions, and identities are individually lived. This approach resulted in a more hetero-geneous analysis, messy and confusing to say the least, but in the end, it offered enriched understandings of people's lives, significant to possibilities for social change.

Hybrid Subjectivities, Connecting Identities

A framing of intersectionality in this study provided insight into how the construction of various intersecting subject positions can create space for connection (or, in some cases, disconnection). Striking is the extent to which religion and/or spirituality was constitutive of identity for many study par-ticipants, as exemplified by the woman who was unable to describe her heritage by any other descriptor than "Sikh" (Reimer-Kirkham 2009). Kwame Appiah (2008, 44) observes that religion is an important "crucible of social identity" and describes this as a feature of diverse societies in particular. In the past, in places with a single dominant religious tradition, religious iden-tity was not as important as a source of social identity, for religious identities, like ethnic identities, are "the product of social boundary formation" (ibid., 45). However, as Manuel Vásquez and Marie Marquardt (2003, 32) observe, "religion is not just about difference and marking boundaries (territorial-izing) but also about mixing and blurring boundaries (deterritorializing)."

Through the lens of intersectionality, we were struck by how religious identity was expressed at the intersection of other social categories such as gender, class, and race in specific locales. These social categories became mutually constitutive, where lived classed, gendered, and raced experiences were shaped by religious situatedness, and in turn, religious expression was shaped by class, gender, nationality, ethnicity, age, and so forth. In the fol-lowing comment by a Sikh woman, an internalized colonialized identity is referenced, akin to Frantz Fanon's (1967) description in *Black Skin, White Masks*, in her contrast between white and brown: "Typically, in India the thinking is 'the grass is always greener on the other side.' White is fair and more beautiful as opposed to brown. But on the other hand, you mature and grow up. Today on the street, if I would see a brown elderly man standing, I would be more likely to help him. It is about trust. If he's wearing a turban, I would think he's religious and will not harm me." Along with what could be understood as a colonized national identity, the strong tie of shared religion (trust based on the visible marker of a turban) is layered onto a fear of harm and a gendered mistrust of men, which is reflected in her comment that he "will not harm me."

This excerpt, then, illustrates the intersection of shared Sikh religion, race, and nation within a gendered and colonial framing, while alluding to the influence of migration on identity. Vásquez and Marquardt (2003, 35) trace the dialectic between globalization and religious identities, positing that global migration results in a loss of the "natural" relation of culture to geographical and social territories, with religion a main protagonist in an "unbinding of culture from its traditional referents and boundaries" and with relocation in new "space-time" locations. By this line of argument, religion can become a main player in the construction of social identity, displacing culture, ethnicity, or nationality. The authors go on to suggest that "religion is a key component in transnational flows and ... contributes to the formation of multiple and hybrid identities at 'borderlands,' sites where two or more life-worlds meet" (ibid., 43).

For participants in this study, these borderlands with intersecting identities became points of connection (Anzaldúa 1987). Whereas individuals might be "outsider" on one social plane, they might well be "insider" on another. Connection through religious identity was not unusual, as explained by one participant: "With Catholics the diversity of cultures is just incredible. From Lebanon, China, Asia, all the continents of the earth. There's the diversity of culture and what unites all of them is the Catholic faith. They know the language of faith and so that makes it easy."

Even when the religious traditions were quite different, devoutness, belief in God, or deep existential experiences could result in profound interpersonal connection. Spirituality and/or religion could thus become a connecting point that served to bridge a variety of social differences. A Sikh spiritual care volunteer recounted being asked to pray with a white Christian woman who was refusing to have surgery until someone had prayed with her. In her words,

> She [referring to the nurse who made this request] said, "It's Good Friday today, all the priests are busy on the outside." And I said, "I'm not Christian and I don't know how to do that prayer." The nurse said, "But you're a very spiritual person, you can do it. Please, this is very important." She took me to those two gentlemen [the patient's sons]. They were, 6'1" or 2", those

guys. They had the black jackets, those bikers, and they had those belts and tattoos ... I said, "Oh my gosh" 'cause I'm not that big ... You know how we judge sometimes people from the outside, they were two amazing gentlemen. I arrived at the hospital room and there were five or six more of their brothers, sisters, their spouses and their kids, the whole family. The surgeon said, "Okay, I'm stepping out and you guys do your job, so then we'll start our job." I just put my hands together. I did a general prayer. That's it. General prayer.

Saying a "general prayer" was her way of tapping into a universal shared humanity through a hybrid and syncretic occurrence of bringing two cultures, two religious traditions together. This participant, herself Sikh, noted the difference in gender (emphasizing the height of the men), ethnicity (she referred to the patient as "white"), and religion ("I'm not Christian") but nonetheless was able to connect through her own sense of a common humanity and belief in the divine. She told this story with an emphasis on a universal shared humanity that included those with beliefs different from her own. Our fieldnotes comment, "She describes herself as humanist. No matter her Sikh religion or culture, love transcends all differences." Her stance then portrays transcendence of difference through love, respect, and an acceptance of the pluralism of (non)belief. Applying an intersectional framing to such a narrative elucidates how identities are shaped by the various social locations one holds (or affiliates with) and how these dimensions of one's identity may be foregrounded or backgrounded as means to negotiate connection with others.

Marginalizing Practices and Resistances

At other times, religion and spirituality were sites of tension and resistance rather than connecting points. Application of the analytic lens of intersectionality draws attention to those practices that maintain inequality and reinscribe marginalization, as evidence of the ways in which "structural influences are always subsumed and internalized in the individual" (Vakulenko 2007, 186). To document both the constructive and destructive, the peaceful and the violent capacities of religion is in keeping with the increasing acknowledgment of the ambivalences and contradictions in how religion is taken up and, most obviously, how the politics of religion occur. A compounding effect results when other axes of marginalization are layered onto religion, in this study pronounced around race, class, and gender.

The concern was raised by participants that Sikh patients did not always receive adequate health care, sometimes due to lack of respect or uncaring communication. At times, they did not receive essential medical information on discharge from hospital, or severe physical symptoms went unnoted due to incomplete assessments. For example, a health care professional might assume a Sikh patient did not speak English and therefore would make little attempt to elicit vital information from the patient. Several Sikh participants felt that racism on the part of health care providers explained why the religious beliefs of Sikh patients were sometimes not honoured (for cleanliness, facilitating prayers, accommodating visitors, or diet). One said, "So I still see racism prevalent at every level in the hospital. And I clearly see it ... 'I don't know who they are,' 'they look so different,' 'they dress so different,' 'everything smells different,' 'everything is different.'" Such observations suggest that patients are marginalized as "different" in a mix of religion, race, culture, and language. Religious garb and brown skin become markers of difference in a move that conflates culture, ethnicity, and race with religion to infer an incommensurability typical of cultural racism. In this conflation, religion is racialized and certain features ("look," "smell") become attached to religion to aggravate the othering of non-white, non-Christian groups (Sikh in this case). In her work on Indian Americans, Khyati Joshi (2006) explains how the racialization of religion results in or exacerbates the oppression of minority groups. Yet, at the same time, the essential nature of the discrimination – racial or religious – becomes disguised or lost entirely. Additionally, the racialization of religions such as Sikhism, Hinduism, and Islam renders these faiths as theologically, socially, and morally illegitimate in the popular eye (ibid.).

However, it would be inaccurate to leave the impression that racialized religion was not resisted. Patients and families continued to practise their Sikh traditions: for example, relatives brought certain foods, and prayers and rituals were conducted. Some large families resisted hospital protocol by taking the time and physical space they needed to care and grieve for a loved one. At one site, a community radio station took calls from patients/families who would report on their hospital experiences. When this same community group raised money for the hospital with a telethon, hospital administration took note with efforts for more culturally and religiously responsive services to the extent that new facilities being planned now have much larger rooms where families can congregate. Spiritual care volunteers from this community often acted as bridges of understanding between patients and health care staff. Countering hegemonic discourse and acting as agents for their own change made marginalization a source of education and progress. Clearly, marginality is more than deprivation; it is "also the site of radical possibility" (hooks 1990, 149).

Class also intersected with religion and spirituality in assumptions regarding who might or might not be "spiritual" based on a constellation of lifestyle choices and resources, especially in the case of street-involved or drug-involved patients. A spiritual care provider told of a man who was palliative but had nowhere to go:

He was essentially homeless. Shelters are not equipped to provide the health care he needed and his behaviours could make it difficult for him to stay at the hospice he is now at. He has associations with a biker gang, used street drugs but now has a terminal condition. This type of patient is very difficult for the staff to look after. There is lots of bias against this type of patient. A lot of staff would not see the spiritual side of a person like this, or seek to connect with him in that way. The staff just can't relate and this can be a bigger barrier than something like a language difference or ethnic differences.

Like many of the Sikh patients, this man resisted the assumptions made about him and his marginalization. As he himself put it, he "did not follow the rules" of either hospital or hospice. He challenged middle-class assumptions about how to die as he gathered several other hospice patients into a "club" to play poker and take motorized wheelchairs out to buy "junk food," fish down at the river, and smoke pot, all with a good-natured camaraderie. Many health care providers were uncomfortable with him, evidence of the "racialization of class division" (hooks 2000, 111). In this story, "Whiteness [is] a shifting designation that is impacted by social class, language, generational status, and religious affiliation" (Joshi 2006, 214). The patient eventually connected with two spiritual care coordinators, who spent time with him. Although describing himself as "not religious," he referred to a spiritual care coordinator as "a life saver," explaining, "I talked to her. I've told her my soul, I've cried in front of her ... I know she's a priest but she's the first priest I've ever interlocked with in my life." He resisted gendered middle-class assumptions of who might be spiritual, who provides spiritual care, and how to die. He pushed the systems of power that keep normative structures in place. Yet his spiritual experience fit within the existential non-religious spirituality typical of hospice (Garces-Foley 2006) and became a route for connection.

The realities of gender and religion also come into focus through an intersectional lens, as alluded to above. Women employed various mechanisms to resist marginalization resulting from their religious and or spiritual affiliation and practices. Clearly, there was a range of gendered experiences, where some women's faith experiences were rooted in institutionalized religion, and those of others were much more expressive of individualized spiritualities. For those affiliated with religious traditions maintained by strong gendered roles, especially in which ecclesiastic positions were occupied by men as priests or imams, health care settings provided a space where women too could "minister" in a reformulated role of spiritual leadership. In the case above, the female Sikh spiritual care volunteer provided the religious ritual of a prayer in the absence of the priests who were all busy with Good Friday church services. There were subversive moves, then, by women against the dominant religious structures and the gendered roles expected of them. Sacralization also occurred in subtle, sometimes subversive, ways, as illustrated by health care providers who quietly enacted spiritual rituals outside of formal religion. For example, a nurse opened the window when a patient died so the spirit could find its way; another nurse touched each patient on the forehead in a spiritual, healing gesture. Intersectional analysis makes visible marginalizing practices and resistances at the junctures of religion, race, class, and gender.

Conclusion: Implications of Intersectional Analysis

In conclusion, data from this ethnographic study offer important insights about intersectionality. For many participants, religion was a vital aspect of life, not something to be left outside the hospital doors so to speak. Religion was constitutive of social identity, in conjunction with other social markers, for many individuals, often resulting in hybrid (re)formulations at "border-lands." Religion and spirituality served as both an avenue for connection across difference and a site of tension, reflecting the politically infused nature of religion. Marginalizing practices at the intersection of religion with race, gender, or class reinscribed lines of social belonging and inequity. Yet religion and spirituality also served as sites of resistance and subversion, where those marginalized exercised their agency. Taken together, these insights restate the case for the inclusion of religion and spirituality in intersectional analysis in health care theorizing and practice.

Our efforts have revealed numerous complexities to be held in tension in these types of intersectional theorizing. First, more nuanced readings of religion and spirituality are needed to account for how they are lived out in gendered, racialized, and classed ways. The variation in values and beliefs located loosely under the umbrella of religion and spirituality is vast. Religion is not to be understood simply by its creed or doctrine but rather by the myriad of interpretations thereof; how it is lived out varies by individual interpretations shaped by class position, location across time and place, gender, and so on. These nuanced readings must also accommodate those who do not affiliate with religion or spirituality. Mindfulness of how other social locations themselves become part of the story of lived religion is paramount. A second challenge is that of leveraging intersectional analyses to create space within health care services (and other public arenas) for these multiple viewpoints.

The historical trajectory of health care services in Canada has seen the shift from hospitals and other health and social services founded by religious orders to the current secular model where the state funds and administers the majority of health care services. A pressing question brought to the fore through critical analysis is that of whether presumed secular health care services are indeed neutral or whether they originate from a hegemonic unnamed Christian centre (Beaman 2003). Intersectional analyses may well assist in the creation of plural spaces where the range of today's religious and spiritual expressions are made welcome. In making the case for the inclusion of religion and spirituality in intersectional analyses, we face a third challenge – the risk of exclusion whereby other intersecting social forces are sidelined in the effort to demonstrate the influence of religion and spirituality. Analysis of simultaneous oppressions is inevitably a formidable task, but the balancing act must be to analyze how "different social divisions are concretely enmeshed and constructed by each other and how they relate to political and subjective constructions of identities" (Yuval-Davis 2006, 205). Given the shifting nature of oppressions, each situation and context must be evaluated to see which social categories are most salient as sites of oppression and when one category might act as a proxy for another.

Finally, our analyses in this chapter have underlined the imperative of maintaining a critical analytic stance that continually holds up relations of power for scrutiny. Relations of power are often attributed to religion, particularly in drawing attention to religion's complicity in colonizing histories, but less so to spirituality (Henery 2003; Pesut et al. 2008). Here again, meticulous intersectional analyses are crucial to untangle the strands of influence and oppression toward ends that decolonize religion and spirituality. These are the types of challenges and complexities that must be sorted out for the progression of intersectional analysis.

In sum, overlooking religion and spirituality, we contend, produces incomplete accounts and possible misrepresentations of people's lived realities. Also overlooked are the processes whereby marginalization operates through religion in conjunction with other social forces. Where religion has been complicit or instigator in subjugation, we need to understand how symbols, rituals, and constructions are working and how they can be disrupted, either by leaving them behind or transforming them (Klassen 2003). Thus, religion must be portrayed as more than solely an oppressor, as co-conspirator with colonization and patriarchy; though it is increasingly politicized in the everyday and undoubtedly the source of oppression and global conflict, more deliberate and inclusive analyses are necessary to account for its role in social cohesion, peace building, and individual meaning making (Banchoff 2008). As intersectional analysis requires us to dwell in the borderlands where hybrid identities are created and to scrutinize marginalizing practices that become pathways for social and health disparities, it also provides a space to decolonize religion and spirituality, and to reclaim them as meaningful in people's lives.

Note

1   We are grateful for funding from the Social Sciences and Humanities Research Council of Canada (SSHRC) for the project "SPIRIT: The Negotiation of Religious and Spiritual Plurality in Health Care," which was conducted from 2006 to 2009. The research team consisted of S. Reimer-Kirkham, B. Pesut (University of British Columbia-Okanagan), R. Sawatzky (Trinity Western University), H. Meyerhoff (Trinity Western University), S. Sharma (health and social sciences researcher), M. Cochrane (research coordinator), L. Thiessen and A. Ingeveld (research assistants), and collaborators S. Thorne (University of British Columbia) and J. Anderson (University of British Columbia). We acknowledge the synergy of this outstanding team, which served as fertile ground for the insights presented in this essay. We are also grateful to members of the project's advisory group and of the Fraser Health Authority Spiritual Care Professional Practice Group who engaged in these types of ideas with us. We are particularly indebted to all the patients, families, spiritual care providers, health care providers, and administrators who graciously shared their views with us.

References

Anderson, L.M., and P. Dickey Young, eds. 2004. *Women and religious traditions.* Toronto: Oxford University Press Canada.

Anzaldúa, G. 1987. *Borderlands/La frontera: The new mestiza.* San Francisco: Aunt Lute Books.

Appiah, K.A. 2008. Causes of quarrel: What's special about religious disputes? In *Religious pluralism? Globalization and world politics,* ed. T. Banchoff, 41-64. New York: Oxford University Press.

Banchoff, T. 2008. Introduction: Religious pluralism in world affairs. In *Religious Pluralism? Globalization and world politics,* ed. T. Banchoff, 3-38. New York: Oxford University Press.

Beaman, L.G. 2003. The myth of pluralism, diversity, and vigor: The constitutional privilege of Protestantism in the United States and Canada. *Journal for the Scientific Study of Religion* 42(3): 311-25.

–. 2006. Introduction. In *Religion and Canadian society: Traditions, transitions and innovations,* ed. L.G. Beaman, ix-xii. Toronto: Canadian Scholars' Press.

Berger, P. 1997. Epistemological modesty: An interview with Peter Berger. *Christian Century* 114(12): 972-78.

Beyer, P., and L.G. Beaman, eds. 2007. *Religion, globalization and culture.* Toronto: Brill.

Bruce, S. 2002. *God is dead: Secularization in the West.* Oxford: Blackwell.

Crenshaw, K. 1991. Mapping the margins: Intersectionality, identity politics, and violence against women. *Stanford Law Review* 43(6): 1241-99.

Daly, M. 1968. *The church and the second sex.* Boston: Beacon Press, 1985.

Dole, C. 2004. In the shadows of medicine and modernity: Medical integration and secular histories of religious healing in Turkey. *Culture, Medicine and Psychiatry* 28: 255-80.

Fanon, F. 1967. *Black skin, white masks.* Trans. C. Markmann. New York: Grove Press.

Fernandes, L. 2003. *Transforming feminist practice: Non-violence, social justice and the possibilities of a spiritualized feminism.* San Francisco: Aunt Lute Books.

Gaines, A., and R. Davis-Floyd. 2003. On biomedicine. In *Encyclopedia of medical anthropology,* ed. C. Ember and M. Ember, 95-108. Yale: Human Relations Area Files. http://www.davis-floyd.com/userfiles/Biomedicine.pdf.

Garces-Foley, K. 2006. Hospice and the politics of spirituality. *OMEGA* 53(1-2): 117-36.

Heelas, P., and L. Woodhead. 2005. *The spiritual revolution: Why religion is giving way to spirituality.* Oxford: Blackwell.

Henery, N. 2003. The reality of visions: Contemporary theories of spirituality in social work. *British Journal of Social Work* 33(8): 1105-13.

hooks, b. 1990. *Yearning: Race, gender, and cultural politics.* Boston: South End Press.

–. 2000. *Where we stand: Class matters.* New York: Routledge.

Joshi, K. 2006. The racialization of Hinduism, Islam, and Sikhism in the United States. *Equity and Excellence in Education* 39(3): 211-26.

Klassen, C. 2003. Confronting the gap: Why religion needs to be given more attention in women's studies. *Thirdspace* 3(1). http://thirdspace.ca.

Lyall, S. 2009. Atheists send a message, on 800 British buses. *London Journal,* 6 January. http://www.nytimes.com/.

McCall, L. 2005. The complexity of intersectionality. *Signs: Journal of Women in Culture and Society* 30(3): 1771-1800.

Micklethwait, J. 2007. In God's name. *Economist,* 3 November, 3-5.

Orsi, R. 2003. Is the study of lived religion irrelevant to the world we live in? Special presidential plenary address, Society for the Scientific Study of Religion, Salt Lake City, November 2, 2002, *Journal for the Scientific Study of Religion* 42(2): 169-74.

Pesut, B., M. Fowler, T. Johnston, S. Reimer-Kirkham, and R. Sawatzky. 2008. Conceptualizing spirituality and religion for healthcare. *Journal of Clinical Nursing* 17(21): 2803-10.

Ruether, R. Radford. 2000. *Christianity and the making of the modern family: Ruling ideologies, diverse realities.* Boston: Beacon Press.

Reimer-Kirkham, S. 2009. Lived religion: Implications for nursing ethics. *Nursing Ethics* 16(4): 406-17.

Reimer-Kirkham, S., and J. Anderson. 2002. Postcolonial nursing scholarship: From epistemology to method. *Advances in Nursing Science* 25(1): 1-17.

Ricketts, B. 2008. The *Komagata Maru* incident. Mysteries of Canada. http://www.mysteriesofcanada.com.

Sharma, A., and K.K. Young. 2007. *Fundamentalism and women in world religions.* New York: Continuum.

Spector, R. 2008. *Cultural diversity in health and illness.* 7th ed. Upper Saddle River, NJ: Prentice-Hall.

Thomas, S. 2005. *The Global resurgence of religion and the transformation of international relations: The struggle for the soul of the twenty-first century.* New York: Palgrave Macmillan.

Tremonti, A.M. 2008. Monia Mazigh interview. *Current,* 29 October. Canadian Broadcasting Corporation. http://www.cbc.ca.

Vakulenko, A. 2007. "Islamic headscarves" and the European convention on human rights: An intersectional perspective. *Social and Legal Studies* 16(2): 183-99.

Vásquez, M., and M. Friedmann Marquardt. 2003. *Globalizing the sacred: Religion in the Americas.* Piscataway, NJ: Rutgers University Press.

Vincett, G. 2008. The fusers: New forms of spiritualized Christianity. In Aune, Sharma, and Vincett 2008, 133-45.

Vincett, G., S. Sharma, and K. Aune. 2008. Women, religion and secularization in the West: One size does not fit all. In *Women and religion in the West: Challenging secularization,* eds. K. Aune, S. Sharma, and G. Vincett, 1-19. Ashgate: Aldershot.

Weber, L., and D. Parra-Medina. 2003. Intersectionality and women's health: Charting a path to eliminating health disparities. In *Advances in gender research.* Vol. 7, *Gender perspectives on health and medicine,* ed. M.T. Segal, V. Demos, and J.J. Kronenfeld, 181-230. Oxford: Elsevier.

Wong, Y.-L. R., and J. Vinsky. 2009. Speaking from the margins: A critical reflection on the "spiritual-but-not-religious" discourse in social work. *British Journal of Social Work* 39(7): 1343-59.

Woodhead, L. 2008. Secular privilege, religious disadvantage. *British Journal of Sociology* 59(1): 53-58.

Yuval-Davis, N. 2006. Intersectionality and feminist politics. *European Journal of Women's Studies* 13(3): 193-209.

Part 2
Intersectionality Research across the Life Course

Edited by Nazilla Khanlou and Olena Hankivsky

6

Navigating the Crossroads: Exploring Rural Young Women's Experiences of Health Using an Intersectional Framework

Natalie Clark and Sarah Hunt

I have resorted to fancy dancing
In order to survive each day
No wonder I have earned
The dubious reputation of being
The world's premier choreographer
Of distinctive dance steps
That allow me to avoid
Potential personal paranoia
On both sides of this invisible border.

– Ipellie (1992)

Within North America, increasing attention has been paid to the need for sex- and gender-based analysis in health research and to the impact of social determinants of health from a gender perspective (Johnson, Greaves, and Repta 2007; Health Canada 2000; Benoit 2006). However, there is growing recognition of the need for health research to expand beyond gender analysis to embrace life course and the special health needs and life circumstances of girls, including the intersections of risk across social determinants of health (Hankivsky 2007; Tyyskä 2006). Regardless of the words used to describe them – whether they are "adolescent female," "girl," "female youth," and "younger woman" – research, policy, and practice within the areas of health and women's health have continued to ignore the unique experiences of this age group. At best, young women are an add-on to the dialogue about women's health, or they are invisible within the categories of children and youth. At worst, their experiences are not considered at all. When girls are taken into account, they "are being represented and simultaneously groomed as consumers, soldiers, HIV carriers, potential victims, virgins, whores, sweatshop workers, drug lord mules, sex workers, mothers, students – transmitting culture, capital, values, virtue and disease" (Torre et al. 2007, 222). Whether girls are invisible or hyper-visible, their lives and voices are not truly present in the discourse on women's health; neither is the complexity of their experiences, which emerges through intersections of socio-political positioning. However, there has been increasing support for young women to play a meaningful role in the discourse on women's health and for the researchers, practitioners, and advocates who work with them to "agitate for counter public spaces in which young women can grow, develop and stretch their critical consciousness toward participatory action and research" (ibid., 224).

In this chapter, we use an intersectional framework in the development of girls' group program models that support the multiple and emergent identities of girls and their relationship to health and wellness, particularly as these models have been implemented in rural and Aboriginal communities in BC. The chapter is guided by the inclusion of our own voices as women, together with those of girls on the margins, whose "subjugated knowledges" have historically been devalued, misinterpreted, excluded, or trivialized (Brown and Strega 2005). We have had the privilege and honour of working with girls in rural communities across BC and have heard their voices in all their complexities. As researchers, practitioners, and educators, we have experienced transformation alongside the girls, as they have come to voice the impacts of intersecting factors in shaping their health and well-being. Simultaneously, in many cases, we have held multiple roles, connecting with the girls as relatives, community members, and mentors. Here we hope to honour these relationships and our own personal growth through sharing both our stories and those we have witnessed in this work with rural girls.

Centering Rural Girls' Health

Research completed in Canada, and in British Columbia, over the last ten years has consistently identified that girls are more likely than boys to feel distressed and that this distress manifests in a number of interrelated health challenges for girls, including substance abuse, risky sexual behaviour, body image and eating disorders, and self-esteem and achievement issues (McCreary Centre Society 2004; Jiwani 1999). Further, girls who are marginalized and disadvantaged are at greater health risk (Smith et al. 2007). For example, McCreary Centre Society research with street-involved youth revealed that Indigenous girls and lesbian, gay, bisexual, transgender, and queer (LGBTQ) girls were overrepresented in street youth populations and were three times more likely to be physically and sexually abused than youth of the same age who were in school (ibid.; Saewyc et al. 2007).[1] Greater health risks are associated with increased violence against Aboriginal girls and women, rooted in colonization (Amnesty International 2004). For example, in Canada, 50 percent of girls have experienced violence; for those who are marginalized, such as Indigenous, immigrant, impoverished, and

LBTQ girls, these numbers are higher (National Council of Women of Canada 1999). Further, there is a growing recognition that the specific health needs of marginalized and disadvantaged girls are not being met through current health policies and that current prevention strategies often fail, as girls do not see themselves or the intersecting oppressions they experience reflected in these policies (Oxfam Canada 2008). At the Alliance of Five Research Centres on Violence, one of the few studies considering rural girls through an intersectional lens identified that "effective programs recognize how gender, race, class, sexuality, disability, and age intersect in particular ways to shape women's and girls' experiences of violence and their access to programs and services" (Blaney 2004, vi; Berman and Jiwani 2003).

The limited research that has been done on the health needs of girls in rural areas indicates the need for more in-depth research and intersectional analysis. In a review of Health Canada statistics from 2000 to 2001, Statistics Canada contrasted the experiences of over seventeen thousand girls in rural and urban areas. It found that only 17 percent of girls in rural areas and 15 percent of those in northern regions identified their health as excellent, whereas 33 percent of girls in major metro centres did so (Statistics Canada 2004). Health issues linked with age, gender, and rurality include increased suicide rates, with girls in rural areas six times more likely to commit suicide (boys were four times more likely) and higher rates of death due to injuries (DesMeules et al. 2006). In a study of the health experiences of Mi'kmaq girls living on-reserve in Nova Scotia, participants identified multiple stressors, including racism in school, violence and abuse, and relationship stress. Aboriginal pride and a strong cultural identity were linked to health, and the absence of cultural identity was seen as a stressor (McIntyre et al. 2001). These finding were echoed in recent research on Aboriginal youth health in BC, which found that intersections of geography and gender have a strong impact; for example, the highest rates of suicide and sexual abuse for Aboriginal females were found in the BC Interior (van de Woerd et al. 2005).

Perhaps more important than the findings of professionals and academics are the voices of rural girls themselves, voices that have long called for a more complex understanding of their experiences of health and wellness. It is no surprise to people working and living in rural communities that girls face a complex web of factors that shape their embodied experiences of power and powerlessness. The impact of intersecting axes of power and privilege is experienced daily, in the bodies and minds of the girls themselves. In a study examining experiences of transitioning to adulthood, which was completed in both rural and urban areas, Natalie Clark interviewed rural girls who described experiencing discrimination while working in the male-dominated industries and resource-based economies that define much of small-town life. As one girl described,

My girlfriend's brother is a drywaller, and I asked him if I could get a part-time drywalling job like doing drywall 'cause I want to take a trade. And he looked at me and said, "I can't do it." And I was like: "Why? 'Cause I am a girl?" And he was just like, "Yeah, and all the other guys wouldn't like having a girl there." And I was like, "That's not fair." And he was like, "Well, that's just how it goes" ... You see girls like in construction sites like doing framing and stuff like that, but a lot of the time they won't even give you a chance. And it is so hard. (Leadbeater, Smith, and Clark 2008, 14)

Our research and writing have consistently highlighted the absence of, and need for, research focused on rural and remote communities, which considers the impact and intersections of gender, culture, sexuality, and geography on the health and service needs of young women living in these communities (Justice Institute of British Columbia 2006, 2002; Bell-Gadsby, Clark, and Hunt 2006). One of the key themes emerging from our research has been the issue of isolation for girls living in rural communities, in particular those who are marginalized due to their racial and cultural identity, class position, gender identity, and/or sexual orientation.

Starting from Where We Stand: Our Personal Positions

Who is speaking and who is listening are key questions to ask in our relationship with girls. Locating ourselves with respect to locations of power and privilege, as well as those where we experience oppression, is important. In their research with girls, Jill McLean Taylor, Carol Gilligan, and Amy M. Sullivan (1995) found that women who are similar to the girls (in race, class, sexual orientation) and who "tell the truth" are key to their formation of healthy and supportive relationships. Other theorists, such as bell hooks (1992) and Tracy Robinson and Janie V. Ward (1991), have identified that a central factor in health of girls of colour is the development of resistance strategies that are liberating and that allow girls to critically engage with the world and systems that oppress them (Ward 2007). Cultivating this resistance strategy, or "oppositional gaze" as hooks described it, is central to the work we do in our research and practice with girls, and has required us to ground in our own experience of adolescence in addition to naming our own intersecting identities. "Talking back" is not only about locating our own voice within the dialogue on girls' and women's health but is also a form of counter-storytelling to create narratives that disrupt dominant spaces such as those within the health field, allowing us to speak alongside the many young women with whom we have worked and built community. Critical race theorists such as Richard Delgado (2000, 61) suggest that these narratives can "shatter complacency and challenge the status quo."

To this end, we have chosen to use auto-ethnography to explore the perspectives we have developed through our multiple roles as researchers, writers, academics, aunties, sisters, mentors, and relatives. Deborah E. Reed-Danahay (1997, 4) writes in the anthology *Auto/Ethnography: Rewriting the Self and the Social* that "double identity and insider/outsider are constructs too simplistic for an adequate understanding of the processes of representation and power." Ethnography helps us to understand "women's subjectivities by insisting that women themselves be the interlocutors of their own lives and experiences" (Inhorn 2006, 367). We also draw on bell hooks's (1989, 9) concept of talking back, which she says "is no mere gesture of empty words, [but] is the expression of our movement from object to subject – the liberated voice." By including aspects of our own stories, we are enacting our previously theorized concept of intersectional research teams, which "implies we not only consider the full complexity of the location of our co-researchers but first begin with who we are and the power, ethics, and diversity of who is on the research team" (Clark and Hunt 2007).

Sarah Hunt

As an Indigenous woman working in the academy and across various communities, I aim to be useful as a tool to those members of my community who do not ordinarily have access to modes of knowledge production within the university setting. Certainly, this is how I have seen myself in my work with girls in rural communities: as someone who can offer a set of tools, bridge differences, and bring their voices forward to decision makers. Gloria Anzaldúa (2002, 4) writes that bridging is "about honoring people's otherness in ways that allow us to be changed by embracing that otherness rather than punishing others for having a different view, belief system, skin color, or spiritual practice." Although I may share similar cultural and gender identities with the girls with whom I've worked, I have never assumed that these points would instantly provide a sense of sameness or similarity. For me, locating myself in all of my multiplicity has been a central part of loosening the boundaries of identity to see the richness of experience that we all bring to our lives. Having worked with sexually exploited youth, having listened to many stories of extreme violence, trauma, and abuse, I believe that it was my compassion and refusal to judge that allowed the girls to connect with me, in addition to my lived understanding of colonialism as an Indigenous person. We must look beyond our fixed notions of identity to those of shared spaces where all of our selves meet, mingle, and experience together. These spaces of grief, anger, despair, repair, healing – they are beyond identity and require a lens of intersectionality if we are to comprehend their fullness. As academics, practitioners, and allies of the youth with whom we work, we must not attempt to slot the lives of girls into boxes but must stand back and witness the richness of their experiences emerge.

An intersectional lens has been important for my own self-awareness and the shifting nature of my identity. I am a member of the Kwakwaka'wakw

First Nation, but I grew up away from my Indigenous community, with my Ukrainian English single mom, so I learned the complexities of identity at an early age. As a girl, I moved between rural and urban areas of BC, and I knew the isolation of being the only Indigenous person on my street, as well as the joy of being on a rural reserve with my Aboriginal relatives. When I look back on my experiences of adolescence, and my view of health and wellness, my understanding emerged out of the spaces I occupied, moving between white and Indigenous communities, rural and urban spaces, on- and off-reserve.

When I was in grade nine, I remember that my sewing teacher was concerned about my weight and suspected I wasn't eating. Because I was Aboriginal, she asked the male Aboriginal counsellor to talk to me. When he called me in to his office, I was terrified and told him I was fine (I was not). This singular view of my identity along the axis of race/culture put me into a box that determined the health services offered to me and ultimately hurt my chances of accessing help. Had I been offered support by a female counsellor with whom I could connect around issues of body image, I might have reached out for support.

I believe that by focusing on the connections, intersections, and interwoven nature of our lived experiences, we are moving beyond identity politics (which puts us in boxes according to race, gender, and so on) to one of building coalitions toward a common goal. As Anzaldúa (2002, 2) puts it, "the knowledge that we are in symbiotic relationship to all that exists and co-creators of ideologies – attitudes, beliefs, and cultural values – motivates us to act collaboratively." I believe that by exposing intersecting axes of power at work in our lived experiences and analytical frameworks, we are ultimately contributing to the goal of decolonizing these same power systems.

Natalie Clark

My previous and ongoing work with young women always calls me to answer the question "who are you and why do you care?" I have had to continuously engage in the process of locating myself and of role modelling for young women the multiple locations and identity moments in one's life. I have shared my stories of intersecting identities of oppression and privilege, and how these change over time and space. I share these not as a point of connection with the girls but as a form of counter-storytelling, or call and response.

One story goes like this: I am in grade ten, an Anglo-European Canadian girl, living on income assistance with my "single mom" in a rural town. I am at school and my basketball coach, whom I have respected, tells me that he "feels sorry for me" because I come from a single-parent home. Basketball was my saviour, a space I could inhabit where I was free to be strong and powerful, and here was my coach taking this from me in one small comment. I go to the counsellor's office, the only time in high school, and I share with the counsellor my anger about this statement. The counsellor encourages me to take my anger, right then and there, interrupt my coach in his teaching, and share how I feel. I still remember the feeling of marching down the quiet hallway, as everyone was in class. I arrive at the classroom where he is teaching and stare through the small window. I knock and ask to speak to him. I tell him how angry I am – that, in fact, my experiences, my daughter-of-a-single-parent identity, have provided me with my gifts, my insights, my strength. He started to cry. I still remember that feeling of challenging his view of me, of "talking back" and replacing his view with my own.

The adolescent young women with whom I have been privileged to work are theorists of identity. They are living in the intersections of societal oppression, and they inhabit the spaces where they are actively being othered, experiencing privilege or oppression depending on their social location. They continue to ask me "who are you and why do you care?" and as my answer to these questions shifts over time, space, and geography, so too does my relationship with the girls. I currently work with girls as a researcher and am a girls' group facilitator in an Indigenous girls' group in the same rural town where I grew up. My identity has shifted since I was an adolescent in this town: I am now a solo-parent of three children, a mixed-race girl and twin boys who are from the Secwepemc Nation; and I learned recently of my own Métis heritage at my maternal grandmother's funeral, something she had long denied. I also work at the university, live in a small city, and no longer live in the poverty that many of the girls I work with do. Sharing my current stories and challenges alongside their own becomes a form of storywork, shared storytelling, and inviting them to challenge the dominant discourses about who they are and how they see themselves.

Colonialism and Intersectionality: The Lives of Indigenous Girls

As previously noted, many examples of the consequences of intersecting oppressions manifest themselves in the lives of Indigenous girls in rural BC. One primary example is the Highway of Tears, or Highway 16 between Prince George and Prince Rupert in northern BC, which came to public attention after reports surfaced that a number of girls and young women had gone missing or been murdered along this stretch of highway. All but one of them were Indigenous. Similar situations exist in communities across the province, as well as nationally, as acknowledged by the Native Women's Association of Canada's Sisters in Spirit campaign. NWAC's research found that more than five hundred Aboriginal girls and women have gone missing from across Canada, many from rural communities. Although both local and national efforts have framed this as an issue facing "Aboriginal women," an intersectional lens might expose the reality that age is a factor, as many of the girls were teenagers at the time they went missing. Indeed, the first nine victims identified by police along the Highway of Tears were between fourteen and twenty-five years old. An intersectional lens illuminates the many risk factors that make Indigenous girls in northern communities particularly vulnerable: geographic location, social isolation, gender, racial background, and lack of financial resources, among other factors, come together in their lives to increase the risks of violence and abduction. Whereas much of the work on this issue provides an analysis of racial and gender violence (using an additive approach of analyzing these two axes of power), an intersectional lens exposes a more nuanced understanding of the lives of rural Indigenous girls in BC.

Indeed, much writing and research about Indigenous women focuses on the impact of racism and sexism in their experiences of health and wellness. Indigenous scholar Emma D. LaRocque (1994, 74) writes that "a direct relationship between racist/sexist stereotypes and violence can be seen ... in the dehumanizing portrayal of Aboriginal women as 'squaws,' which renders all Aboriginal female persons vulnerable to physical, verbal and sexual violence." In her "squaw poems," Marilyn Dumont (1996, 19) reflects on the impact of the squaw stereotype on her lived experience as an Indigenous girl: "I would become the Indian princess, not the squaw dragging her soul after laundry, meals, needy kids and abusive husbands. These were my choices. I could react naturally, spontaneously to my puberty, my newly discovered sexuality or I could be mindful of the squaw whose presence hounded my every choice." These stereotypes and images are powerful examples of the ways in which racism and sexism have affected the lives of Indigenous girls and women. However, colonialism has affected their lives much more deeply than these two axes of power.

Sarah

Indigenous world views have been forever affected by the imposed set of power systems and institutions that force Indigenous people to speak about our lives as fractured into many pieces. We have internalized the power systems embedded in concepts of race, gender, class, ability, sexuality – the list goes on and on. Like Dumont, we are hounded and haunted by the ideologies of colonialism. On a more practical level, in order to access services, we must fracture ourselves into many pieces: mental, physical, spiritual, emotional. Outside of traditional Indigenous systems of holistic health, few spaces account for the many aspects that make up our lived experiences of health and wellness.

This fracturing is exacerbated for girls in rural areas, particularly on First Nations reserves, where communities face a general lack of resources. In many rural areas, health services are not available locally, and if they are, they are very limited. Many services or programs in nearby cities or towns are designed with one specific axis of identity in mind. A girl may choose to access a program for GLBTQ youth in order to explore her sexuality but may find that she continues to experience marginalization because the other youth in the program are white. Communities are challenged to design programs that account for the complex nature of rural girls' experiences and emerging identities, which continue to be in flux across their lifetime. Girls' groups are one model that we have found capable of responding to this need.

Girls' Groups: A Model for Exploring the Crossroads

We have developed a girls' group model and framework that provides marginalized and at-risk pre-adolescent and adolescent females with a space to explore a wide range of issues that affect their daily lives. The groups give the girls the opportunity to explore their experiences of abuse, sexual exploitation, body image, and violence, as well as their strengths and daily lived realities in a safe and non-threatening environment. The model we developed (in collaboration with other practitioners over the years), together with our current and past research with marginalized girls in rural communities, centres rural girls' health experiences within an intersectional framework that considers multiple axes of difference (race/ethnicity, socioeconomic status, sexual orientation, geography, ability, age, and migration status). Girls' groups centre the girls' own voices, speaking directly to the experiences of health and well-being that form the paradigm (or context) for the groups and for this chapter.

According to the Canadian Women's Foundation report *Girls in Canada* (2005, 55), a gender-specific girls' program is defined as "a single-sex program intentionally designed to respond to the specific needs and strengths of the girls it serves ... There is no one experience of being a girl. Gender combines with race, socioeconomic status, sexual orientation and dis/ability status to shape girls individually and collectively, and programs for girls reflect such diversity." The research of Stephanie Covington and Barbara Bloom (2003, 13) has found that wraparound models such as the girls' group are key as girls have been socialized to value relationships; therefore, service delivery approaches "that are based on ongoing relationships, that make connections among different life areas, and that work within women's existing support systems are especially congruent with female characteristics and needs."

Girls' groups provide a space for connection at a time when girls are disconnecting from key relationships – from society, family, peer groups, culture, school, community, and themselves (ibid.). Silencing themselves or being silenced by others can become more apparent when girls encounter racism, sexism, homophobia, and any intersections of these in their lives. As they come into girlhood, key strategies of disconnection include substance misuse, self-harming behaviours such as cutting, and disordered eating. These coping mechanisms and survival strategies are not honoured for their creativity or meaning; instead, girls who utilize them are further labelled and pathologized within the health care system.[2]

Making Their Strengths Visible

As noted earlier, discussions of girls' health tend to focus on problems, particularly on resistance strategies that manifest in eating disorders and other self-harming activities. Therefore, in order to shift and counter this, girls' group activities and relationships between girls and adult facilitators emphasize making the girls' strengths visible. This is done through displaying art, encouraging publishing of writing, and invitations to contribute to community projects. For example, in one of the groups that Natalie facilitated, the girls painted birdhouses to raise funds for a local neighbourhood house.

Another core concept that guides girls' group activities in this model is the link between individual problems, coping mechanisms, and society. Girls are encouraged to name and centralize the location of the problem outside of themselves. For example, with respect to eating disorders, girls use collage to explore the messages they are given about how they should look and act; they are encouraged to resist these through creating a collage of images and words that embody what girls really look like and are (including representing the diversity of girls in the group, those with glasses, those who are size sixteen, girls of colour, bi-racial girls, and so on). Within the group, they are given the analytical tools to situate themselves within larger power systems and institutions, and to problematize ideals around girlhood, health, and other norms. Through this process, they can identify the ways in which their lives are shaped by intersecting societal processes and can explore creative ways to question or undermine the hold of these processes. Rather than asking "what is wrong with me and how can I better fit in to society's ideals?" the girls are encouraged to ask "what is wrong with societal norms, and what ideals do I hold true for my own vision of health?"

Understanding the Context of Trauma and Violence

Trauma is a constant presence in the lives of most rural girls. High rates of violence, daily acts of sexual harassment, racism, abuse, and trauma are statistically within the daily range of experience for most of the girls with whom we work. We have found that most of this abuse and trauma goes undisclosed and untreated, resulting in high-risk behaviours such as suicide attempts and self-harming. It is at this key time that girls are developing a new relationship as health consumers, and it is often in their first encounters with medical professionals, including those who work in mental health, that their health is defined as a problem and when individual medical solutions are provided to structural issues. With statistics indicating that over 53 percent of girls experience sexual harassment and body-based harassment on a daily basis in schools (McCreary Centre Society 2004), health care practitioners need to recognize that trauma extends beyond direct experiences of violence to include racism, sexism, and the intersections of these in the girls' lives. In a study of violence and young women of colour in BC, the majority of the girls identified racism as the number-one form of violence they experienced; many of them, particularly in rural communities, had few safe places or services to access (Jiwani 2006).

Many of the girls who have attended our girls' groups describe experiences of seeking help and being prescribed medications for depression. In our research with sexually exploited youth and violence (Justice Institute of BC 2006), many girls shared stories of not reporting violence, because their first experiences of doing so had been negative. They further told us that, if they were to disclose abuse or violence, they would do so in a relationship with a trusted adult or a friend. Girls' groups are places and relationships where the complexity of who they are is present, and therefore their stories of violence and abuse can be present without reducing them to those experiences. Further, in our research, participants disclosed abuse by people in positions of trust, including police, justice system staff, health care providers, or chief and council. Young women in such situations must often choose between leaving their communities or staying to face further violence. The combination of these factors makes it unlikely that they will access help from people in positions of power; instead, they will seek support from a trusted adult, such as a girls' group facilitator.

Much of the literature on girls' health locates problems within the girls themselves, whereas girls' groups such as the ones we developed locate the source of the girls' challenges within systemic problems (such as racism, poverty, sexism) and the intersections of these in their lives. They support the young women in healthy resistance to these oppressions. Researchers and practitioners writing from post-colonial feminist perspectives have also argued that it is "critical to avoid decontextualized discussions of health statistics" and that these must be seen within a socio-political understanding of the intersection of "social, historical and economic determinants" (Browne, Smye, and Varcoe 2007, 132).

Intersectionality and Rural Girls' Health: Implications
Our research with girls, our clinical and frontline practice experience with them, and our own experiences growing up as rural girls taught us that the most marginalized and labelled girls are absent from programs, and their strengths and experiences of community building are not reflected in health programs and policies. Grounded in the reality that girls' lives and voices

have been overlooked and/or marginalized in research and that identity constructs such as sexual orientation and rurality cannot be hived off from gender, intersectional theory is a cutting-edge framework that allows for the development of a better understanding of the process of marginalization for girls. It further situates girls' health within the historical, social, and political contexts in which they live (Varcoe, Hankivsky, and Morrow 2007; Blaney 2004; Brown and Strega 2005; De Vault 1999; Kirby, Greaves, and Reid 2006; Lather 1991). Their embodiment of multiple positionalities affects their experiences of health, calling for the inclusion of "voices from the margins" in order to "produce insights that are intended to interrupt dominant discourses about race, class, gender relations and feminism" (Anderson 2002, 18, quoted in Brown, Smye, and Varcoe 2007, 127).

Health programs based on Western value systems serve only to further colonize girls' bodies and identities. The health of marginalized girls – and Indigenous girls in particular – must be accounted for in models based in more nuanced concepts of wellness. Indigenous traditions and belief systems may provide localized strategies for incorporating spiritual, emotional, and other axes of self in programming for girls. Rather than promoting any one model with a fixed concept of indigeneity, gender role, sexuality, or other aspects of identity, programs that are able to respond to the unique needs and experiences of local girls will have the capacity to foster resilience and community connectedness much more meaningfully. In addition, mainstream health programs have failed to provide access to safe spaces outside of home and school; nor do they address the overall lack of safety that girls experience in their communities. Our research found that girls were frequently putting themselves at risk in order to seek health services. Although this is not unique to rural girls – indeed, due to a general lack of transportation, rural boys are also forced to take risks in moving between communities – girls face much higher rates of vulnerability to violence. Some communities have created solutions by providing space at band offices for drop-in health care, counselling, recreation, and other services on a rotating basis. However, most of these services cannot be accessed anonymously, and so girls will continue to leave town to deal with traumatic issues. Girls' groups may provide one model that can be implemented in rural areas, creating spaces for girls to find support for their healthy development and complex identities.

Closing Thoughts: Application of an Intersectional Lens

Natalie

I have had the privilege and honour of working with girls in rural communities across BC and have heard their voices, in all their complexities. As a researcher, practitioner, and now social work educator, I am experiencing transformation alongside the girls, students, and communities. As they have come to voice the impacts of intersecting factors in shaping their health and well-being, it is imperative that I too share my own experiences here. Through auto-ethnography and storytelling about my own challenges and personal growth, both as a rural girl and now as a woman, I hope to encourage health educators, practitioners, and policy makers to explore the richness brought about by an intersectional lens and critical engagement with other processes of "talking back." Without the inclusion of a diversity of voices in the health field, health policies and programs will continue to reinscribe harmful power dynamics that serve to disempower girls rather than empower them. As a practitioner, researcher, advocate, and former rural girl, I remain committed to fundamentally reorienting the ways in which health provision for girls is framed and ultimately operationalized.

Sarah

The embodiment of intersectionality, as manifested in our experiences of health and wellness in the context of colonial society, is difficult to put into words. As an Indigenous woman, and someone who has worked alongside girls in negotiating their complex identities in rural and urban contexts, I am reminded of the gap between embodied knowledge and the theoretical frameworks we use to give voice to it. As a community-based researcher, academic, and social justice advocate, I remain committed to exploring the space between our assumptions about girls' lives and the multiple ways they express and name their realities, including the messages they send about what they truly need to cultivate spaces of health and wellness in our communities. I see this work as very much grounded in the seven-generations model, making decisions today that will have a positive impact on the seven generations ahead, as we reframe and reconceptualize our relationship to systems of power and privilege, as manifested in our work with girls in our communities.

Intersectional frameworks, and the movement toward social justice on which these frameworks are centred, have policy implications for girls' health and girls' health research. We join the voices of others privileged to stand with young women at the crossroads and call for the reform of health policy and practices, starting with the critical interrogation of these policies for their impact on young women (see Blaney 2004; Jackson and Henderson 2006; Janovicek 2001). The potential benefits of this approach are that the voices of girls on the margins will be made more audible to each other and to society, health and social service agencies will have a better sense of how to provide health services to vulnerable young women, and researchers will be able to develop research proposals that reflect the perspectives of this population and involve it as collaborators. We are committed to addressing the needs of girls and influencing health policy and programming that are sensitive to race, language, culture, and geography.

When one applies an intersectional approach to the ways in which policies affect girls, particularly those in rural and Aboriginal communities, one should always ask the following question: How does this policy affect a young Indigenous female living in rural British Columbia? Further, when young women are involved in research that is centred in intersectional frameworks and that employs a participatory action research agenda, they can "critically investigate the social policies that construct and constrict their lives, interrogating policies that ravage their communities and threaten their imaginations" (Torre et al. 2007, 238). As practitioners, researchers, advocates, and former rural girls, we urge our colleagues to explore the richness brought about by an intersectional lens in order to fundamentally re-orient the ways in which girls' and women's health is framed.

To this end, we leave the following questions for future investigation in this area: What key components of policy, programming, and practice are identified by marginalized girls, such as those in Aboriginal girls' groups, in meeting their health and health-related needs? What unique health experiences are faced by marginalized girls in rural and isolated areas, First Nations reserves, and small cities? How are their lives shaped by mainstream institutions and ideas of health that exclude cultural, gendered, and spatial experiences of their health and wellness, and the intersections of these in their lives? How can I strategically use my position of voice, power, or authority as an ally to marginalized girls in creating opportunities for their needs and experiences to be centralized in making decisions at the levels of policy, analysis, program development, and frontline service?

Notes

1   We use the terms "Indigenous" and "Aboriginal" to include all First Nations, Métis, and Inuit peoples. It is important to note that, as the commonly used acronym GLBTQ suggests, transgender youth are often lumped in with gay, lesbian, bisexual, and queer youth, but they may face very different issues. Transgender identity is based in gender identity, whereas gay, lesbian, and bisexual identities are typically referring to sexuality. Additionally, the term "two-spirit" is generally used to refer to Aboriginal GLBTQ people.

2   For more information on the girls' group model, see Bell-Gadsby, Clark, and Hunt (2006).

References

Amnesty International. 2004. *Stop violence against women, stolen sisters: Discrimination and violence against Indigenous women in Canada, a summary of Amnesty International's concerns.* Ottawa: Amnesty International.

Anzaldúa, G.E. 2002. Preface: (Un)natural bridges, (un)safe spaces. In *This bridge we call home: Radical visions for transformation,* ed. G.E. Anzaldúa and A. Keating, 1-5. New York: Routledge.

Bell-Gadsby, C., N. Clark, and S. Hunt. 2006. *It's a girl thang: A manual on creating girls groups.* Vancouver: McCreary Youth Foundation.

Benoit, C. 2006. *Health determinants: Summary and notes, WHRN workshop.* Vancouver: Women's Health Research Network. http://www.whrn.ca.

Berman, H., and Y. Jiwani, eds. 2003. *Violence prevention and the girl child, phase two report: In the best interests of the girl child.* Vancouver: Alliance of Five Research Centres on Violence.

Blaney, E. 2004. *PRISM: Probing rural issues – Selecting methods to address abuse of women and girls: (E)valu(at)ing "better" practices and reflexive approaches.* Fredericton: Muriel McQueen Fergusson Centre for Family Violence Research.

Brown, I., and S. Strega, eds. 2005. *Research as resistance: Critical, Indigenous, and anti-oppressive approaches.* Toronto: Canadian Scholars' Press.

Browne, A., V.L. Smye, and C. Varcoe. 2007. Post-colonial feminist theoretical perspectives and women's health. In *Women's health in Canada: Critical perspectives on theory and policy,* ed. M. Morrow, O. Hankivsky, and C. Varcoe, 124-43. Toronto: University of Toronto Press.

Canadian Women's Foundation. 2005. *Girls in Canada.* Toronto. http://www.cdnwomen. org.

Clark, N., and S. Hunt. 2007. "The empress has no clothes": Exposing the truth of inter-sectional research with marginalized populations. Invited lecture at the Institute for Critical Studies in Gender and Health, Simon Fraser University, Vancouver, BC, 26 April 2007.

Covington, S.S., and B.F. Bloom. 2003. Gendered justice: Women in the criminal justice system. In *Gendered justice: Addressing female offenders,* ed. B.E. Bloom, 1-20. Durham: Carolina Academic Press. http://www.stephaniecovington.com/pdfs/4.pdf.

De Vault, M.L. 1999. *Liberating method: Feminism and social research.* Philadelphia: Temple University Press.

Delgado, R. 2000. Storytelling for oppositionists and other: A plea for narrative. In *Critical race theory: The cutting edge,* ed. R. Delgado and J. Stefancic, 60-70. Philadelphia: Temple University Press.

DesMeules, M., R.W. Pong, C. Lagace, D. Heng, D. Manuel, J.R. Pitblado, R. Bollman, J. Guernsey, A. Kazanjian, and I. Koren. 2006. *How healthy are rural Canadians? An assessment of their health status and health determinants.* Ottawa: Canadian Institute for Health Information.

Dumont, M. 1996. *A really good brown girl.* London, ON: Brick Books.

Hankivsky, O. 2007. More than age and biology: Overhauling lifespan approaches to women's health. In *Women's health in Canada: Critical perspectives on theory and policy,* ed. M. Morrow, O. Hankivsky, and C. Varcoe, 64-93. Toronto: University of Toronto Press.

Health Canada. 2000. *Health Canada's gender-based analysis policy.* Ottawa: Health Canada.

hooks, b. 1989. *Talking back.* Boston: South End Press.

–. 1992. *Black looks: Race and representation.* Boston: South End Press.

Inhorn, M.C. 2006. Defining women's health: A dozen messages from more than 150 ethnographies. *Medical Anthropology Quarterly* 20(3): 345-78.

Ipellie, A. 1992. Walking both sides of an invisible border. In *An anthology of Canadian Native literature in English.* 2nd ed., ed. D.D. Moses and T. Goldie, 324. Oxford: Oxford University Press.

Jackson, M.A., and A.D. Henderson. 2006. Restorative justice or restorative health: Which model best fits the needs of marginalized girls in Canadian society? *Criminal Justice Policy Review* 17: 234-51.

Janovicek, N. 2001. *Reducing crime and victimization: A service providers' report.* Vancouver: FREDA Centre for Research on Violence against Women and Children.

Jiwani, Y. 1999. *Violence prevention and the girl child, phase one report.* Vancouver: FREDA Centre for Research on Violence against Women and Children.

–. 2006. Racialized violence and girls and young women of colour. In *Girlhood: Redefining the limits,* ed. Y. Jiwani, C. Steenbergen, and C. Mitchell, 70-88. Montreal: Black Rose Books.

Johnson, J.L., L. Greaves, and R. Repta. 2007. *Better science with sex and gender: A primer for health research.* Vancouver: Women's Health Research Network.

Justice Institute of British Columbia. 2002. *Commercial sexual exploitation: Innovative ideas for working with children and youth.* New Westminster, BC: Justice Institute of BC.

–. 2006. *Violence in the lives of sexually exploited youth and adult sex workers: Provincial research final report.* New Westminster, BC: Justice Institute of BC.

Kirby, S., L. Greaves, and C. Reid. 2006. *Experience, research, social change: Methods beyond the mainstream.* 2nd ed. Peterborough: Broadview Press.

LaRocque, E.D. 1994. *Violence in Aboriginal communities.* Ottawa: National Clearinghouse on Family Violence.

Lather, P. 1991. *Getting smart: Feminist research and pedagogy with/in the postmodern.* New York: Routledge.

Leadbeater, B., A. Smith, and N. Clark. 2008. *Listening to vulnerable youth: Transitioning to adulthood in British Columbia.* Victoria: Centre for Youth and Society, University of Victoria.

Lewis, T. 1999. *Living beside: Performing normal after incest memories return.* Toronto: McGilligan Books.

McCreary Centre Society. 2004. *Healthy youth development: Highlights from the 2003 Adolescent Health Survey III.* Vancouver: McCreary Centre Society.

McIntyre, L., F. Wien, S. Rudderham, L. Etter, C. Moore, N. MacDonald, S. Johnson, and A. Gottschall. 2001. *An exploration of the stress experience of Mi'kmaq on-reserve female youth in Nova Scotia.* Halifax: Maritime Centre of Excellence for Women's Health.

McLean Taylor, J., C. Gilligan, and A.M. Sullivan. 1995. *Between voice and silence: Women and girls, race and relationship.* Cambridge: Harvard University Press.

National Council of Women of Canada. 1999. *Girls/young women and violence project.* Funded by Status of Women Canada. Winnipeg: National Council of Women of Canada. http://www.ncwc.ca.

Oxfam Canada. 2008. Blueprint for action on women and girls and HIV/AIDS: Report card backgrounder: Canada August 2008. http://www.womensblueprint.org.

Reed-Danahay, D.E. 1997. *Auto/ethnography: Rewriting the self and the social.* New York: Oxford University Press.

Robinson, T., and J.V. Ward. 1991. A belief in self far greater than anyone's disbelief: Cultivating healthy resistance among African American female adolescents. In *Women, girls, and psychotherapy: Reframing resistance,* ed. C. Gilligan, A.G. Rogers, and D. Tolman, 87-103. Binghamton, NY: Harrington Park Press.

Saewyc, E., C. Poon, N. Wang, Y. Homma, A. Smith, and the McCreary Centre Society. 2007. *Not yet equal: The health of lesbian gay and bisexual youth in BC.* Vancouver: McCreary Centre Society.

Smith, A., E. Saewyc, M. Albert, L. MacKay, M. Northcott, and the McCreary Centre Society. 2007. *Against the odds: A profile of marginalized and street-involved youth in BC.* Vancouver: McCreary Centre Society.

Statistics Canada. 2004. Health status and behaviours of Canada's youth: A rural-urban comparison. *Rural and Small Town Canada Analysis Bulletin* 5(3). http://www.statcan.ca.

Torre, M.E., M. Fine, N. Alexandra, and E. Genao. 2007. Don't die with your work balled up in your fists: Contesting social injustice through participatory research. In *Urban girls revisited: Building strengths,* ed. B. Leadbeater and N. Way, 221-42. New York: New York University Press.

Tyyskä, V. 2006. The health of girls and young women. Special issue, *Women's Health and Urban Life: An International and Interdisciplinary Journal* 5(2): 3-7.

van de Woerd, K.A., et al. 2005. *Raven's children II: Aboriginal youth health in BC.* Vancouver: McCreary Centre Society.

Varcoe, C., O. Hankivsky, and M. Morrow. 2007. Introduction: Beyond gender matters. In *Women's health in Canada: Critical perspectives on theory and policy,* ed. M. Morrow, O. Hankivsky, and C. Varcoe, 3-32. Toronto: University of Toronto Press.

Ward, J.V. 2007. Uncovering truths, recovering lives: Lessons of resistance in the socialization of black girls. In *Urban girls revisited: Building strengths,* ed. B. Leadbeater and N. Way, 243-60. New York: New York University Press.

7

Exploring Health and Identity through Photovoice, Intersectionality, and Transnational Feminisms: Voices of Racialized Young Women

Jo-Anne Lee and Alison Sum

This chapter examines identity, health, and well-being from the perspectives of racialized young women who live transnational lives. It explores selected findings from a participatory action research study that used photovoice, a methodology that employs photos, narratives, stories, and discussions to assist research participants in describing and reflecting on their experiences. The racialized women who participated in our study experience health and well-being in ways that have yet to be fully acknowledged and theorized. To make sense of their narratives, we integrated transnational and post-colonial feminist theories and concepts into an intersectional feminist analysis. We suggest that health researchers investigating the lives of racialized minority women will find it useful to incorporate these concepts into their analytical frameworks of women's health issues.

Our interest in exploring health and wellness from the perspectives of racialized women who live in and across multiple national and cultural borders was prompted by several concerns. First, few health researchers question the raced, classed, and gendered construction of the nation, or how these nationalizing processes intersect to shape health policies and programs and women's health experiences (Anderson and Reimer-Kirkham 1998). Second, many researchers investigating cultural or racial inequities in health still rely on essentialist notions to interpret study findings (Reimer-Kirkham 2003). This is partly because dominant nationalist cultural norms are left unquestioned. In reality, ideologies and discourses of nationalism and national belonging play a central role in constructing social hierarchies and identities (Beck 2002; Wimmer and Schiller 2003). Further, recent health studies have found that many Canadian women and girls from ethnic and racial minority backgrounds confront interlocking systems of oppression that move across cultural and political boundaries (Jiwani 2001; Reimer-Kirkham 2003; Harding 2005). Hence, to dismantle exclusionary policies and practices in health care, there is an urgent need to transcend essentialist views that portray non-Western cultures as traditional and passive, thus inherently negative, and Western cultures as modern and active, thus positive (Browne, Smye, and Varcoe 2007).

In contrast to mainstream essentializing discourses, our findings demonstrate that racialized women who move across national boundaries and territories do not simply passively comply with hegemonic structures that render them invisible. They have the capacity and ability to act as conscious agents, creating and re-creating strategies of survival, negotiation, and resistance in their everyday lives (Rattansi 1992; Hall 1994; Ong 2003). Following Antonio Gramsci (1971), we understand hegemonic systems of domination not as unidirectional, fixed, and rigid but as dynamic, adaptive, and responsive to pressures from diverse sources that, in turn, compel individuals and groups to also change and adapt. These dynamic processes generate distinctive forms of social exclusion and inclusion of varying intensities and effects.

Thus, our research sought to address a number of questions: What effects do historically and globally dynamic, intersecting, and emergent structures of inequality have on women and girls from families and communities that have moved across numerous borders and cultural worlds to arrive in Canada, only to be relegated to the nation's margins (Grewal and Kaplan 1994)? Is there a need to think differently about health and well-being to better comprehend these experiences? How do racialized young women who live transnational lives understand their own health and well-being? How do their perceptions of health shape their ability to achieve a positive state of health and well-being for themselves and their families?

In the sections that follow, we introduce some key concepts and theories that guided our approach, describe the methodology of photovoice, present and discuss selected images and narratives, and conclude by drawing implications for intersectional health research.

Conceptual Framework

Destabilizing Identities: The Analysis of Women's Health

Transnational Feminist Frameworks
Our research questions were informed by studies that have documented embedded inclusion and exclusion in Western health discourses and practices (Reimer-Kirkham 2003; Anderson 2006). We also drew on Chandra Mohanty (2003) and others who have observed flawed logic in Western feminist scholarship that ascribes agency and complexity to those positioned as Western but denies women from non-Western backgrounds these same qualities. Similar bias is found in mainstream public health delivery, where racial minority women are often positioned in a monolithic category of otherness and where the norms against which otherness is defined are taken

as natural (Anderson and Reimer-Kirkham 1998; Grove and Zwi 2006). Importantly, Patricia Hill Collins's (2009) recently revised edition of *Black Feminist Thought* now acknowledges the importance of thinking transnationally about black women in the diaspora, given global influences in women's lives. Collins (2009) argues that it is necessary to theorize transnational experiences and contexts to further develop our understandings of intersectional systems of oppression. Transnational feminist scholars including Avtar Brah and Ann Phoenix (2004) and Nira Yuval-Davis (2006) also make a case for incorporating postmodern, post-structural, post-colonial, and transnational theories of difference and subjectivities into feminist intersectional frameworks. In our analysis, we draw from post-colonial and transnational feminist theories. Concepts such as diasporic spaces, cultural hybridity, and transnational positionality, among others, deepen and broaden our analyses of interlocking systems of oppression that travel across time, space, and place – an increasingly common context confronting women in this era of globalization. Although these concepts have their own conceptual baggage and debates, they nonetheless help guard against overpsychologized, individualized, nationalized, and abstracted views of socially constructed identities (Reimer-Kirkham 2003; Verloo 2006).

Feminist Post-Colonial Theory

Feminist post-colonial theory decolonizes Eurocentric thought by deconstructing binary logics and cultural essentialisms. Joan Anderson (2002) calls for the integration of post-colonial feminist theory and methodology in nursing scholarship. Alongside a critique of capitalism, feminist post-colonial thought reveals how borders of inclusion and exclusion work by using biological and cultural differences to distinguish between self and other. In revealing colonialism's long reach into present-day realities, feminist post-colonial theorists and scholars (Said 1979; Spivak 1987; McLintock 1993) argue that colonizing ideologies continue to rework and reproduce unequal social relations in ways that mirror master/slave and metropole/periphery binaries that existed in colonial times. The "post" in post-colonialism does not mean that colonialism has passed: it refers to the continuing salience of colonial ideologies long after formal colonialism, as a military, political, administrative, and imperial practice, declined. For example, colonial ideologies of race, class, gender, sexuality, and ethnicity produced in the justification of European domination and exploitation of the non-European world are today reproduced in ideologies of nationalism that position those deemed to be natural citizens as deserving of protection and social goods, and justify the treatment of those deemed to be aliens as non-citizens or proto-citizens who are begrudgingly offered limited rights (Stasiulis and Bakan 1997; Lee and Cardinal 1998).

Multiple Scattered Hegemonies

In taking apart ideologies of nationalism and their liberal discourses of universality and equality, transnational feminist investigations of diaspora and migration suggest that nation-state formations give rise to structural inequality as well as myriad contradictory, paradoxical experiences of citizenship and belonging (Westwood and Phizacklea 2000). Individuals who cross national and cultural boundaries possess consciousness of belonging and non-belonging to multiple hegemonies and cultural worlds. They are constituted and constitute themselves as culturally hybrid citizen-subjects. Residence in a nation-state does not necessarily erase attachments to non-hegemonic cultures and ethnic communities internal and external to the territorially bounded nation. The term "scattered hegemonies" names the way power relations travel and mutate in new ways in new sites of settlement, intermingling with existing hegemonic cultural norms. In other words, individual and collective migrant subjects confront and respond to scattered hegemonies, or hegemonic structures and processes that are mobile, adaptable, transient, and responsive structures of inequality (Grewal and Kaplan 1994).

Diaspora

Another highly productive concept is that of "diasporic space," understood as a space of mobility, displacement, and emplacement, linked to power. The term "diaspora" analyzes the mobility of cultures, peoples, commodities, capital, and information flow in the context of transnationalism and globalization, yet it acknowledges that embodied subjects are always grounded in particular places and spaces (Brah 1996; Werbner and Modood 1997; Prazniak and Dirlik 2001). Some feminist analysts of diaspora understand the concept of diasporic space not only through the intersections of socio-economic, political, and cultural "differences" in their variable forms but also by emphasizing emotional and psychic dynamics of difference (Brah and Phoenix 2004, 83). This latter insight allowed us to "hear" the personal stories and images produced by our co-researchers/participants.

Cultural Hybridity

Finally, the concept of cultural hybridity acknowledges the active, productive, and constructive practices of living diasporically across national and cultural borders. Derived from post-colonial theory, the notion of cultural hybridity names the agency of the colonized when confronted with colonial domination. It focuses on how individuals actively negotiate, utilize, and make sense of diverse ways of being when living within oppressive systems. Colonized and nationalized subjects create alternative ways of being that allow them to retain their humanity as they manoeuvre between and across cultural worlds, despite pressures to comply as subordinated Others to dominant cultural formations (Werbner and Modood 1997).

Together, these concepts help to advance intersectionality-type research in women's health in the millennial period by directing research and analytical attention toward diasporic spaces where mobile and fluid hybrid identities and subjectivities are formed. They insist that researchers look for contradictions and complexity, refuse unidimensional, unidirectional, reductionist, and singular determinations, and link the personal with the structural. These conceptualizations of the social serve to extend feminist intersectional critiques of essentializing discourses of race, class, gender, and sexuality, among other markers of difference. They offer counter-explanations to conventional analyses of racialized women's health that too often erase, silence, and deny the complexity and diversity of racialized women's and men's diasporic lives (Reimer-Kirkham and Anderson 2002). We deploy these concepts to guard against stereotyping racialized women and to advance more nuanced, complex, and robust intersectional frameworks for comprehending transnational racialized women's diverse experiences of health and well-being.

Exploring Multiple Exclusions: A Photovoice Project

Context of the Research

This research study is an integral part of our ongoing involvement in feminist participatory action research (FPAR) and community development with young racialized and indigenous girls and women in Victoria, BC. When FPAR is explicitly combined with community development, community-engaged researchers are more able to translate feminist anti-racist theories and analyses into meaningful, sustainable, grassroots community initiatives. FPAR supports research participants in taking action on knowledge that they collectively produce about the inequalities they experience in their lives (Lee and de Finney 2005; Lee 2006). Because racialized women and girls are usually excluded from modes of knowledge and policy production, we selected photovoice as a research methodology to amplify their voices and project their self-representations. Within an FPAR approach, photovoice offered young women the space to critically reflect on their experiences of health and well-being by telling stories and sharing intimate interpersonal encounters in the context of belonging and not belonging to multiple diasporic spaces.

Participants

The project began with the formation of a group of eight self-identified heterosexual racialized young women who were interested in exploring health and identity through creative means of expression. Participants ranged in age from twenty-one to twenty-eight, and only one, who identified as Métis, was born in Canada. The others had moved to Canada from elsewhere and had lived there for between four and fifteen years. Four participants spoke English as a first language; the others spoke Hokkien, Cantonese, Pahadi, or Farsi as a first language. Six knew three or more languages. Three identified with more than one nationality, although seven had Canadian citizenship, and one held dual Indian and Canadian citizenship. All had some post-secondary education. When asked to indicate their class background, one identified as lower middle class, three as middle class, and four as upper middle class.

The majority of participants were recruited from a grassroots organization called antidote, a multiracial girls' and women's network for racialized and indigenous girls and young women (www.antidotenetwork.org). Most belonged to a subgroup of young women within antidote's intergenerational structure, informally called the "Sistahs." Two had no prior affiliation with antidote and were recruited by word of mouth by other study participants.

There were four inclusion criteria for recruitment: potential participants had to be between the ages of eighteen and thirty, self-identified as racialized or indigenous, available for the duration of the project (one week total), and willing to express and share their thoughts and ideas with others.

About Photovoice

Photovoice is "an innovative participatory action research method based on health promotion principles and the theoretical literature on education for critical consciousness, feminist theory, and non-traditional approaches to documentary photography" (Wang 1999, 185). This methodology facilitates self-reflexivity, critical existence, and reimagination. Photovoice allows people to listen to and learn from the participants' own portrayals of their lives (ibid.).

We followed several stages in our use of photovoice. The first stage involved brainstorming meanings associated with health and well-being at different points in the women's lives. This was followed by a storytelling session in which participants shared stories and anecdotes prompted by the brainstorming session. This stage allowed our co-researchers time and space to talk about experiences that had affected their lives and wellness.[1] The exercise also encouraged women to build a sense of solidarity and connectedness with one another by hearing each other's experiences and stories. In the third phase, participants took pictures of places, people, objects, scenes, or symbols that reflected their experiences of health and well-being. They were asked to take approximately five photos each day over the course of a week and to keep a self-reflexive journal of their thoughts and feelings while they did so. They could either focus on the themes and issues that surfaced throughout the workshop or simply take pictures of their everyday realities and let themes emerge afterward. One week later, they emailed their digital photos to Alison Sum (research facilitator), who printed the photos and brought them to a second meeting.[2] During this session, participants reflected on their photos and told stories to the group, which opened up discussion on various topics.

Discussion of Findings

In the following sections, we share selected findings from our collaborative and participatory research study. We highlight four themes that emerged in connection with identity, health, and well-being: self-understandings of health; mobility, identity, and health; living between worlds; and finding balance.

Self-Understandings of Health

Rather than defining the research participants by their "health status," we set out to discover how they defined health and well-being in their own words and how these understandings were derived from their personal experiences and knowledge. Although some racialized women may experience violence or illness and may be conventionally classified as physically and/or mentally "unhealthy," it is important not to pathologize all racialized minority women or assume that the experiences of some women can be unproblematically generalized to all racialized women from similar backgrounds.

Our own experiences as relatively "healthy" individuals, and listening to stories shared among our peers in antidote, suggested that we question common Western definitions of what counts as health in order to make room for our own personal understandings.

As indicated by the growing number of health researchers who are concerned with how minoritized and marginalized women perceive health, feminist health researchers are increasingly dissatisfied with dominant discourses of health, which they perceive as unresponsive to and disconnected from marginalized women's realities (Reid 2002). There is growing consensus that ideas of health are shaped by cultural, economic, biological, environmental, social, and political factors, and that the imposition of "objective" definitions, however useful for managing data, actually limits our understanding of health (ibid.; Anderson 2006). Rather than imposing Western biomedical definitions of health, we encouraged participants to converse about health in ways that were personally meaningful and relevant to them. The following quote by research participant Dawn provides an example of how health can be subjectively defined transnationally, cross-culturally, and cross-contextually:

Health is so very personal, not just in experience but in design. And what we consider healthy/unhealthy changes with age, values, social class, community, cultural context, and myriad other things. For example, an overweight person is generally perceived as unhealthy in North America, but perhaps not so in other parts of the world. A little extra flesh doesn't necessarily spell "unhealthy" if the individual has a healthy attitude and lifestyle. On the other hand, there are some universal benchmarks that ensure adequate health and well-being for a person, such as food, water, safety, shelter, and belonging. Is that survival or health? How is health linked to survival?

Dawn's statement demonstrates a conscious critique of prescribed definitions of health that reflect Eurocentric, Western, masculinized, gendered, and able-bodied norms of dominant groups, which ultimately circumscribe and reinscribe systemic inequalities. In this regard, this research study follows a path established by other racialized women's health research studies that have revealed large gaps between standard biomedical prescriptions of health, socially, politically, and economically determined understandings of health, and women's own self-conscious perceptions of dominant health discourses (Mullings and Schulz 2006; Varcoe, Hankivsky, and Morrow 2007; Women's Health in Women's Hands 2003).

These gaps are further demonstrated by another participant, Monica. In the following text, written in conjunction with Figure 7.1, she draws important links among her health, the instability of her identity due to her family's colonial history in South Africa, and her need to find a place of belonging in Canada:

My feet remain grounded but still unsteady. I am calmed and connected to the passing tide, my love of the ocean and my longing for it comes from my longing of my homeland. Also there is my ancestral ties to the ocean – it symbolically represents where I'm from. My forefathers come from coastal towns in India swept to coastal towns in Africa. Twice removed we find ourselves drawn to similar places in Canada. The ocean conveys a collective memory of past and community. The image of my feet being touched by the waves can also represent cleansing, washing away of the old, a rejuvenation. Health, to me, is formed by who I am and how I feel – my identity is reflected by my connection to the sea, which I associate with where I come from.

Here, Monica references multiple generational migrations and homelands – a genealogy of diasporic spaces as lived reality. She recalls romanticized memories, a time of happiness and connectedness to family and community, a time when inclusion was never in doubt. Her sense of health and wellness is linked to memories of belonging, which now seems unstable as she searches for inclusion and a place to call home. Her next statement, however, describes how the bond her family has tried to maintain with their original homeland does not sufficiently provide her with a sense of belonging: "[We're an] im-

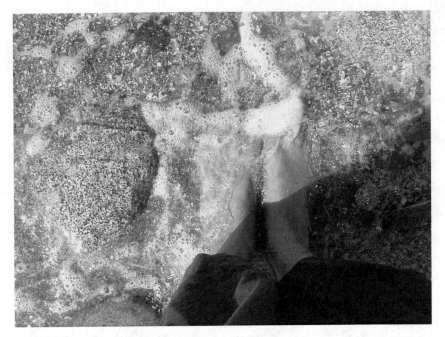

Figure 7.1 **Longing**
Source: Monica, age twenty-three.

migrant family from Africa, [but] we hold strong cultural ties to India because that's where our forefathers were taken from as indentured labourers to South Africa. And growing up in South Africa, you're constantly aware of who you are and your identity because of our past with racial exclusion. And I don't know, I just have trouble ever finding home, I think, because I don't have one set place."

Monica's narratives describe a constant state of ambivalence and contradiction that arises from paradoxical experiences of inclusion and exclusion when living in multiple locations. Without a strong sense of ancestral identity, Monica struggles to find balance in her life, which ties into her health. Although these struggles present momentary obstacles for her, she also speaks of ways in which she reclaims her health and identity by sharing food and culture with her family and by learning about her history through storytelling with her grandparents.

These forms of resistance, acknowledgment, and self-determination can be considered health-seeking behaviours that are unique to Monica (Smith 1999). Her expressions of longing for her "homeland," after being displaced by the forces of colonization and migration, can be understood through the concept of diasporic hybridity, which is explored in the following section.

Mobility, Hybrid Identity, and Health

Several of our co-researchers expressed a common theme revolving around metaphors of place, mobility, liminality, negotiations, and multiplicity. Their narratives of identity and health suggest that it is important to be specific about changing social locations in intersectional research. For example, when one considers which intersecting forces are important and how they are experienced, internalized, managed, questioned, negotiated, and resisted, it is essential to attend to dimensions of time, place, and space, as well as to socio-structural factors. Participants critically reflected on their lives in different times and locations, and discussed how they learned to understand their health and wellness as they moved and lived in, between, and across various geographic, political, and cultural spaces.

Jenna, a twenty-one-year-old participant who identifies as Filipina Canadian, was raised in the southern United States for most of her life. Her struggles as a dark-skinned mixed-race girl began in grade one, when she was forced to identify her ethnicity as either black, white, or other on a standardized school test. The following excerpt from her narrative illustrates one aspect of locational fluidity and specificity concerning mixed-race identity, culture, and health: "It was the first standardized test I'd ever really took and I asked my teacher ... 'what do I do because my mom is Filipina and my

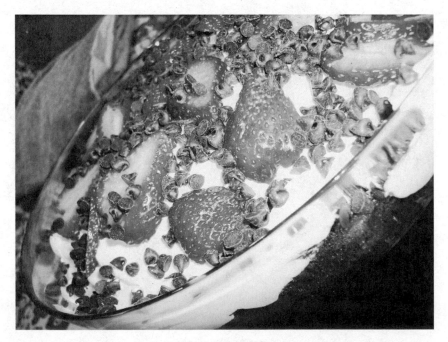

Figure 7.2 **Trifle**
Source: Jenna, age twenty-one.

dad is White?' I said something like, 'I'm both.' She was like, 'oh, just do whatever your dad is' ... So from grade 1 through maybe grade 7 or 8, I checked White for every single standardized test that I did and like, look at me! I'm not even White!" Jenna learned at a young age that it was more acceptable to fit into a predetermined category of normativity than to identify as an other. Because she identified as white on paper for so many years, she "ignored the fact that [she] was different" until recently.

Jenna's photovoice image (Figure 7.2) and her accompanying text illustrate the potential limitations of linear models of intersectionality. In contrast to these, her representation of her identities does not consist of nodal points that exist on lines that cross. She describes her multiple identities as woven together, layered and transformed into a unique work of art, yet constituting pieces, or ingredients, that are sifted or mediated through the societies and cultures in which she has lived:

> This picture represents my favourite foods. It has chocolate chips, straw-berries, whipped cream and brownie mix. I find that this somehow reaches me due to my ethnicity as a mixed-race young woman. I feel that my multiple identity as both 'White' and 'racialized' or 'brown' makes it impossible to mix both models or both cultures, even though I try to. I find that I end up layering each identity on top of each other.

In reference to this piece, Jenna talks about the inability to find her own space: "I just found it really complex, just like skin politics, how people categorize you. It's like there's no grey area, there's no area where I felt like I could fit 'cause it's like I can't be Filipina because I have all these other features, but yet I can't be White ... It's like well I can't be White, I can't be other, per se, or racialized 'cause I'm somewhere in between and it's like there wasn't an area left, there's no little space for me."

Here, Jenna defines her health and wellness spatially and makes reference to a "space" of nowhereness. This in-between space that she describes is associated with feelings of ambiguity and exclusion, which ultimately affect her self-esteem and overall well-being. Again, this space of nowhereness is a concept that cannot be fully theorized by metaphors of linear intersec-tionality converging into a single point of integration. To enhance our understandings of young transnational women's health and well-being, there is an urgent need for conceptual frameworks that theorize the layering, blending, and multiplicity of identities that do not fit into singular, homo-geneous, and tightly bordered categories or vectors.

Living between Worlds

Many minority women experience paradoxical and ambiguous feelings of belonging and not belonging to multiple national and ethnic communities

(Dossa 2004; Reimer-Kirkham 2003). Contradictory and conflicting realities of living as marginalized subjects in Canada are experienced not only through suffering but also through personal strategies of healing. The notion of living a "double life" was brought forth by Dawn, a participant who is familiar with the complexities of transnational migration, cultural adaptation, being part of a second-generation diasporic community, and having more than one ethnic/cultural influence in her life.

Dawn's descriptions of her experiences with migration differ from dominant immigrant female youth discourses, which often embody a dualistic "cultural orientation" or "acculturation/assimilation" perspective (Handa 2003). For example, cultural psychology studies often place Asian "collectivist" and North American "individualist" cultures in binary opposition with one another (Phinney, Ong, and Madden 2000; Salant and Lauderdale 2002; Zhou and Xiong 2005). Dawn's description of living a double life must be carefully distinguished from these dichotomous views of culture. Her photovoice piece below explains how the notion of living a double life is linked to the idea of liminality and negotiation, or living in an in-between space (Figure 7.3):

> I love the fact that the compass is situated in between the two tall buildings. This, in my mind, is the perfect symbolism for my journey – living in the liminal. The liminal space is where I sit, speak, thrive, trash, ponder, explode, and sometimes just breathe. What I mean by liminal is that it is basically the in-between, the just-there-but-not-quite, the "this and that." It is where uncertainty dwells. In the liminal space, one is inclined to be lost because the boundaries are not well-defined. Such is true for my life, where the path is not so certain. It can be, but it also can't. My identity is divided, and so are my decisions, inclinations, relationships.

In this picture, the liminal space between two buildings would not exist without the concrete structures of the skyscrapers. Metaphorically, this image can represent the enclosing and exclusive boundaries that surround social categories. Those who dwell in spaces outside these categories can be said to occupy spaces in between. Dawn explains how leading a double life and living in a liminal space involve psychological division, which can lead to negative effects on her health:

> The whole sense of being between two worlds ... I find for myself that it's something that I deal with every single day ... I think that for me that's probably the single most important thing that I have to deal with, and it affects a number of areas in my life that ultimately affect my health ... just being psychologically divided, and how do we negotiate that ... By virtue of being racialized, you're going to experience that psychologically, and it has

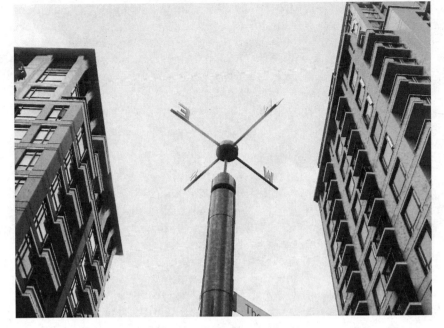

Figure 7.3   **Compass in the Sky**
Source: Dawn, age twenty-four.

implications on our health. Like, most obviously mental health, but there's also social health, and then, and in some senses, our relationships as well.

She elaborates: "If, say, my mom and I are not doing so good, I tend to feel down and, like, confused and sad and kind of helpless as to what to do, and I tend to not feel very good about myself." Dawn's transnational, diasporic, and culturally hybrid background has shaped her shifting identity, leading to intergenerational tensions and conflicts within her family. Although manifestations of these tensions were most outwardly expressed through a conflictive relationship with her mother, Dawn was empathetic regarding the situation, understanding that her mother had primary responsibility for parenting while her father lived in the Philippines. She acknowledged that the tensions between them stemmed from the interconnecting pressures brought forth by forces of migration, family and cultural values, social expectations from the different communities of which they had become a part, her parents' gendered and ethnicized ideals and values, the dominant society's gendered and raced norms, and the racisms and oppressions that she faced on a day-to-day basis. These intersecting realities are much more complex and global than processes that are commonly analyzed at the intersections of race, class, and gender.

The in-between space that Dawn speaks about highlights the need for frameworks that can validate the lived experiences of those who may not fit neatly inside socially constructed categories. Such lived experiences are historically and locationally specific and emergent. Hence, they cannot be fully comprehended at the level of theory. In order to understand the lives of individuals and groups whose mobility and diaspora bring them into contact with scattered hegemonies, both theory and empirical research are needed.

Finding Balance

Collins (2009) has suggested that racialized women's sexuality requires deeper theorization. She sees the troubles and pain that black women experience regarding their sexuality as having to do with negotiating states of rejection and abjection of black peoples. The narratives of many of the women in our study who were involved in relationships with men from the dominant culture reveal the accuracy of this observation. Mixed-race heterosexual love relationships were the source of much frustration and tension among our co-researchers (Ifekwunigwe 2004). As mentioned above, these are not simply interpersonal relationship problems having to do with sexuality as separate from other markers of difference. For racialized minority women, sexuality and intimacy in personal relationships are also linked to and mediated by structural marginalizations based on multiple dimensions of oppression. Furthermore, transnational racialized women's needs for closeness, acceptance, and intimacy are also intertwined with negotiations within culturally hybrid and diasporic spaces, which contribute another dimension of the inclusion/exclusion matrix.

Rebecca's photo (Figure 7.4) and accompanying narrative address these issues:

> The photo of the videos, to me, represents taking time for self-care. The stresses of academic life tend to throw my life out of balance. As a result I forget about me. A very important part of my life is my involvement with the Aboriginal community, on campus and off campus ... The creative self was hiding and now I am finally exploring my creativity ... I had a previous relationship where my partner did not want to accept that I was Métis and an artist. This had a negative impact on my health. I internalized everything and forgot to take care of myself. My life was out of balance and now I'm trying to find that balance. The image is blurred because sometimes I feel like I am living a dream. I am finally waking up from a deep sleep.

Rebecca affirms that not being fully accepted as a Métis and an artist by her ex-partner took a toll on her health and well-being. She found herself unable to have a relationship with someone who would not allow her to express

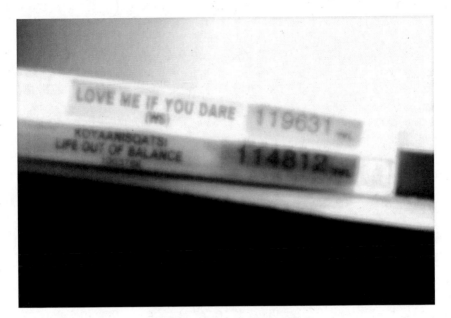

Figure 7.4 **Love Me If You Dare**
Source: Rebecca, age twenty-seven.

all sides of herself. The prolonged suppression of her identities brought to a conscious level the issues that she had subconsciously struggled with throughout her life. Her eventual break-up with her boyfriend became a conscious act that brought to the forefront the realities of living within a history of colonization. She began to acknowledge the generations of alcoholism in her family, abuse, and low self-esteem that, until this point, had been buried in shame. She uses the words "waking up" and "finding balance" to describe her process of coming to consciousness – a concept that Paulo Freire (1970) associates with becoming liberated through activism and serious reflection.

Rebecca's narrative exemplifies the compartmentalization of multiple and contradictory selves, and its ensuing emotional and psychological stresses. The tendency to keep certain parts of her life and identities separate and unintegrated is a demand created by the dominant culture, and this eventually took a toll on Rebecca's mental and emotional health. Behavioural health models that suggest that individuals simply need to make "good choices" to achieve health and well-being fail to consider how societal norms and expectations mediate paths that are available to different individuals.

The pain of living "in between" is not a result of personal or interpersonal inadequacies but a legacy of cultural subordination. Living under intersecting structures of domination, racialized women can pretend only for so long to be what they are not for the sake of others. These young women may be conditioned to hide parts of their racial and ethnic identities from others and from themselves so as not to raise discomfort and conflict. Often motivated by a fear of powerlessness, they paradoxically hide their differences (if they can) in order to be accepted by the mainstream, while simultaneously desiring acceptance of their differences.

Rebecca's story poignantly demonstrates an internal struggle that many mixed-race and racialized women encounter in their relationships with men and women from the dominant culture who "just don't get it." Their partners often unfairly ask them to deny their double consciousness and multiple selves – to be more like them, to separate from the racialized part of themselves, or to split themselves in two – impossible tasks when multiple identities overlap and intertwine. These demands are extremely stressful, and ultimately, as Rebecca states, "it had a negative impact on my health. I internalized everything and forgot to take care of myself."

Conclusion

The stories and photos shared by these young women offer empirical evidence for rethinking conceptualizations of health, social exclusion, and intersectionality in the context of multiple migrations and national belongings. Self-narrations highlight the importance of theorizing the health and well-being of racialized minority women through frameworks that acknowledge multi-levelled, multi-layered interconnectedness (Nash 2008). As shown in participants' images and texts, the shifting historical and cultural contexts through which unstable social identities of otherness are constituted must not be reduced to economic factors, as is often the case in Canadian discourses of social exclusion and social determinants of health (Galabuzi 2004; Shaw, Dorling, and Smith 2006).

Moreover, alternative metaphors for intersectionality are needed. Treating race, gender, sexuality, and class as social variables that intersect in a linear fashion does not address the complexity and mutability of these structural forces in racialized women's diverse lives. The stories and photos that co-researchers generated help reveal how macro-social structures such as nation, culture, and borders, among others, have diverse, generative, layered, co-constitutive, and interactive effects on the personal intimate aspects of their everyday lives. They suggest a need to integrate transnational mobility, citizenship status, multiple and shifting belongings and non-belongings to national and diasporic communities, cultural hybridity, translocational positionality, and relationality into intersectional analyses of women's health (Brah 1996; Mohanty 2003; Anthias 2006, 2008).

Finally, the stories and photos that we share in this chapter represent women who have found and created spaces for healing – women who are not yet totally confined, disciplined, and constrained by social power. The "in between" can be understood as a contingent site for marginality and creative possibility, and a place of imagined well-being. The narratives contribute to mounting evidence concerning the limitations of mainstream conceptualizations and methodologies used to comprehend health inequalities and inequities in Canada (Reimer-Kirkham 2003; Anderson 2006; Grove and Zwi 2006).

Notes

1 We use the term "co-researchers" to describe our study participants because they documented their own lives, critically reflected on their images, and identified and selected themes for analysis. However, they are not listed as co-authors, because they were not involved in the transformation of their stories using the theoretical concepts that underpin this chapter.
2 The research was primarily undertaken by Alison as part of her master's research study. She was a member of antidote, and her lived experiences informed this study.

References

Anderson, J.M. 2002. Toward a post-colonial feminist methodology in nursing research: Exploring the convergence of post-colonial and black feminist scholarship. *Nurse Researcher* 9(3): 7-27.
–. 2006. Reflections on the social determinants of women's health. Exploring intersections: Does racialization matter? *Canadian Journal of Nursing Research* 38(1): 7-14.
Anderson, J.M., and S. Reimer-Kirkham. 1998. Constructing nation: The gendering and racializing of the Canadian health care system. In *Painting the maple: Essays on race, gender, and the construction of Canada,* ed. V. Strong-Boag, S. Grace, A. Eisenberg, and J. Anderson, 242-61. Vancouver: UBC Press.
Anthias, F. 2006. Belongings in a globalising and unequal world: Rethinking translocations. In *The situated politics of belonging,* ed. N. Yuval-Davis, K. Kannabiran, and U. Vieten, 17-31. London: Sage.
–. 2008. Thinking through the lens of translocational positionality: An intersectionality frame for understanding identity and belonging. *Translocations* 4(1): 5-20.
Beck, U. 2002. The cosmopolitan society and its enemies. *Theory, Culture and Society* 19(1-2): 17-44.
Brah, A. 1996. *Cartographies of diaspora: Contesting identities.* London: Routledge.
Brah, A., and A. Phoenix. 2004. Ain't I a woman? Revisiting intersectionality. *Journal of International Women's Studies* 5(3): 75-83.
Browne, A.J., V.L. Smye, and C. Varcoe. 2007. Postcolonial-feminist theoretical perspectives and women's health. In *Women's health in Canada: Critical perspectives on theory and policy,* ed. M. Morrow, O. Hankivsky, and C. Varcoe, 124-42. Toronto: University of Toronto Press.
Collins, P.H. 2009. *Black feminist thought: Knowledge, consciousness and the politics of empowerment.* 2nd ed. New York: Routledge Classics.
Dossa, P. 2004. *Politics and poetics of migration: Narratives of Iranian women from the diaspora.* Toronto: Canadian Scholars' Press.
Freire, P. 1970. *Pedagogy of the oppressed.* Trans. M.B. Ramos. New York: Continuum.
Galabuzi, G.-E. 2004. Social exclusion. In *Social determinants of health: Canadian perspectives,* ed. D. Raphael, 235-52. Toronto: Canadian Scholars' Press.
Gramsci, A. 1971. *Selections from the prison notebooks.* Ed. and trans. Q. Hoare and G. Nowell Smith. London: Lawrence and Wishart.
Grewal, I., and C. Kaplan. 1994. *Scattered hegemonies: Postmodernity and transnational feminist practices.* Minneapolis: University of Minnesota Press.
Grove, N.J., and A. Zwi. 2006. Our health and theirs: Forced migration, othering and public health. *Social Science and Medicine* 62(8): 1931-42.
Hall, S. 1994. Cultural identity and diaspora. In *Colonial discourse and post-colonial theory,* ed. P. Williams and L. Chrisman, 392-403. New York: Columbia University Press.

Handa, A. 2003. *Of silk saris and mini-skirts: South Asian girls walk the tightrope of culture.* Toronto: Women's Press.

Harding, A.S., ed. 2005. *Surviving in the hour of darkness: The health and wellness of women of colour.* Calgary: University of Calgary Press.

Ifekwunigwe, J., ed. 2004. *Mixed race studies.* London: Routledge.

Jiwani, Y. 2001. *Intersecting inequalities: Immigrant women of colour, violence and health care.* Vancouver: FREDA Centre for Research on Violence against Women and Children. http://www.vancouver.sfu.ca.

Lee, J. 2006. Locality, participatory action research, and racialized girls struggle for citizenship. In *Girlhood: Redefining the limits,* ed. Y. Jiwani, C. Mitchell, and C. Steenbergen, 89-108. Montreal: Black Rose Books.

Lee, J., and L. Cardinal. 1998. Hegemonic nationalism and the politics of multiculturalism and feminism in Canada. In *Painting the maple: Essays on race and gender in Canada,* ed. V. Strong-Boag, S. Grace, A. Eisenberg, and J. Anderson, 215-41. Vancouver: UBC Press.

Lee, J., and S. de Finney. 2005. Using popular theatre for engaging racialized minority girls in exploring questions of identity and belonging. In *Working relationally with girls: Complex lives/complex identities,* ed. M. Hoskins and S. Artz, 95-118. Toronto: Haworth Press.

McLintock, A. 1993. *Imperial leather: Race, gender and sexuality in the colonial context.* London and New York: Routledge.

Mohanty, C.T. 2003. *Feminism without borders: Decolonizing theory, practicing solidarity.* Durham, NC: Duke University Press.

Mullings, L., and A.J. Schulz. 2006. Intersectionality and health: An introduction. In *Gender, race, class and health: Intersectional approaches,* ed. A.J. Schulz and L. Mullings, 3-17. San Francisco: Jossey-Bass.

Nash, J.C. 2008. Rethinking intersectionality. *Feminist Review* 89: 1-15.

Ong, A. 2003. *Buddha is hiding: Refugees, citizenship, the new America.* Los Angeles: University of California Press.

Phinney, J.S., A. Ong, and T. Madden. 2000. Cultural values and intergenerational value discrepancies in immigrant and non-immigrant families. *Child Development* 71(2): 528-39.

Prazniak, R., and A. Dirlik. 2001. *Places and politics in an age of globalization.* Oxford and New York: Rowan and Littlefield.

Rattansi, A. 1992. Changing the subject? Racism, culture and education. In *Race, culture and difference,* ed. J. Donald and A. Rattansi, 11-48. London: Sage.

Reid, C. 2002. *A full measure: Towards a comprehensive model for the measurement of women's health.* Vancouver: British Columbia Centre of Excellence for Women's Health.

Reimer-Kirkham, S. 2003. The politics of belonging and intercultural health care. *Western Journal of Nursing Research* 25(7): 762-80.

Reimer-Kirkham, S., and J. Anderson. 2002. Postcolonial nursing scholarship: From epistemology to method. *Advances in Nursing Science* 25(1): 1-17.

Said, E. 1979. *Orientalism.* London: Vintage.

Salant, T., and D.S. Lauderdale. 2002. Measuring culture: A critical review of acculturation and health in Asian immigrant populations. *Social Science and Medicine* 57(1): 71-90.

Shaw, M., D. Dorling, and H.D. Smith. 2006. Poverty, social exclusion, and minorities. In *Social determinants of health,* ed. M. Marmot and R.G. Wilkinson, 196-223. New York: Oxford University Press.

Smith, L.T. 1999. *Decolonizing methodologies: Research and indigenous peoples.* London: Zed Books.

Spivak, G.C. 1987. *In other worlds: Essays in cultural politics.* New York: Methuen.

Stasiulis, D., and A.B. Bakan. 1997. Negotiating citizenship: The case of foreign domestic workers in Canada. *Feminist Review* 57: 112-39.

Varcoe, C., O. Hankivsky, and M. Morrow. 2007. Introduction: Beyond gender matters. In *Women's health in Canada: Critical perspectives on theory and policy,* ed. M. Morrow, O. Hankivsky, and C. Varcoe, 3-30. Toronto: University of Toronto Press.

Verloo, M. 2006. Multiple inequalities, intersectionality and the European Union. *European Journal of Women's Studies* 13(3): 211-28.

Wang, C.C. 1999. Photovoice: A participatory action research strategy applied to women's health. *Journal of Women's Health* 8(2): 185-92.

Werbner, P., and T. Modood, eds. 1997. *Debating cultural hybridity: Multicultural identities and the politics of anti-racism.* London: Zed Books.

Westwood, S., and A. Phizacklea. 2000. *Trans-nationalism and the politics of belonging.* London: Routledge.

Wimmer, A., and N.G. Schiller. 2003. Methodological nationalism, the social sciences, and the study of migration. An essay in historical epistemology. *International Migration Review* 37(3): 576-610.

Women's Health in Women's Hands Community Health Centre. 2003. *Racial discrimination as a health risk for female youth: Implications for policy and healthcare delivery in Canada.* Toronto: Canadian Race Relations Foundation. http://www.whiwh.com/Research/ ePub_RacialDiscrimination.pdf.

Yuval-Davis, N. 2006. Intersectionality and feminist politics. *European Journal of Women's Studies* 13(3): 193-209.

Zhou, M., and Y.S. Xiong. 2005. The multifaceted American experiences of the children of Asian immigrants: Lessons for segmented assimilation. *Ethnic and Racial Studies* 28(6): 1119-52.

8

An Intersectional Understanding of Youth Cultural Identities and Psychosocial Integration: Why It Matters to Mental Health Promotion in Immigrant-Receiving Pluralistic Societies

Nazilla Khanlou and Tahira Gonsalves

The integration of immigrants is gaining increasing attention around the world, with growing numbers of migrants moving to Western countries. Despite varying levels of integration among immigrants, it is generally expected that their children (the second generation) will be more deeply and effectively integrated into the "host" society. Although this model of linear assimilation or integration might apply in some cases, it is not necessarily the reality for all immigrant or second-generation youth in Western countries today. For these youth, their particular life stage, gender, racialized status, and their or their parents' immigrant status create unique sets of intersections.

This chapter will focus on the psychosocial integration of immigrant and second-generation youth into Western, and particularly Canadian, society. Psychosocial integration is influenced by both identity formation of youth at the individual psychological level, as well as by such factors as migrant status and racialization at the societal level. The broader socio-political context also affects changes in identity, as when racialized youth are "othered" in the post-9/11 context, for example. We will argue that using an intersectional approach in understanding youth cultural identities and psychosocial integration matters in re-visioning youth mental health promotion in immigrant-receiving pluralistic societies.

As definitions of terms can vary across disciplines, we define what we mean by the terms "second generation," "host country," "gender," and "racialization." We will also define our understanding of the term "intersectionality" and provide definitions for cultural identity, psychosocial integration, mental health, and mental health promotion in later sections of the chapter.

The second generation is usually considered to consist of the offspring of one or both parents born outside of the host country. However, we recognize that definitions can differ across countries and studies. Above, we have used the term "host country," but we recognize that it is a problematic term, which may indicate that members of the second generation are forever "guests" in the country of their birth (Kobayashi 2008, 4). Gender is a social construction and an identity marker that fundamentally intersects with youth's other identities. We use the term "racialization" to signal a process by which so-called visible minority groups are set apart and often discriminated against on the basis of their skin colour or other markers that are thought to differentiate them from the white European middle-class mainstream of Canada.

Why Intersectionality?

Intersectionality as a theoretical framework emerged through the work of second-wave feminists, when women of colour challenged mainstream feminism and its domination by white, educated, and middle-class women. Intersectionality emphasized the importance of race as a salient aspect of identity, and proponents argued that mainstream feminism did not speak for women of colour (see Shields 2008). Given its origins, much of the work on intersectionality has tended to focus on women and specifically women of colour. The term "women of colour" is at times contested by those to whom it is applied, recognizing that all humans have colour and that the term may further marginalize groups.

Due to its cross-disciplinary appeal, intersectionality can also encompass many different approaches. For instance, Floya Anthias (2008, 5) applies the term "translocational positionality" to intersectionality and describes it as "an intersectional frame [that] moves away from the idea of given 'groups' or 'categories' of gender, ethnicity and class, which then intersect ... and instead pays much more attention to *social locations and processes* which are broader than those signaled by this" (emphasis in original). She further problematizes the tendency in academic scholarship to treat "identity as a possessive attribute of individuals and groups," but she argues that her frame "also avoids the rabid deconstructionism of some post-modern approaches to belonging and identity" (ibid., 5-6). In another example, Michelle Fine and Selcuk R. Sirin (2007, 31) use what they term a "hyphenated selves" framework, which they argue "is a radical departure from 'fixed,' and in most cases dichotomous notions of identity that favor 'group comparisons' in favor of more fluid and contextual, hybrid notions of identity."

Although these two approaches problematize the very notion of fixed categories of gender, ethnicity, and class, policy documents and organizational approaches to intersectionality tend to treat these categories in more stable ways. The United Nations uses an intersectional approach to discussing discrimination and outlines it as follows: "An intersectional approach to analyzing the disempowerment of marginalized women attempts to capture the consequences of the interaction between two or more forms of subordination. It addresses the manner in which racism, patriarchy, class oppression and other discriminatory systems create inequalities that structure the relative positions of women, races, ethnicities, classes, and the like. Moreover, intersectionality addresses the way that specific acts and policies operate together to create further disempowerment" (Working Group on Women and Human Rights no date).

It is important to factor gender into any analysis, as has been attempted by departments within the Canadian government through such practices as gender-based analysis (GBA). However, simply differentiating between genders may not capture their "complexity and interaction with other determinants" (Hankivsky and Christoffersen 2008, 273). It is not enough to understand how men and women differ but how they differ in relational terms. Gender as a category also assumes certain standards or norms from which those who "deviate" are excluded. The norm is usually that of the white middle-class heterosexual man or woman (ibid.; Guthrie and Low 2006, 10).

However, gender itself is a socially constructed category and cannot be assumed to be fixed and stable across cultural groups or life stages. In fact, there is nothing particularly innate about gender or culture, and interrogating the constituent parts of any of these categories requires a relational analysis of them. Precisely because intersectionality examines how multiple identity markers of an individual interact, it allows for an analysis of how gender is also cultured (Allen 1996, 98). As Ramaswami Mahalingam, Sundari Balan, and Jana Haritatos (2008, 328, 332) point out in their "idealized cultural identities" model, idealized patriarchal beliefs around femininity and masculinity are often used as boosters of ethnic pride. For instance, many women in the Asian communities they studied took pride in patriarchal identity constructions, as these were a symbol of their cultural integrity and in opposition to "western values." Intersectionality thus permits a critical gender analysis without prejudging cultural practices through particular feminist lenses.

A relational understanding, which unpacks the assumed stability of categories, may be possible in theory, but when research is conducted on the ground, theoretical abstractions may be difficult to sustain. Research may begin with assumptions of stable identity categories, as in the case of adolescent second-generation racialized youth, but throughout the research process (especially the emergent process embedded in qualitative research), participants frame their identities in language that makes sense to them. Barbara J. Guthrie and Lisa Kane Low (2006, 8) contend that the best way to understand the health history of adolescents is to ask *them* questions. These self-definitions show the fluidity and dynamicity of categories. In this chapter, we draw from two studies with female and male youth to explicate our argument.

Study 1, titled "Immigrant Youth and Cultural Identity in a Global Context" (Khanlou, Siemiatycki, and Anisef 2003-6), examined cultural identity, self-esteem, and migration experiences of youth. Participants came from four cultural groups, including those from both traditional and new source countries of migration to Canada. A prospective comparative longitudinal design was applied, and quantitative and qualitative methods were utilized to collect data. The sample of forty-five participants consisted of English-speaking female and male youth who were immigrants or descendants of immigrants and were between the ages of seventeen and twenty-two. Traditional immigration source countries included Italy (eleven participants) and Portugal (eight youth). Recent immigration source countries included Afghanistan (nine youth) and Iran (seventeen youth). (For further details, see Khanlou 2008; Khanlou, Koh, and Mill 2008.)

Study 2, titled "Mental Health Services for Newcomer Youth: Exploring Needs and Enhancing Access," focused on newcomer female and male youth (those who had arrived in Canada within the last five years and who were between the ages of fourteen and eighteen) from Afghan, Colombian, Sudanese, and Tamil communities (Khanlou, Shakya, and Muntaner 2007-9). A mixed-method participatory research approach, which included qualitative and quantitative methods, was utilized. Data were collected through six focus groups and six interviews with youth from the above communities, one focus group and five interviews with service providers who serve these communities, and five interviews with parents from these communities. Fifty-six questionnaires were also administered to youth.

Youth Identities and Psychosocial Integration
According to Katherine Rossiter and Marina Morrow (see Chapter 16 this volume), age is among the excluded categories in intersectional scholarship (the others are sexual orientation, gender identity, and physical disability). We also add that though various disciplinary approaches have been used to understand intersections of identity markers such as gender, race, and class, little work exists on these markers with reference to migrant status and life stage. Whether an individual is a new immigrant, older immigrant, refugee, or without legal papers (precarious status) also affects her/his particular engagement with other individuals and with society. The layers of intersectionality are complexified even further when identity markers of gender, race, class, and migrant status are juxtaposed with a particular life stage of an individual, such as adolescence.

Youth Cultural Identities
Adolescence marks an important stage of identity development, and for immigrant and second-generation youth, cultural identity may become an

important part of their overall identity development. Cultural identity "refers to a complex set of beliefs and attitudes that people have about themselves in relation to their cultural group membership," and these come to the fore when people are in regular contact with others who do not belong to their cultural group (Berry 2001, 620). John W. Berry (ibid.) also discusses cultural identity as "a parallel approach to understanding acculturation strategies" used by immigrants. Acculturation is defined as "a process that entails contact between two cultural groups, which results in numerous cultural changes in both parties" (Redfield, Linton, and Herskovits 1936, quoted in ibid., 616).

Scholars have made further distinctions around cultural identity. For instance, Berry (ibid.) divides cultural identity into identification with one's own heritage (which others have referred to as ethnic identity) and identification with the majority or dominant group in society (which has been referred to as civic identity). In a study of Turkish adolescents in Norway and Sweden, Erkki Virta, David L. Sam, and Charles Westin (2004) highlight identity as one of the important factors in the adaptation process. They further divide identity into ethnic minority and majority identities.

Different groups of youth have varied aspects of identity that they regard as salient in their lives. For example, for certain racialized groups (such as blacks), racial identity tends to be more salient than cultural identity because of the visibility of markers of difference (skin colour) and the exclusions and barriers that result from it. Although cultural identity is also significant for some groups (including blacks), the extent to which certain racialized groups are able to integrate will depend more on visible signifiers than on cultural ones.

For immigrant and second-generation youth, self-identified markers of identity depend in part on the host country context. Given that cultural identity becomes prominent in the presence of those who are culturally different, identity and cultural identity must be contextually understood in a globalized world (Khanlou 2007). Cultural identity, as a particular part of identity, emerges "through living in a multicultural context as a member of a major or a minor group ... through daily contact with other cultures, [and through awareness] of the cultural component of the self" (Khanlou 2005, 12). Individual identities are thus formed in relation to the social context and may perform a protective function whereby individuals can feel a sense of belonging to both their own culture and the mainstream culture. For example, in Study 1, cultural identity emerged as a central theme for the Afghan youth across the focus groups, interviews, and self-journal writings. The Afghan youth were aware of their identity as "Afghans," as "teens," as "Muslims," and as newcomers to Canada in the process of adjusting to a new culture. They were aware of the complexities of cultural identity that include the influences of family and parents, religion, personal responsibility, and experiences of ethnocultural discrimination and stereotypes. They were also aware of the contextual and temporal nature of identity, and for a few participants, the notion of a dual or hybrid Afghan Canadian identity was revealed.

Identity construction in the post-9/11 context for Muslim first- and second-generation youth is an important example, as it demonstrates that this is a fluid and context-bound process, which is also historically and structurally situated (Khanlou 2008; CRIAW 2006). The process continually influenced by global political and economic events, as they mutate over time. Despite prevailing stereotypical images of fixed identities, youth in Canada move quite comfortably between self-definitions that are based on cultural, ancestral, national, hyphenated, racial, and/or migrant identities (Khanlou and Crawford 2006; Khanlou, Koh, and Mill 2008).

Again, as Study 1 revealed, it is important to note that not all participants embraced the concept of cultural identity. Within the Afghan, Iranian, and Portuguese groups, some participants questioned the notion of cultural identity. For example, one of them (an Afghan female) rejected the label of cultural identity as she felt it was too confining and irrelevant since no one can choose his or her birthplace. For this participant, the label of identity created barriers, invoking notions of "difference," and she felt that she could not "reduce" herself to one identity label (Afghan female participant, journal entry). She questioned what can be defined as Afghan identity since so much cultural diversity exists within the country. With rapid migration of Afghans around the world, she argued that Afghan identity is continually changing as it is mixed with other cultural milieus. Her articulation of cultural identity, or resistance to an ascribed one-dimensional cultural identity, underscores the relevance of an intersectional, multi-dimensional understanding of identity and the fluidity embedded in it.

In their study with Muslim American youth, post-9/11, Fine and Sirin (2007) also discuss how subjectivities are created within politically and culturally difficult contexts. They propose a conceptual theoretical framework of the "hyphenated self," which is based on their research with over two hundred young Muslims from varied origins in the US. As they put it, the hyphen is "theorized as a dynamic social-psychological space where political arrangements and individual subjectivities meet." Fine and Sirin (ibid., 21) explain that "the psychological texture of the hyphen is substantially informed by history, media, surveillance, politics, nation of origin, gender, biography, longings, imagination, and loss – whether young people know/ speak this or not."

In Study 2, we interviewed both youth and parents. During one interview, an adolescent spoke of his struggle with being stereotyped and his challenges to that stereotype: "When I first came here, everyone was making jokes about Afghanistan and terrorists. So every time I told them I was Afghan, they'd ask me if I was a terrorist. So, like, that really hurt. So after that, every time people would ask me questions like that, I'd start asking them questions. So if they'd ask me if I was a terrorist, I'd say, 'Do you see a bomb on me?'" (Afghan male participant, interview).

In diverse cities such as Toronto, newcomers respond favourably to the multiculturalism they encounter but can also struggle with their own and other's preconceptions. During an interview, a Colombian mother from a fairly homogeneous home culture discussed her attempts to become comfortable with the diversity she saw in Toronto: "The different conceptions or misconceptions that we have regarding – for example ... about the colour, about the smells and about the cultural costumes and even the difference in dress and difference in appearance. And it's difficult ... that's why maybe racism comes more strong. We grow up with [these] conceptions" (Colombian mother, talking about diversity in Canada, interview).

Psychosocial Integration
In psychosocial research, integration has been discussed under the terms "acculturation," "assimilation," "settlement," and "adaptation." The latter two generally refer to the initial stages of adjustment to a new country but do not necessarily capture the more layered and longer process of integration. Whereas acculturation considers the longer and complex process of integration, there also tends to be "embedded in it the notion that the acculturating individuals, or groups, acquire the mainstream culture and, at the same time, lose some level of their original cultural identity" (Khanlou 2005, 13). The term "assimilation" tends to imply a process, whereby immigrants are expected to embrace the dominant cultural and national identities of the host country.

There are other models of integration (bidimensional or transcultural) that do not assume that identification with and adaptation to a particular culture indicates a loss of the original cultural identification (Khanlou 2005). The acculturation model of John W. Berry et al. (1989, 188) includes integration as one of the four modes of acculturation, and integration here "implies the maintenance of the cultural integrity of the group, as well as the movement by the group to become an integral part of a larger societal framework." There may not be a "best" way to acculturate, but evidence suggests that "double cultural involvement (in both one's heritage cultures and the society of settlement) is the most positive strategy" for how well someone can adapt to the new society (Berry 2008, 50). An orthogonal model (Salant and Lauderdale 2003; Oetting and Beauvais 1991) similarly allows for multiple and complex modes of cultural identification that are also fluid.

In recent years, debate around the integration of racialized immigrants into Western countries has tended to be influenced by stereotypical constructions of "unassimilable others" and monolithic notions of various Western national identities (see Kobayashi 2008). Since they are often seen as a cultural bridge between their parents and the host society, second-generation youth are "a prime locus for understanding the complexities of multicultural society" (ibid., 3). The second generation is expected to adapt and integrate as well as those whose families have a long history in the country.

In Study 1, unlike the Afghan and Iranian youth, the Italian and Portuguese participants discussed experiences of discrimination primarily in terms of anecdotal and historical evidence from their parents and relatives who had previously migrated to and settled in Canada (except for one who was born in Portugal, the Italian and Portuguese participants were all born in Canada).[1] For example, a female participant of Italian background noted that the "[first Italian immigrants] were more segregated only because even with my mom, when she says we were considered WOPS, people, you know everybody thought we smelled" (interview).

As the youth reflected on discriminatory experiences, they often appeared to rationalize them. In an interview, one participant from an Italian background reported that many Italian immigrants changed their names as a way to hide their Italian identity. Although he explained this phenomenon as a clear result of discrimination – "A lot of them changed their name when they came here because no one would hire someone with an Italian last name" (interview) – he did not seem to reflect on this as a troubling concern for cultural identity. He appeared to rationalize the need to hide their identity by changing their names because "they came half way around the world to change their life. They will change their name for sure ... I don't think a name is that important to who you are. I think you can still remember your roots if you had a different name."

The above interpretation by youth from Italian backgrounds may be partially due to the successful cultural, economic, and political integration of Italian descendents in Canada and the United States (Khanlou 2008). Notably, in the same study, youth from a Portuguese background spoke about the lack of educational integration of many of their Canadian Portuguese peers and, as a result, a sense of marginalization from mainstream Canadian society (ibid.).

As the following quote from Study 2 indicates, for immigrant youth the effects of racism can be particularly dire, given that they may already feel excluded in other ways from mainstream society: "When I go to school I wear the bindi and I braid my hair ... So most people look at me weirdly wearing a bindi and going to school braided ... One of my grade six teachers ... told me, 'Who does the braids for you?' And I told him, 'My mom.' He told me 'When you're coming to school, wear your braids. And when you're in school, take them off and be Canadian, and after school, braid it back so your mom won't find out'" (Tamil female participant, focus group).

For racialized second-generation youth who are often negotiating two or more identities, that of their parents and that of the majority community in their host country, experiences of racism may also affect their identity and integration. Further, global political events may produce a sense of transnational belonging and affiliations for them. The notion of a pan-identity and transnational belonging is seen in the following quote from Study 2: "I see myself as first Ismaili because it's bigger than Afghan, because it's the whole world: Ismailis are spread everywhere, where Afghans are only in Afghanistan. So I see myself first as my religion, then where I'm from" (Afghan female participant, interview).

More research is required that compares the experiences of second- and subsequent-generation Canadian youth from racialized backgrounds to those who are not racialized and to those of immigrant youth.

Revisioning Youth Mental Health Promotion: Cultural Identity and Psychosocial Integration Matter

Cultural identity and psychosocial integration matter to youth mental health promotion in pluralistic societies. When a broad and inclusive perspective is taken toward enhancing the mental health and well-being of diverse populations, opportunities to promote mental well-being are not confined to one service sector or one disciplinary approach. Multidisciplinary understandings of mental well-being become paramount as do efforts directed at multiple levels, including individuals, their families, their communities, and society at large. Practice and policy recommendations arising from intersectional analysis and interpretation become more reflective of diverse needs under this approach.

The role of cultural identity in mental health is gaining attention beyond academic venues. In *Toward Recovery and Well-Being: A Framework for a Mental Health Strategy for Canada*, put forth by the Mental Health Commission of Canada (2009, 13), cultural identity was recognized as a "potential source of resilience, meaning and value." We have defined cultural identity above, and here it is useful to describe what we mean by "mental health." We draw from the World Health Organization's (WHO 2007) definition, which considers mental health as "a state of wellbeing in which the individual realizes his or her own abilities, can cope with the normal stresses of life, can work productively and fruitfully, and is able to make a contribution to his or her community."

The WHO (ibid.) further argues that, without mental health, there is no health. Mental health promotion (MHP), in turn, is "the process of enhancing the capacity of individuals and communities to take control over their lives and improve their mental health. [MHP] uses strategies that foster supportive environments and individual resilience, while showing respect for culture, equity, social justice, interconnections and personal dignity" (Centre for Health Promotion 1997 as cited in Willinsky and Pape 1997, 3). This definition of MHP aligns well with an intersectional approach to understanding the factors and processes that promote or challenge the mental well-being of individuals and communities.

Overall mental well-being is buttressed by self-esteem, which is the evaluative part of a person's self-concept, or the sense of his or her self-worth (Khanlou 2004). Good self-esteem supports resiliency, and this is associated with other positive mental health outcomes and patterns of health behaviour among youth (see ibid.; Khanlou and Crawford 2006; Virta, Sam, and Westin 2004). The concept of resilience has the underlying recognition of the presence of adaptation and coping in response to risk, adversity, and challenges of life (see Barankin and Khanlou 2007). When a systems approach is applied, individual, familial, and social environmental factors promote youth resilience (ibid.). These factors do not operate in isolation from one another, and an intersectional lens allows for a better understanding of their interactions.

Studies that look at racialized immigrant populations tend to consider the lack of successful integration due to economic circumstances, barriers to employment, and discrimination, among others. Often, the resiliency and resourcefulness demonstrated by many immigrants are not fully considered. Where the second generation is successfully integrated, as measured by broader economic and social indicators, their own resiliency or that of their immigrant parents may not be accorded a due share of credit.

Mental health promotion models and approaches grounded in majority-culture-based research may be limited in that they do not necessarily take into account multiple cultural, linguistic, and systemic barriers to maintaining and promoting health in the post-migration and resettlement context. Understanding, developing, and implementing culturally sensitive MHP principles and strategies offers important opportunities for enhancing the mental well-being of diverse segments of society.

An intersectional approach to MHP can assist in connecting existing Western clinical psychological perspectives, where the focus tends to be placed on an individual's own ability to develop good self-esteem and a positive sense of self (James and Prilleltensky 2002; Fernando 2003), to other ways of understanding the self and its connection to mental well-being. Among various immigrant communities in Western immigrant-receiving contexts, the sense of self is often deeply embedded within the collective, and self-esteem depends in large part on the societal or collective evaluation of the individual. This is not to say that there are binary distinctions between "Eastern" and "Western" values but that loose patterns can be found that correspond to the culturally embedded nature of self-understanding and being in the world.

Cultural sensitivity or competency refers to attitudes and policy decisions that evolve within a particular system and facilitate thereby an understanding of how to work in multicultural or cross-cultural circumstances (Cross et al. 1989). Earlier notions of cultural competence were restricted to focusing on cultural differences at the individual level and their implications for clinical practice. Such approaches have been criticized for not considering multiple oppressions faced by non-mainstream groups and implications for health disparities at group and community levels. More recent approaches to cultural competence recognize the influence of power in clinical cultural competence. For example, Rani Srivastava (2007, 58) proposes a culture care framework and considers the overlap between cultural sensitivity, cultural knowledge, and cultural resources in providing culturally congruent care. Cultural sensitivity requires understanding the concept of culture and one's own culture, "including values, biases, and prejudices," as well as "understanding the dynamics of difference and relationships."

Proponents of cultural competency approaches in health care and proponents of anti-oppression practice in the community often find themselves disagreeing (at times even refusing to dialogue with one another) due to differences in underlying beliefs and models. However, we argue that, in mental health promotion practice with diverse populations, practitioners would benefit from an understanding and application of both: cultural competence to best address the strengths and challenges of individuals/families within the practice context, and anti-oppression approaches to recognize the social and systemic contexts of mental well-being, and advocacy for best policies to address health disparities.[2] We also recognize that cultural competence models need to integrate a gender-sensitive approach in addressing competent care. To this end, application of intersectional approaches would be of particular benefit in providing care that recognizes differences without stereotyping them.

Combining our knowledge from cultural competency and anti-oppression practice would allow for best practices and policies that recognize that health disparities experienced at the individual level are intimately connected to such social determinants of health as class, gender, and racialized and migrant status, and need to be contextualized within an analysis of prevailing systems. Understanding these intersections allows for the recognition that certain groups of individuals are often multiply marginalized: having one factor of marginality – such as a disability, for instance – can indicate the existence of other factors such as poverty, compromised health, and poor housing.

Conclusion
This chapter began by discussing youth identities and psychosocial integration in pluralistic and immigrant-receiving settings and ended by making suggestions for mental health promotion, referring to cultural competence and anti-oppression practice. Although at first glance the two topics may seem remotely related, we argue that mental health promotion scholarship,

practice, and policy can benefit from recognizing the importance of both. Being able to successfully negotiate the intersections of identities is important for the mental health and well-being of immigrants and their children. A particularly useful approach to link the two and address health disparities is the application of an intersectional lens.

Disciplinary approaches to understanding identity tend to remain in their silos. Intersectionality provides a space for interdisciplinarity and cross-fertilization of ideas. It recognizes the connection between the psychological and social aspects of identity, where institutional practices (including hiring policies and how they may affect the second generation), and global structures (in particular, large financial institutions that regulate banking and governmental policies that control the flow of migration), inscribe individual and collective identities. And these collective identities in turn influence broader global processes.

Intersectionality can provide a way to examine the positions of oppression and of relative privilege or power that are carved out by immigrants and their second-generation children. In other words, intersectionality can position us to understand how agency (or resiliency and resourcefulness within the MHP approach) is negotiated within structures of the host society. Indeed, one of the key aspects of an intersectional framework is not to essentialize notions of power and privilege or oppression and marginalization.

Scholars have observed that intersectionality focuses on fluidity rather than rigidity (Anthias 2008; CRIAW 2006), without losing sight of power as a crucial theoretical component (Hankivsky and Christoffersen 2008). We suggest that the next steps for scholarship in this field are to further elucidate how this fluidity is experienced by individuals (for example, negotiated cultural identities by immigrant or second-generation youth) or groups (for example, intergroup relations) and to propose research approaches that would best capture the fluidity embedded in such experiences (for example, through multi-method longitudinal studies influenced by multi-theoretical and interdisciplinary scholarship) and its link to mental well-being.

Acknowledgments
Study 1 – Immigrant Youth and Cultural Identity in a Global Context – was funded by the Social Sciences and Humanities Research Council of Canada under its standard research grants. Study 2 – Mental Health Services for Newcomer Youth: Exploring Needs and Enhancing Access – was funded by the Provincial Centre of Excellence for Child and Youth Mental Health at the Children's Hospital of Eastern Ontario. Nazilla Khanlou holds Echo's OWHC Chair in Women's Mental Health Research at York University, which is supported, in part, by Echo: Improving Women's Health in Ontario, an agency of the Ministry of Health and Long-Term Care.

Notes
1 For a full discussion of findings on experiences of prejudice and discrimination among Afghan and Iranian youth in Study 1, see Khanlou, Koh, and Mill (2008).

2   Beiser and Stewart (2005, S4) observe that "despite Canada's generally high standard of living and despite a system that promises universal access to high quality care, disparities in health remain a pressing national concern."

References

Allen, D.G. 1996. Knowledge, politics, culture, and gender: A discourse perspective. *Canadian Journal of Nursing Research* 28(1): 95-102.

Anthias, F. 2008. Thinking through the lens of translocational positionality: An intersectionality frame for understanding identity and belonging. *Translocations* 4(1): 5-20.

Barankin, T., and N. Khanlou. 2007. *Growing up resilient: Ways to build resilience in children and youth.* Toronto: Centre for Addiction and Mental Health.

Beiser, M., and M. Stewart. 2005. Reducing health disparities: A priority for Canada. *Canadian Journal of Public Health* 96(Suppl. 2): S4-S5.

Berry, J.W. 2001. A psychology of immigration. *Journal of Social Issues* 57(3): 615-31.

–. 2008. Acculturation and adaptation of immigrant youth. *Canadian Diversity* 6(2): 50-53.

Berry, J.W., U. Kim, S. Power, M. Young, and M. Bujaki. 1989. Acculturation attitudes in plural societies. *Applied Psychology: An International Review* 38: 185-206.

CRIAW. 2006. *Intersectional feminist frameworks: An emerging vision.* Ottawa: Canadian Research Institute for the Advancement of Women.

Cross, T., B. Bazron, K. Dennis, and M. Isaacs. 1989. *Towards a culturally competent system of care.* Vol. 1. Washington, DC: Georgetown University Child Development Center, CASSP Technical Assistance Center.

Fernando, S. 2003. *Cultural diversity, mental health and psychiatry: The struggle against racism.* New York: Brunner-Routledge Taylor and Francis Group.

Fine, M., and S.R. Sirin. 2007. Theorizing hyphenated selves: Researching youth development in and across contentious political contexts. *Social and Personality Psychology Compass* 1(1): 16-38.

Guthrie, B.J., and L.K. Low. 2006. Moving beyond the trickle-down approach: Addressing the unique disparate health experiences of adolescents of colour. *Journal for Specialists in Pediatric Nursing* 11(1): 3-13.

Hankivsky, O., and A. Christoffersen. 2008. Intersectionality and the determinants of health: A Canadian perspective. *Critical Public Health* 18(3): 271-83.

James, S., and I. Prilleltensky. 2002. Cultural diversity and mental health: Towards integrative practice. *Clinical Psychology Review* 22: 1133-54.

Khanlou, N. 2004. Influences on adolescent self-esteem in multicultural Canadian secondary schools. *Public Health Nursing* 21(5): 404-11.

–. 2005. Cultural identity as part of youth's self-concept in multicultural settings. *International Journal of Mental Health and Addiction* 3(2): 1-14.

–. 2007. Youth and post-migration cultural identities. In *Diasporic ruptures: Globality, migrancy, and expression of identity.* Vol. 2, ed. A. Asgharzadeh, E. Lawson, K.U. Oka, and A. Wahab, 81-94. Rotterdam: Sense.

–. 2008. Psychosocial integration of second and third generation racialized youth in Canada. *Canadian Diversity* 6(2): 54-57.

Khanlou, N., and C. Crawford. 2006. Post-migratory experiences of newcomer female youth: Self-esteem and identity development. *Journal of Immigrant and Minority Health* 8(1): 45-55.

Khanlou, N., J.G. Koh, and C. Mill. 2008. Cultural identity and experiences of prejudice and discrimination of Afghan and Iranian immigrant youth. *International Journal of Mental Health and Addiction* 6(4): 494-513. http://www.springerlink.com.

Khanlou, N., Y. Shakya, and C. Muntaner. 2007-9. Mental health services for newcomer youth: Exploring needs and enhancing access. Study funded by the Provincial Centre of Excellence at Children's Hospital of Eastern Ontario. Data in possession of the principal investigators.

Khanlou, N., M. Siemiatycki, and P. Anisef. 2003-6. Immigrant youth and cultural identity in a global context. Data in possession of the principal investigators.

Kobayashi, A. 2008. A research and policy agenda for second generation Canadians: Introduction. *Canadian Diversity* 6(2): 3-6.

Mahalingam, R., S. Balan, and J. Haritatos. 2008. Engendering immigrant psychology: An intersectionality perspective. *Sex Roles* 59: 326-36.

Mental Health Commission of Canada. 2009. *Toward recovery and well-being: A framework for a mental health strategy for Canada*. Draft for public discussion. http://www.mentalhealthcommission.ca/SiteCollectionDocuments/Key_Documents/en/2009/Mental_Health_ENG.pdf.

Oetting, E.R., and F. Beauvais. 1991. Orthogonal cultural identification theory: The cultural identification of minority adolescents. *International Journal of the Addictions* 25(5A-6A): 655-85.

Salant, T., and D.S. Lauderdale. 2003. Measuring culture: A critical review of acculturation and health in Asian immigrant populations. *Social Science and Medicine* 57(1): 71-90.

Shields, S. 2008. Gender: An intersectionality perspective. *Sex Roles* 59: 301-11.

Srivastava, R. 2007. *The healthcare professional's guide to clinical cultural competence*. Toronto: Mosby Elsevier.

Virta, E., D. Sam, and C. Westin. 2004. Adolescents with Turkish background in Norway and Sweden: A comparative study of their psychological adaptation. *Scandinavian Journal of Psychology* 45: 15-25.

WHO. 2007. Mental health: Strengthening mental health promotion. Fact Sheet 220. World Health Organization. http://www.who.int.

Willinsky, C., and B. Pape. 1997. *Mental health promotion*. Social Action Series. Toronto: Canadian Mental Health Association.

Working Group on Women and Human Rights. No date. Background briefing on intersectionality. http://www.cwgl.rutgers.edu.

9

Adopting an Intersectionality Perspective in the Study of the Healthy Immigrant Effect in Mid- to Later Life

Karen M. Kobayashi and Steven G. Prus

The application of an intersectionality perspective to the study of immigrant health underscores the importance of understanding the multi-dimensional nature of health inequality in vulnerable populations. Indeed, adequately addressing health inequities in such populations behooves us to move beyond an analysis of one or two possible predictors to an exploration of the influence of a number of markers of difference such as age, gender, socio-economic status, ethnicity/race, marital status, and sexual orientation, to name a few. The movement to examine and understand the intersecting relations between these factors then represents a necessary acknowledgment of the complexity inherent in the "production" of health among adult immigrants.

This chapter focuses primarily on the relationship between immigrant status – whether one is foreign- or native-born – and health, with a particular emphasis on the "healthy immigrant effect" (HIE) literature, given that, historically, research on this phenomenon has used an intersectional-type approach to address issues of health inequality. Over time, the number of key inequality markers examined in immigrant health studies has grown beyond socio-economic status, ethnicity, and gender to include age (that is, adult life course stages) (Gee, Kobayashi, and Prus 2004) and subjective social status (Leu et al. 2008), thereby broadening our understanding of the nature of health inequality and strengthening the case for the application of an intersectionality perspective to studies in this area.

In this chapter, we provide an example of a recent study to highlight the use of intersectionality as an appropriate conceptual framework and, concomitantly, Leslie McCall's (2005) intercategorical approach as a suitable methodology by which to research the healthy immigrant effect.[1] Like Jennifer Black and Gerry Veenstra (Chapter 3 this volume), we use this methodology to examine the impact of a number of intersecting factors, both biological and socially constructed, on the health of immigrants, paying particular attention to age (mid-life, older adult), gender (male, female), and visible minority status (visible, non-visible). In staying true to this approach and with the objective of addressing a gap in the literature on intersectionality in the health domain, we analyze data from the 2005 Canadian Community Health Survey "to explore inequalities within and across social groups" (Hankivsky and Cormier 2009, 6). Providing a segue into a discussion of the study, we first present a demographic profile of immigrants in the Canadian population, followed by a comprehensive review of the literature on the HIE and a rationale for examining the HIE according to age and gender.

A Profile of Immigrants in the Canadian Population

According to the 2006 census, 19.8 percent (6,186,950) of the Canadian population is foreign-born, the highest proportion in seventy-five years. This figure, up from 18.4 percent in 2001, reflects the increasing number of immigrants entering Canada, particularly in the past two and a half decades. Further, of those who were born outside of the country, 17.9 percent (1,110,000) are recent immigrants who arrived between 2001 and 2006.

In addition, the makeup of the foreign-born population according to country of birth has changed. Until the early 1970s, the primary sources of immigrants were European countries. In the last decade, however, immigrants are most likely to be from Asia, with India and China being the major source countries. Concomitantly, an increasing proportion of new immigrants are allophones – neither English nor French mother tongue – and the proportion with English mother tongue has been on the decline.

A breakdown of the adult (twenty and older) immigrant population in Canada by age and gender in 2006 indicates that 34.0 percent (the rate is 34.5 percent for males and 33.5 percent for females) are mid-life (forty-five to sixty-four years) individuals, whereas approximately 19.6 percent (18.9 percent for males and 20.3 percent for females) are older adults (sixty-five years and up). Further, recent immigrants (less than ten years since immigration) comprise 17.1 percent (the rate is 17.9 percent for males and 16.4 percent for females) of the mid-life immigrant population but only 4 percent (3.6 percent for males and 4.3 percent for females) of the later-life group.

An examination of adult immigrant men and women (excluding refugees) and their length of residence in Canada is important in that it may provide vital preliminary insights into the intersecting nature of the trajectories of education and work, family, and health for individuals in these groups. For example, it is assumed that recent middle-aged immigrant women have moved to Canada to join spouses and/or adult children (for family reasons), whereas men in this category may still be seeking further education/training and/or gainful employment opportunities (for economic reasons). Longer-term immigrant males (more than ten years of residence) in mid-life have probably completed any necessary training and secured employment; that is, they are well on their way to establishing themselves socio-economically in their new home country. This may not be the case for women, who, like recent immigrant women, have probably migrated for family reasons and, like their Canadian-born counterparts, have experienced disruptions in their occupational trajectories due to family commitments related to the transitions to marriage, parenthood, and/or grandparenthood in the post-immigration period. For older immigrant men and women, particularly those of colour, who have come to join their adult children and/or relatives, their formal work life is over and, depending on their financial resources, they have entered into a life course stage that may revolve around informal child care responsibilities for their grandchildren. Given the diversity of experiences according to age, gender, and ethnicity among the foreign-born, it is important to recognize the different ways in which these variables intersect to influence the health of immigrant populations over time.

With regard to health, mid- to later life adulthood (forty-five and older) is an important life course stage(s) to examine, given that great physical and psycho-emotional changes are likely to occur and continue during this period, particularly for women. Do the recent changes in Canada's immigrant population – its size and composition – have implications for the health status and/or health care utilization patterns of visible minority men and women in mid-life onward? An examination of the healthy immigrant effect by gender and visible minority status responds to this inquiry. Such an undertaking is important because the literature has not explored the effect of these variables on differential experiences.

The Healthy Immigrant Effect

The healthy immigrant effect hypothesis maintains that recent immigrants are healthier (and subsequently, that they use the health care system less) than their Canadian-born counterparts but that over time this health status advantage decreases. It is believed that the effect is strongest among new immigrants for two reasons: healthier (and younger, better educated) individuals self-select into the immigration process; and the health requirements in the Immigration Act for entrance into Canada tend to disqualify people with serious medical conditions (Oxman-Martinez, Abdool, and Loiselle-Léonard 2000). It is thought that the decline in health status over time can be attributed to immigrants' adoption of mainstream Canadian beliefs, attitudes, and lifestyle behaviours (such as smoking, dietary changes, and increased alcohol consumption), resulting in a convergence in health status (and health care utilization) between the foreign- and non-foreign-born populations (Ali 2002; Chen, Ng, and Wilkins 1996; Gee, Kobayashi, and Prus 2004; Hull 1979; McDonald and Kennedy 2004; Newbold 2005; Pérez 2002; Zambrana et al. 1997). This argument is supported by Canadian studies comparing immigrants by time that has elapsed since immigration, which tend to show that longer-term immigrants are not as healthy as newly arrived individuals, due to deteriorations in their health over time.

Using data from the 1994-95 National Population Health Survey, Jiajian Chen, Edward Ng, and Russell Wilkins (1996) find the following support for the HIE: immigrants, particularly recent immigrants, are less likely than the Canadian-born population to have chronic conditions or disabilities. Further, their results indicate that the effect is strongest for those from non-European regions (such as China, Hong Kong, Taiwan, and India), individuals who constitute the majority of recent immigrants to Canada.

Research by Claudio Pérez (2002) and Jennifer Ali (2002) provides further support for the healthy immigrant effect in Canada. In examining health status and health behaviour in the Canadian population, Pérez (2002) compares the physical health (incidence of heart disease, diabetes, high blood pressure, and cancer) of immigrants with that of the Canadian-born, whereas Ali (2002) focuses on variations in mental health (incidence of depression and alcohol dependence). Both studies observe the HIE with respect to selected physical and mental health indicators. In addition, the findings indicate that time since immigration is also related to variations in the health of immigrants; that is, the longer their period of residence in Canada, the more likely their health status is to converge toward the Canadian norm. Additionally, these findings remain significant when a number of demographic, socio-economic, and lifestyle factors are held constant.

Several Canadian studies over the past fifteen years, using differing measures of health (such as disability, dependency, life expectancy), also find evidence for the HIE in Canada (Chen, Ng, and Wilkins 1996; Dunn and Dyck 2000; Hyman 2001; McDonald and Kennedy 2004; Newbold and Danforth 2003; Parakulam, Krishnan, and Odynak 1992). These studies support the previously reported findings that length of residence in Canada (along with country of birth and demographic/socio-economic factors) contributes to variations in the health of immigrants.

Finally, in a recent American study on Asian immigrant mental health, Janxin Leu and his colleagues (2008) examine the influence of subjective social status – operationalized as the self-perception of an individual's socio-economic status (SES) relative to others in the US and in his/her "community" – in addition to a number of traditional markers of inequality (gender, SES) and find that age at immigration moderates the relationship between social status and mood dysfunction. Specifically, although there is no association among immigrants who migrated at younger ages, a strong association exists for those who did so at or after the age of twenty-five. This study represents a recent trend in the immigrant health literature to include subjective assessments of class as a marker of inequality, which is based on the salience of such indicators in previous American studies on health inequality in adult populations (Adler et al. 2000; Ostrove et al. 2000; Singh-Manoux, Adler, and Marmot 2003). Unfortunately, these measures are not available on Canadian health surveys, limiting the analysis of population data in this country to more traditional markers.

The Healthy Immigrant Effect, Age, and Gender

In a study on the health care utilization patterns of immigrants, Steven Globerman (1998, 31) concludes that "age is the strongest single determinant of health problems" regardless of immigrant status; in fact, his research suggests that immigrants and the Canadian-born utilize health care resources in similar ways at all stages of the life course including in old age. According to Globerman, the HIE does not exist with regard to the use of health care services even in later life. In an attempt to interrogate this statement further, Ellen Gee, Karen Kobayashi, and Steven Prus (2004) use a population health perspective to examine the relationship between length of residence in Canada (time since immigration) and health status in mid- to later-life individuals. Such a perspective recognizes that the immigrant, socio-economic, and demographic characteristics of individuals (such as age, gender, ethnicity, and language), rather than "medical care inputs and health behaviours" (Dunn and Dyck 2000, 1574), are the most salient predictors of health status over the life course. The findings from this study indicate that there are indeed differences between recent, longer-term, and non-immigrant Canadians according to age on global measures of health status; specifically, there is evidence of a healthy immigrant effect for recent immigrants in mid-life (forty-five to sixty-four) but not for older adults (sixty-five and older).

Although the significance of age in relation to the HIE has been established, few studies have focused on it and/or other important socio-demographic markers such as gender and ethnicity/visible minority status; that is, few have moved beyond the inclusion of such variables as controls in their analyses. One recent study that attempts to address this gap is Bruce Newbold's (2005) examination of these and other socio-demographic, socio-economic, and lifestyle factors in relation to the risk of transition to poor health. Using longitudinal data from the National Population Health Survey (1994-95 and 2000-1), he finds that females and young adults (aged twenty to thirty-four years) have a lower risk of declining health status relative to males and other age groups, and that blacks have a greater likelihood than other racial groups of moving from healthy to unhealthy status. These findings prompt us to further explore the significance of these factors alone and in intersection in any future study of immigrant health in Canada.

Intersectionality and Immigrant Health: The 2005 CCHS

The current study takes up this challenge by using an intercategorical approach (McCall 2005) to answer the questions "Do gender, age, and ethnicity matter in assessing the health of immigrants? And, if so, in what ways?" Such an approach is appropriate in that it recognizes that "pre-existing categories of difference" (Hankivsky and Cormier 2009, 6) can be useful in exploring within- and between-group inequalities in health. Further, in an attempt to move beyond the typical research triumvirate of ethnicity-class-gender in connection with immigrant health, we also include age as a salient marker of inequality in this study.

Although quantitative in its methodological approach, the study makes a significant contribution to the literature on intersectionality and health in that its key objectives are to identify and propose a response (in the policy domain) to health inequalities among the immigrant population in Canada. Indeed, by using an intercategorical approach to secondary data analysis to answer our research questions, we are acknowledging the potential of this type of analysis to transform the health and health care experiences of visible minority immigrant men and women at different stages of the adult life course. Further, findings from this study can then be explored qualitatively through in-depth interviews, focus groups, and/or participant observation with mid-life and older visible minority immigrant men and women to provide insights into the self-reported and functional health statuses of individuals in these groups. Such a mixed methods approach is a good fit with an intersectionality perspective for studies on immigrant health.

Methods for the Study

The results of this study are based on data from the public-use microdata file of the 2005 (Cycle 3.1) Canadian Community Health Survey (CCHS). The sample consists of 132,221 Canadians aged twelve or older living in private dwellings, with an overall response rate of approximately 85 percent. Adjusted sample weights were used to account for unequal probabilities of selection and non-response in the multi-stage stratified cluster sampling design employed in the CCHS.

The independent variable, country of birth, is dichotomized as Canadian- and foreign-born. The foreign-born are further classified by length of time in Canada since initial immigration (zero to nine years and ten or more years) and cultural/racial origin (non-white and white).

Three self-reported indicators of overall health are used as dependent variables. First, self-rated health, which provides a respondent's assessment of his/her overall health, is dichotomized into poor/fair versus good/very good/excellent. Second, "chronic condition" indicates whether the respondent has one or more chronic health conditions that have lasted six months or more and been diagnosed by a health professional or has at least one chronic condition versus no chronic condition. Third, "activity restriction" classifies respondents according to their need for help for health reasons with instrumental activities of daily living: needs help with at least one task versus does not need help. Restriction of activities is often considered a broad measure of functional limitation and disability.

Other variables used in the analysis include age in years (and age square), education (less than a high school diploma versus high school diploma or higher), household income (before taxes), number of years as a smoker (for current daily smokers only; all others are coded as 0); and body mass index (under- or overweight = BMI of less than 18.50 or greater than 24.99 versus other). Education and income have a large number of missing cases than do

Table 9.1

Sample characteristics by age and gender

	Male		Female	
	45-64	65+	45-64	65+
Poor/fair health	13.4%	26.3%	14.0%	26.4%
Chronic condition	72.7%	88.4%	80.6%	92.9%
Activity restriction	10.0%	26.6%	19.9%	44.3%
Immigrant status				
FB, <10 yrs	3.4%	1.0%	3.1%	1.2%
FB, 10+ yrs	20.4%	27.8%	19.7%	23.9%
CB	76.2%	71.2%	77.2%	74.9%
Visible minority				
(non-white)	13.6%	12.8%	8.6%	9.0%
Mean age in years	53.6	73.2	53.5	74.1
(SD)	(5.4)	(5.5)	(5.4)	(5.8)
Mean age square	2,905	5,392	2,892	5,524
(SD)	(596)	(820)	(592)	(858)
Education				
<High school	15.7%	36.7%	15.4%	43.2%
Missing	2.8%	5.3%	2.7%	4.9%
Mean income in dollars	$73,592	$44,226	$65,586	$36,003
(SD)	(36,520)	(27,867)	(36,549)	(25,645)
Unacceptable weight	66.4%	60.5%	52.5%	53.8%
Years smoking	6.9	5.0	5.9	3.8
(SD)	(14.3)	(15.7)	(13.2)	(13.5)
n	20,090	8,519	20,550	10,627

Notes: FB, <10 yrs: foreign-born, less than ten years in Canada
    FB, 10+ yrs: foreign-born, ten or more years in Canada
    CB: Canadian-born
    SD: Standard Deviation
Source: Canadian Community Health Survey 2005 (weighted data).

the other variables. A linear regression substitution approach was used to handle missing income data. A regression was used to predict what a missing score "should be" on the basis of other variables in the dataset (such as age, sex, marital status, and labour force status). The missing income data were then replaced with these predicted scores. A dummy variable was constructed to indicate missing versus non-missing education data. Table 9.1 provides information on all variables used in the study.

Logistic regression is used to model health outcomes for adults (forty-five years and older) across immigrant/visible minority groups. Three models are progressively developed. Model 1 shows the main effects of immigrant status (new immigrant, long-term immigrant, and Canadian-born) on each health measure. Model 2 further distinguishes between visible minority statuses: white and non-white. The inclusion of this variable allows us to examine if any immigrant status disparities in health observed in Model 1 are due to visible minority status – that is, to examine if a healthy immigrant effect actually reflects visible minority differences in health. Model 3 repeats the analysis in Model 2 with controls for age, age square, education, income, BMI, and years of smoking. Controlling for these factors allows us to see their impact on immigrant/visible minority differences in health. The Pearson chi-square goodness-of-fit test, X^2, is used to assess the overall fit of the model.

The models are developed for each of the dependent variables. Table 9.2 looks at immigrant/visible minority differences in "poor/fair" (condition of interest) versus "good/very good/excellent" self-rated health. Table 9.3 examines "having a chronic condition" (condition of interest) versus "not having a chronic condition," and Table 9.4 details "needing help with daily tasks" (condition of interest) versus "not needing help." With the Canadian-born set as the reference category in the tables, an odds ratio of less than one indicates that a group is less likely than Canadian-born to report a health problem. An odds ratio of greater than one indicates that a group is more likely than Canadian-born to report a health problem. The analysis is done separately for males and females, as well as for ages forty-five to sixty-four years and sixty-five and up. We stratify by age, given that health and reasons for immigration to Canada differ by age.

Results of the Study

Mid-Life: Forty-Five to Sixty-Four Years of Age

Males

There is evidence of the HIE among mid-life males. Recent immigrants in this age group who have been in Canada for less than ten years are healthier than their Canadian-born counterparts. They are significantly less likely to report fair/poor health (OR = 0.256, $p < .01$), a chronic condition (OR = 0.398,

Table 9.2

Odds ratios for immigrant/visible minority status differences in poor/fair self-reported health, by age and gender

Immigrant/visible minority status	45-64			65+		
	(1)	(2)	(3)	(1)	(2)	(3)
Male						
FB, <10 yrs	0 .256[a]			2.112[a]		
White		0.647[c]	0.739		1.006	1.312
Non-white		0.145[a]		0.153[a]	2.369[a]	3.033[a]
FB, 10+ yrs	1.040			0.960		
White		1.112[c]	1.199[a]		0.979	1.095
Non-white		0.968	1.116		0.930	1.172
CB		1.000	1.000		1.000	1.000
χ^2	71.0[a]	86.7[a]	1228.0[a]	9.8[a]	11.9[b]	485.4[a]
Female						
FB, <10 yrs	1.463[a]			0 .706		
White		1.758[a]	2.289[a]		1.904[c]	2.221[b]
Non-white		1.361[b]	1.407[b]		0.457[b]	0.566
FB, 10+ yrs	1.372[a]			1.426[a]		
White		1.240[a]	1.346[a]		1.235[a]	1.276[a]
Non-white		1.589[a]	1.965[a]		2.052[a]	2.354[a]
CB		1.000	1.000		1.000	1.000
χ^2	48.9[a]	60.0[a]	1482.6[a]	51.0[a]	85.2[a]	564.0[a]

Notes: FB, <10 yrs: foreign-born, less than ten years in Canada (white and non-white)
   FB, 10+ yrs: foreign-born, ten or more years in Canada (white and non-white)
   CB: Canadian-born (reference category)
   Model 1 (1) shows effect of immigrant status on health
   Model 2 (2) shows effect of immigrant/visible minority status on health
   Model 3 (3) repeats Model 2, controlling for age (and age square), education, income,
     BMI, and years of smoking.
   a = p <0.01, b = p <0.05, c = p <0.10.
Source: Canadian Community Health Survey, 2005 (weighted data).

p <.01), and a limitation of daily activities compared to Canadian-born persons (OR = 0.406, p <.01). See Model 1 in Tables 9.2 to 9.4 respectively.

A further examination of these results suggests that there is a gradient of deterioration in health with time after immigration (that is, a convergence in health differences between immigrants and Canadian-born persons). In self-rated health or restriction of activity, there is no significant difference between longer-term immigrant males (those who have been in Canada for ten or more years) and Canadian-born males (Model 1 in Tables 9.2 to 9.4).

Turning our attention to Model 2 in Tables 9.2 to 9.4, we see that immigrant status differences in health do reflect visible minority status. The health advantage of recent immigrants is particularly strong for non-whites. For

Table 9.3

Odds ratios for immigrant/visible minority status differences in having a chronic condition, by age and gender

Immigrant/visible minority status	45-64			65+		
	(1)	(2)	(3)	(1)	(2)	(3)
Male						
FB, <10 yrs	0.398[a]			0.366[a]		
White		0.480[a]	0.534[a]		1.012	1.071
Non-white		0.375[a]	0.452[a]		0.322[a]	0.385[a]
FB, 10+ yrs	0.882[a]			0.836[b]		
White		0.951	0.874[a]		0.822[b]	0.799[a]
Non-white		0.780[a]	0.814[a]		0.867	0.966
CB		1.000	1.000		1.000	1.000
χ^2	130.9[a]	141.4[a]	517.4[a]	15.4[a]	17.4[a]	158.6[a]
Female						
FB, <10 yrs	0.613[a]			0.273[a]		
White		1.259	1.363		0.531	0.531
Non-white		0.477[a]	0.616[a]		0.234[a]	0.489[b]
FB, 10+ yrs	0.954			1.065		
White		1.116[c]	1.045		1.046	0.998
Non-white		0.776[a]	0.855[b]		1.105	1.377[c]
CB		1.000	1.000		1.000	1.000
χ^2	26.1[a]	66.7[a]	549.9[a]	26.7[a]	28.7[a]	139.8[a]

Notes: FB, <10 yrs: foreign-born, less than ten years in Canada (white and non-white)
FB, 10+ yrs: foreign-born, ten or more years in Canada (white and non-white)
CB: Canadian-born (reference category)
Model 1 (1) shows effect of immigrant status on health
Model 2 (2) shows effect of immigrant/visible minority status on health
Model 3 (3) repeats Model 2, controlling for age (and age square), education, income, BMI, and years of smoking.
a = p <0.01, b = p <0.05, c = p <0.10.
Source: Canadian Community Health Survey, 2005 (weighted data).

example, the odds of reporting poor/fair health for recent non-white immigrants are 85.5 percent lower relative to Canadian born persons (OR = 0.145, p <.01), whereas the odds for recent white immigrants are just 35.3 percent lower compared with Canadian-born persons (OR = 0.647, p <.10). Hence, the results indicate that the HIE observed in Model 1 can be attributed, in part, to the exceptionally good health of recent non-white immigrants.

Interestingly, the inclusion of socio-demographic and behavioural controls (Model 3 in Tables 9.2 to 9.4) also has very limited impact on health differences between immigrant/visible minority status groups. The health advantage of new immigrant men aged forty-five to sixty-four is not accounted for by differences in age, socio-economic status, or health behaviours between the immigrant/visible minority status groups. These findings seem to contradict the argument that a healthier immigrant population stems from advantages in socio-demographic, SES, and lifestyle factors, at least for males.

Females

The findings for females aged forty-five to sixty-four are less consistent with a healthy immigrant effect. Looking first at foreign-born females who have been in Canada for less than ten years, we see that they are significantly less likely than their Canadian-born counterparts to have a chronic condition; however, they are just as likely to experience an activity restriction and more likely to report fair/poor health (see Model 1, Tables 9.2 to 9.4).

Table 9.4

Odds ratios for immigrant/visible minority status differences in needing help with daily tasks, by age and gender

Immigrant/visible minority status	45-64			65+		
	(1)	(2)	(3)	(1)	(2)	(3)
Male						
FB, <10 yrs	0.406[a]			0.731		
White		0.542[c]	0.568[c]		0.976	1.248
Non-white		0.366[a]	0.342[a]		0.692	0.796
FB, 10+ yrs	0.946			0.990		
White		1.128[c]	1.224[a]		0.969	1.044
Non-white		0.723[a]	0.791[b]		1.004	1.428[a]
CB		1.000	1.000		1.000	1.000
χ^2	29.4[a]	45.9[a]	738.9[a]	1.2	1.6	808.7[a]
Female						
FB, <10 yrs	0.889			1.024		
White		0.856	0.983		1.083	0.914
Non-white		0.903	0.921		1.007	2.232[a]
FB, 10+ yrs	1.229[a]			0.991		
White		1.203[a]	1.192[a]		0.947	0.922
Non-white		1.269[a]	1.445[a]		1.126	1.410[a]
CB		1.000	1.000		1.000	1.000
χ^2	26.6[a]	25.2[a]	494.3[a]	0.1	3.6	1139.2[a]

Notes: FB, <10 yrs: foreign-born, less than ten years in Canada (white and non-white)
   FB, 10+ yrs: foreign-born, ten or more years in Canada (white and non-white)
   CB: Canadian-born (reference category)
   Model 1 (1) shows effect of immigrant status on health
   Model 2 (2) shows effect of immigrant/visible minority status on health
   Model 3 (3) repeats Model 2, controlling for age (and age square), education, income, BMI, and years of smoking.
   a = p <0.01, b = p <0.05, c = p <0.10.
Source: Canadian Community Health Survey, 2005 (weighted data).

These disparities are largely affected by visible minority status. Model 2 (in Tables 9.2 to 9.4) shows that, compared to the Canadian-born, only non-white recent immigrants are less likely to have a chronic condition (OR = 0.477, p <.01). And though this group is moderately (36 percent) more likely to report poor/fair health compared to the Canadian-born (OR = 1.361, p <.05), their white counterparts exhibit a much higher level of poor/fair health (OR = 1.758, p <.01).

For foreign-born females who have been in Canada for ten years or more, the findings show that, unlike their male counterparts, they exhibit a disadvantage in health in comparison to the Canadian-born; that is, they are 1.4 and 1.2 times more likely to report poor/fair health and a chronic condition respectively (Model 1, Tables 9.2 and 9.4). Further, these disparities are similar for whites and non-whites (Model 2) and not affected after controlling for socio-demographic, SES, and lifestyle factors (Model 3).

Later Life: Sixty-Five and Older

Males

The last three columns of Tables 9.2 to 9.4 show the relationship between immigrant/visible minority status and health for persons aged sixty-five and older. Among foreign-born males who have been in Canada for ten years or more, the results do not differ from those reported for ages forty-five to sixty-four; that is, these men are significantly less likely than their Canadian-born counterparts to have a chronic condition (OR = 0.836, p <.05) (Model 1 for age sixty-five and up in Table 9.3).

However, across the two age groups, the results do differ in a few important ways. Recent non-white male immigrants aged sixty-five or older are significantly more likely to report poor/fair health than are the Canadian-born (OR = 2.369, p <.01) (Model 2, Table 9.1); this is in opposition to the findings reported for their younger counterparts. On the other hand, recent male immigrants of sixty-five or older, again non-whites, are significantly less likely to have a chronic condition compared to the Canadian-born (OR = 0.322, p <.01). These results are relatively unaffected by controls for socio-demographic, SES, and lifestyle factors (Model 3).

Females

Non-white older female immigrants who have been in Canada for less than ten years fare better than their male counterparts. Specifically, they are less likely to rate their health in a negative manner (OR = 0.475, p <.05) (Model 2, Table 9.2) or to have a chronic condition relative to older Canadian-born females (OR = 0.234, p <.01) (Model 2, Table 9.3).

When the data are adjusted for socio-demographic, SES, and lifestyle differences, however, their health becomes more comparable to that of older

Canadian-born females. In particular, the odds of reporting poor/fair health for older foreign-born non-white females who have been in Canada for less than ten years become statistically insignificant (OR = 0.566, $p >.10$), and their risk of activity restriction becomes significantly higher relative to the Canadian-born (OR = 2.232, $p <.01$). Foreign-born non-white females who have been in Canada for ten or more years are similarly disadvantaged after controlling for these factors (see Model 3 in Tables 9.2 and 9.4 respectively).

Conclusions of the Study

One of the key findings from the current study is that the HIE applies to mid-life males in Canada. Specifically, recent – those who migrated less than ten years ago – immigrant men between the ages of forty-five and sixty-four have better functional and self-rated health than the Canadian-born. And, on further examination, the results suggest that there is a convergence in health differences between foreign- and Canadian-born men in mid-life. Interestingly, the health advantage of recent immigrants is especially strong for visible minorities, suggesting that the observed HIE for middle-aged men is due, in part, to the exceptionally good health of recent visible minority immigrants. Finally, it should be noted that this advantage is not accounted for by differences in age, SES, or health behaviours between the immigrant/ visible minority groups, contradicting the argument that a healthier immigrant population can be attributed to advantages arising from such factors.

For mid-life women, the findings are less consistent with a healthy immigrant effect, and the disparities are significantly influenced by visible minority status. Further, the study finds that unlike mid-life men, longer-term immigrant women between the ages of forty-five and sixty-four are actually disadvantaged in health (on both self-reported measures) compared to the Canadian-born, and that these differences are similar for visible and non-visible minorities even after controlling for socio-demographic, SES, and lifestyle factors.

A different picture emerges in later life for men, particularly for visible minority men, as recent immigrants aged sixty-five and older are most likely to be disadvantaged vis-à-vis self-reported health even after controlling for key factors. On the other hand, recent visible minority immigrant women in the later stages of the life course fare much better on self-reported health measures. However, this advantage does disappear when the data are adjusted for other differences. The same holds true for longer-term visible minority immigrant women who are similarly disadvantaged when socio-demographic, SES, and lifestyle factors are held constant.

Based on these findings, a key implication for Canadian health care policy and program planning for immigrant men and women in mid- to late adulthood, individuals who make up over one-half of the foreign-born adult population, is noteworthy here. In particular, the study findings underscore the necessity for policy makers to address the differential health care needs of immigrant adults by gender and age group. Recent immigrant visible minority men in mid-life and, to a lesser extent, their later-life female counterparts may have fewer needs for services and programs in the early years of their residency in Canada, whereas certain new immigrant subgroups – namely, older men and mid-life women of colour – may actually have increased needs for services due to poor health status. This increased need is likely to continue for these women as they age in Canada. In response to this reality, policies and programs must be developed at both the federal and provincial levels, particularly in Ontario (Toronto), Quebec (Montreal), and British Columbia (Vancouver), provinces in which the majority of immigrants choose to reside. These policies and programs must target mid-life immigrant and certain subgroups of older immigrant women as they age over time and must respond to the needs of an older immigrant male population from the outset.

Limitations of the Study

Although the Canadian Community Health Survey (CCHS) provides information on the health status and health care needs of older adult Canadians, there are a number of limitations in using its data for this study. First, though its data do allow for an examination of health status and health care utilization among immigrant arrivals, the CCHS does not collect information on immigrant status or on the reasons for immigrants' entry into Canada. Hence, a more detailed analysis of immigrant men's and women's health is not possible; that is, important variations in health status among naturalized citizens, landed immigrants, refugees, and non-permanent men and women cannot be examined in this study. Further, differences in health care utilization between immigrants in the "family reunion" (spouses, children, and parents of Canadian citizens/residents), "refugee," and "investment and independent" (skilled workers and business persons) categories cannot be determined. This study, therefore, cannot provide specific mid- to later life insights into Pérez's (2002) findings that refugees, regardless of gender, are more likely than any other type of immigrant to be disadvantaged in health.

Second, it is important to note that, though CCHS respondents who could not understand English or French were interviewed in their own language, linguistic (as well as cultural) barriers faced by new immigrants may prevent them from consulting health care professionals, resulting in an underdiagnosis of health problems (Laroche 2000; Pérez 2002). Relatedly, cultural factors such as adherence to traditional values and beliefs may influence individuals' willingness to report health problems (Ali 2002; Kopec et al. 2001) as there may be differences in their fundamental conceptualizations of health and illness (Saldov 1991). Overall, the extent to which cultural and language differences in the Canadian population influence the interpretation and reporting of health problems is not well known. However, the magnitude of the differences in men's and women's health status between immigrant and Canadian-born populations, as reported here, makes it unlikely that cultural factors exclusively may explain these results.

Third, despite evidence of a healthy immigrant effect among the forty-five to sixty-four age group, longitudinal data are needed to verify a true convergence in health status between immigrants and Canadian-born persons over time. It is not possible with the cross-sectional data used here to rule out a cohort effect, whereby differences in men's and women's health among immigrant groups are partly due to the country of birth. For instance, longer-term immigrants are more likely to be from Europe and recent immigrants from non-European regions, both of which vary in terms of general population health – today's immigrants may make up a healthier cohort than cohorts who immigrated earlier – and in the type and quality of health care systems. Additionally, health requirements for entry into Canada have changed, becoming more stringent over time (Pérez 2002). Further, as we are unable to acquire standardized health status and utilization data pre-immigration from all source countries, the validity of findings on the HIE may be called into question even if longitudinal data were collected post-immigration.

Finally, using the CCHS public-use microdata file (PUMF) as our primary data source imposed limits on our study because the CCHS categorized respondents in five-year groups (such as forty-five to forty-nine years) and did not record their actual age. Subsequently, some of the key variations between immigrants and non-immigrants may be due to small differences in the average age of respondents within each age cohort group. Further, another limitation of the PUMF is that it does not allow for the consideration of key variables such as ethnicity (country of birth) as both a control and independent variable in the current analyses.

Chapter Conclusion/Discussion
As evidenced in a review of the literature, despite the adoption of an intersectionality-type perspective in a number of key studies, much of the research on the healthy immigrant effect has been exclusively quantitative in nature. This was true also for the study that we undertook to highlight the applicability of an intersectionality perspective to the study of the HIE. Although appropriate for an intercategorical analysis, quantitative methods alone allow only a limited exploration of the myriad ways in which salient markers of difference intersect to produce inequalities in health. In particular, we acknowledge that micro- and meso-level factors are much better identified and their meanings probed with qualitative research methods such as in-depth

open-ended interviews, focus groups, and/or participant observation. Indeed, information collected via qualitative methods is necessary to avoid the homogenization or essentialization of immigrant groups vis-à-vis their health status and/or health care access. Despite this, however, we should not negate the important contributions that quantitative research has made to an understanding of immigrant health to date, specifically with reference to the HIE. From this literature, for example, researchers wanting to apply an intersectional perspective and, concomitantly, an intercategorical approach to the study of health inequities can find interesting starting points from which to build exploratory research problems and questions. They can also look to population research findings to identify the characteristics of participants (such as mid-life visible minority immigrant men) for inclusion in their phenomenological or ethnographic studies, underscoring the importance of quantitative research to the sampling process for qualitative work, the type of research that would benefit from a more intracategorical approach to the study of immigrant health.[2]

Given what we know about the nature of research on the HIE to date, what type of overall methodological framework would fit well with an intersectionality perspective in further studying this effect? First, we suggest that if this perspective is to be applied to population health data in a meaningful way, it needs to be integrated with a macro-level conceptual framework like that of the life course perspective; such an integration, a marriage of macro- and micro-level perspectives, would allow for a more comprehensive exploration of underlying power relationships (from two levels of analysis) in studies on immigrant health. A merging of the key concepts of intersectionality and the life course at the theoretical level provides a guiding framework with which to examine the influences of social structural, cultural, political, and historical exigencies on individuals over space and time.

Second, we believe that the most appropriate overall methodological approach for such an integrated framework would ultimately be a mixed methods strategy. Specifically, a sequential transformative approach (Cresswell 2009) would best be able to provide the data/information necessary to speak to the key concepts and their interrelationships in the application of an integrated intersectionality life course theoretical framework to research on the HIE. That is, a two-phase strategy that employs a theoretical lens to guide the sequential procedures from quantitative to qualitative (or vice versa) recognizes the need to include both deductive and inductive processes in the construction and generation of responses to research questions. Further, this strategy "creates sensitivity to collecting data from marginalized or underrepresented groups, and ends with a call for action" (ibid., 212), making it a most appropriate methodological framework for intersectionality research on the HIE.

Finally, we would like to conclude with a strong statement of support for an intersectional perspective as a tool for transformation in the context of research on the health of immigrant populations. The transformatory power of the intersectionality approach can only be strengthened in integration with the macro-level perspective of the life course, leading us to recommend its application to future research on the healthy immigrant effect.

Notes

1   An intercategorical approach focuses on empirically analyzing the relationships of inequality that exist among social groups. Its aim is to explicate these relationships – which are complex and ever-changing – by interrogating the analytical categories (such as gender, class, and ethnicity) that make up these groups (McCall 2005).

2   An intracategorical approach takes a more critical stance toward understanding the salience and meaning of categories by focusing on those social groups that are often neglected in more traditional forms of inquiry (such as population-based surveys). The objective of this approach is to "reveal the complexity of lived experience within such groups" (McCall 2005, 1774).

References

Adler, N.E., E.S. Epel, G. Castellazzo, and J.R. Ickovics. 2000. Relationship of subjective and objective social status with psychological and physiological functioning: Preliminary data in healthy white women. *Health Psychology* 19: 586-92.

Ali, J. 2002. Mental health of Canada's immigrants. *Health Reports* 13 (Statistics Canada Catalogue 82-003). http://www.statcan.ca/english/freepub/82-003-SIE/2002001/pdf/82-003-SIE2002001.pdf.

Chen, J., E. Ng, and R. Wilkins. 1996. The health of Canada's immigrants in 1994-95. *Health Reports* 7(4): 33-45.

Cresswell, J.W. 2009. *Research design: Qualitative, quantitative and mixed methods approaches.* Thousand Oaks, CA: Sage.

Dunn, J.R., and I. Dyck. 2000. Social determinants of health in Canada's immigrant population: Results from the National Population Health Survey. *Social Science and Medicine* 51(11): 1573-93.

Gee, E., K.M. Kobayashi, and S. Prus. 2004. Examining the "healthy immigrant effect" in mid- to later life: Findings from the 2001 Canadian Community Health Survey. *Canadian Journal on Aging* 23(Suppl. 1): 61-69.

Globerman, S. 1998. *Immigration and health care utilization patterns in Canada.* RIIM Working Paper Series 98-08. Vancouver: Research on Immigration and Integration in the Metropolis.

Hankivsky, O., and R. Cormier. 2009. *Intersectionality: Moving women's health research and policy forward.* Vancouver: Women's Health Research Network.

Hull, D. 1979. Migration, adaptation and illness. A review. *Social Science and Medicine* 13A: 25-36.

Hyman, I. 2001. *Immigration and health.* Ottawa: Health Canada. http://ceris.metropolis.net/Virtual%20Library/WKPP%20List/WKPP2007/CWP55.pdf.

Kopec, J.A., J.I. Williams, T. To, and P.C. Austin. 2001. Cross-cultural comparisons of health status in Canada using the Health Utilities Index. *Ethnicity and Health* 6(1): 41-50.

Laroche, M. 2000. Health status and health services utilization of Canada's immigrant and non-immigrant populations. *Canadian Public Policy* 26(1): 51-73.

Leu, J., I.H. Yen, S.A. Gansky, E. Walton, N.E. Adler, and D.T. Takeuchi. 2008. The association between subjective social status and mental health among Asian immigrants: Investigating the influence of age at immigration. *Social Science and Medicine* 66(5): 1152-64.

McCall, L. 2005. The complexity of intersectionality. *Signs: Journal of Women in Culture and Society* 30(3): 1771-1800.

McDonald, T., and S. Kennedy. 2004. Insights into the "healthy immigrant effect": Health status and health service use of immigrants to Canada. *Social Science and Medicine* 59(8): 1613-27.

Newbold, K.B. 2005. Self-rated health within the Canadian immigrant population: Risk and the healthy immigrant effect. *Social Science and Medicine* 60(6): 1359-70.

Newbold, K.B., and J. Danforth. 2003. Health status and Canada's immigrant population. *Social Science and Medicine* 57(10): 1981-95.

Ostrove, J.M., N.E. Adler, M. Kuppermann, and A.E. Washington. 2000. Objective and subjective assessments of socioeconomic status and their relationship to self-rated health in an ethnically diverse sample of pregnant women. *Health Psychology* 19: 613-18.

Oxman-Martinez, J., S. Abdool, and M. Loiselle-Léonard. 2000. Immigration, women and health in Canada. *Canadian Journal of Public Health* 91(5): 394-95.

Parakulam, G., V. Krishnan, and D. Odynak. 1992. Health status of Canadian-born and foreign-born residents. *Canadian Journal of Public Health* 83(4): 311-14.

Pérez, C.E. 2002. Health status and health behaviour among immigrants. *Health Reports* 13: 89-100.

Saldov, M. 1991. The ethnic elderly: Communication barriers to health care. *Canadian Social Work Review* 8(2): 269-77.

Singh-Manoux, A., N.E. Adler, and M.G. Marmot. 2003. Subjective social status: Its determinants and its association with measures of ill health in the Whitehall II study. *Social Science and Medicine* 56(6): 1321-33.

Zambrana, R.E, S.C.M. Scrimshaw, N. Collins, and C. Dunkel-Schetter. 1997. Prenatal health behaviors and psychosocial risk factors in pregnancy in women of Mexican origin: The role of acculturation. *American Journal of Public Health* 87(8): 1022-26.

10
Intersectionality in the Context of Later Life Experiences of Dementia
Wendy Hulko

Feminists and critical gerontologists brought an intersectionality and inter-locking oppressions paradigm to the field of aging studies some time ago (Brotman 1998; Calasanti 1996; Dressel 1991; Dressel, Minkler, and Yen 1997; McMullin 2000), arguing for a more complex approach to understand-ing the poor health and low incomes experienced by older women and older racialized and ethnic minority people. Despite a recognition within the gerontological literature of the ways in which age intersects with other identity categories such as gender, class, race, ethnicity, and marital status, intersectionality theorists rarely include either age or (dis)ability in their lists of social identity categories (Hulko 2009b; see also Hopkins and Pain 2007; Krekula 2007). Age as an identity category or a social division undoubt-edly structures lived experiences across the life course, yet it tends to be more salient for those at either end of the age continuum (Hockey and James 1993). An intersectionality and interlocking oppressions paradigm is ex-tremely relevant to older persons. Whether or not age is the most significant identity category at this stage of the life course, the lives of older adults continue to be shaped by social divisions based on gender identity and gender expression, race and racialization, ethnocultural group membership, social class, sexual orientation, faith and religious affiliation, (dis)ability and marital status.

Intersectionality – "a metaphor for the entanglement and interaction of multiple and complex identity categories" (Hulko 2004, 236) – draws on the image of a traffic intersection (Crenshaw 1989, 1994) to indicate the ways in which different strands of our identities run alongside and across one another. The theoretical or research paradigm (see Hancock 2007) of inter-sectionality and interlocking oppressions calls attention to "the differential attributions of power that result from such varied configurations, and the need to view intersectional beings holistically rather than try to tease apart different strands of identity" (Hulko 2009b, 48; see Bannerji 1995; Brah and Phoenix 2004; Combahee River Collective 1983; Lorde 2007). This paradigm is invaluable to understanding marginalization and privilege, as it "remind[s] us that oppression can not be reduced to one fundamental type, and that oppressions work together in producing injustice" (Collins 2000, 18).

"Intersectionality" and "interlocking oppressions" have been distinguished from one another by reference to micro and macro sociological processes, in terms of the level at which these concepts operate (Collins 1995, cited in Dressel, Minkler, and Yen 1997, 583-84), although this is far from consistent in the literature (see Hulko 2009b). In my earliest writing on dementia and intersectionality, I stated that "intersectionality is used to point to the ways in which multiple and complex identity categories such as gender, 'race,' ethnicity, class, age, able-bodiedness, sexual orientation and faith/religion interact to shape individual life experiences ... [and] interlocking oppressions [constitute] the structural framework that shapes and constrains the identities and the experiences of people with dementia as they try to make meaning of their lives as intersectional beings" (Hulko 2002, 233-32). More recently, I expanded on this distinction: "The term *intersectionality* is used in conjunction with identities and categories, whereas the term *interlocking oppressions* applies more to processes and systems" (Hulko 2009b, 47, emphasis in original). Racism, sexism, and ageism are examples of interlocking systems of oppression, whereas race, gender, and age are the identity categories on which these forms of oppression are based.

Researchers have responded to calls to situate dementia within a broader socio-cultural context and to ensure greater diversity among research participants as part of a broader movement to ascertain the views of people with Alzheimer's disease and other forms of dementia about their "illness experiences" (Kleinman 1988; see Harman and Clare 2006). Because they confined themselves to a narrow range of people, these efforts have been limited in scope, and to date only a few researchers have applied an intersectional lens to their work (Hulko 2002, 2004, 2009a; O'Connor, Phinney, and Hulko 2010; Price 2008). Focusing on a younger Aboriginal woman of lower socioeconomic status who had atypical vascular dementia and who lived with her same-sex partner, Deborah O'Connor, Alison Phinney, and Wendy Hulko (2010) used intersectionality theory in their case study analysis of her experiences of dementia and her interactions with support services. In her preliminary analysis of in-depth interviews with twenty gays and lesbians who cared for persons with dementia, Elizabeth Price (2008) highlighted the intersectionality of a non-heterosexual identity, increasing age, and dementia. In her analysis of published accounts of people living with dementia, Wendy Hulko (2002, 246) found evidence of intersectional thinking regarding the indivisibility of age and gender as well as of gender, age, and class, and noted that most accounts examined a middle-aged (forty to sixty years old), well-educated, white, married professional in the early stages of dementia, with strong religious or ideological beliefs and a supportive family.

A small group of researchers seeks to redress this imbalance in the literature, shifting the focus from white, middle-class, Anglo-Saxon, heterosexual members of the mainstream who are in the early stages of dementia (Downs 1997; Hulko 2002; Marshall and Tibbs 2006; O'Connor et al. 2007; Steeman et al. 2006). Moreover, they are concerned with foregrounding power when using concepts such as gender, race, and class, and treating these and other identity categories as complex, contingent, and indivisible. As there have been few serious attempts to diversify the respondents (persons with dementia), and to analyze the influence of social location, the core description of the dementia experience – as an overwhelming challenge to be struggled with, defeated by, or succumbed to – remains largely unshaken. Yet, as is demonstrated by the grounded theory research reported here, when intersectionality is applied to the context of later life experiences of dementia, a rather different portrait emerges – one that is far from uniform and that varies depending on the social location of the individual. Indeed, we cannot say there is one experience; instead, there are a multitude of experiences that reflect the degree of privilege and oppression to which people with dementia are subject, based on their gender, racial, ethnic, and class backgrounds – irrespective of their shared status as persons living with dementia.

The grounded theory arising from this research posits that social location shapes how older people with dementia experience this disabling condition, the extent to which they are othered or marginalized by it, and the theories on which they draw to make sense of what is happening to them. This chapter starts with a description of the empirical research from which the data were derived and the grounded theory emerged; it then discusses the range of subjective experiences of dementia and analyzes the links between these and the social locations of the participants. It concludes with implications for future research and theory building related to dementia and intersectionality.

Research Design
This research was exploratory and qualitative. Qualitative research is well suited to investigating lived experiences, teasing out participants' perspectives on the role and influence of social location in their lives and developing theoretical insights into the phenomenon under investigation (Kirby, Greaves, and Reid 2006; Mama 1995). The specific methodology was grounded theory (Charmaz 2006; Glaser and Strauss 1967) informed by feminist and anti-oppression perspectives on research (Brown and Strega 2005; de Vault 1999; Fine et al. 2000; Kirby, Greaves, and Reid 2006). Anti-oppression research takes seriously Patti Lather's (1991, 172) challenge that "those of us who do empirical research in the name of emancipatory politics must discover ways to connect our research methodology to our theoretical

concerns and political commitments." Given this, research relationships take on a markedly different form, with researchers striving to research "with," rather than "on" or "about," acknowledging their social location and subjectivity, and facilitating the voice and inclusion of participants.

Grounded theory aims to go beyond the description of a phenomenon toward an explanation of it (Glaser and Strauss 1967) and has been referred to as "systematic inductive guidelines for collecting and analyzing data to build middle-range theoretical frameworks that explain the collected data" (Charmaz 2000, 509). Key strategies – which I used in this research – include the simultaneous collection and analysis of data, constant comparative method of data analysis, theoretical sampling, and memo writing (Charmaz 2006). The project asked the following research question: What are the relationships between the experiences of older people with dementia and the intersections of race, ethnicity, class, and gender? Over a nine-month period in 2003 and 2004, participants were recruited through theoretical sampling, and data collection and analysis occurred simultaneously, until theoretical saturation was reached (ibid.; Glaser and Strauss 1967).

Data Collection and Analysis

The data were collected through a series of interviews and observation sessions over a one- to two-month period with each of the eight primary research participants, their family members, and other members of their social worlds. In addition to the eight older people with dementia, fifty people signed consent forms for the use of their words and/or images captured during the observation sessions and focus groups. These included family members, neighbours, friends, service users, service providers, and employees who were present during the observation sessions, as well as family members who took part in the focus groups at the end.[1]

The participants and the observation sessions (settings, timing, activities, and people) were selected based on the data analysis; the goals were to confirm or disconfirm the working hypotheses and build the theoretical framework (Glaser and Strauss 1967). Data collection also involved photography and photo elicitation (see Becker 1974; Grady 2001; Harper 2000), which have been recommended for research involving people with dementia (Allan 2001) and older people (Wenger 2002), as questions about photographs or objects can provide a good starting point for discussion and make it easier to talk about sensitive subjects. Visual methods are said to be congruent with grounded theory, as both forms of research enable the comparison of emic (insider) and etic (outsider) perspectives and use an iterative process of data collection and analysis (Prosser and Schwartz 1998).

The forty-three data collection points included twenty-four in-home interviews lasting between forty and ninety minutes, seventeen observation sessions of two to three hours at various settings, including a church group, staff meeting, birthday party, pub, doctor's office, family cottage, art class, and adult day program, and two focus groups with the participants and one of their family members to get feedback on the preliminary findings. The interview questions, observation sites, and research participants were determined initially by theoretical sensitivity (Glaser 1978). As the iterative process of data collection and data analysis progressed, decisions were based on testing (confirming or refuting) the working hypotheses, with participants being recruited on an ongoing basis.

The interviews, which were dialogical, were structured around the individual's self-identity, social location, and experiences of living with cognitive impairment. Questions were designed to evoke subjective reflections on living with cognitive impairment as a person of a particular race, ethnicity, gender, and class, and they made use of conversation aids, such as varied images of older people and third-person questioning (Allan 2001; Dewing 2002). Initial interview questions included the following: What words describe you as a person? When you think of yourself, what image comes to mind? Tell me about your memory. What does it mean to you to have Alzheimer's disease? How does your being a [insert participant's words] shape your experience of living with memory problems?

The observation sessions took place in a setting or at an event that held significance for the person with dementia, negotiated at the end of the first or second interview, sometimes with the involvement of a family member. As a participant-observer, I interacted as appropriate: engaging in informal interviewing, taking photographs as permitted, and making brief notations. Immediately afterward, I wrote up my notes in full for coding. The observations provided additional, and sometimes conflicting, information to that garnered through the interviews (see Hubbard, Downs, and Tester 2003; Lambert and McKevitt 2002). They also allowed for recording of non-verbal communication and interactions with others, shown to be meaningful and purposive for people with dementia (Hubbard et al. 2002; Seman 2002). Further, observation provided another means to assess the influence and interaction of gender, class, race, and ethnicity on the participants' experiences of dementia, often not easily articulated in the interviews. This combination of methods was key to the emergence and development of the second category of the grounded theory: othering dementia.

Throughout the research, I made use of process consent (Allan 2001; Dewing 2002, 2007; Hubbard, Downs, and Tester 2003; Reid, Ryan, and Enderby 2001), which required the ongoing negotiation of consent or assent from the persons with dementia, as well as the procurement of informed consent from their substitute decision makers for those who were incapable of providing it themselves. The participants selected their own pseudonyms, and their words are presented verbatim below. Interpreters were used with two participants (Ester Hernandez and Julianna Molnar), whose words should be read as spoken in their native languages (Tagalog and Hungarian respectively), unless otherwise noted.

Consistent with grounded theory methodology, the data analysis activities included preparing the data, reading and repeatedly examining it, coding line by line, forming two levels of codes (concepts and categories), comparing within and across cases, writing theoretical memos, developing working hypotheses, diagramming relationships, and sorting the analysis into a coherent theoretical framework (Charmaz 2000, 2002; Glaser and Strauss 1967). Three categories emerged: experiencing dementia, othering dementia, and theorizing dementia, which together form my grounded theory of dementia and intersectionality. "Experiencing dementia" captures the diversity of older people's experiences of dementia, which range from "not a big deal" to "a nuisance" to "hellish," with multiply privileged older people holding the most negative views of dementia and multiply marginalized older people largely dismissing its significance. "Othering dementia" refers to the marginalization to which people with dementia are subject: it is shown to be a marked feature of life with dementia and to be connected to social location, with multiply privileged people being othered more often and more marginalized participants demonstrating resilience. "Theorizing dementia" refers to people with dementia actively creating meaning about life with the condition. The outcome of this is shown to relate to social location: only the most privileged participants viewed dementia as a brain disease; all the others made strategic use of normal aging theory to avoid marginalization due to dementia. Through an in-depth exploration of the experiences of a diverse group of older people with dementia, their significant others, and other members of their social worlds, I was able to confirm the connection between social location and subjective experiences of dementia hinted at in published accounts (see Hulko 2002) and to develop a grounded theory as to the nature of these relationships.

Limitations

As the findings reported here are derived from exploratory research with a small sample of community-dwelling older people with dementia, they should be interpreted with caution. Except for their age, the multiply privileged participants in this study were highly similar to those described in the studies discussed above, and they alone viewed dementia in negative terms. However, this finding cannot be generalized to all older people with dementia who share a similar social location. This research demonstrates that, with a diverse sample, only a minority of the views expressed may conform to our present understandings of life with dementia, from the perspectives of people with dementia themselves. Exploratory research of this nature should be replicated in another social context to determine the transferability of

Table 10.1

Socio-demographic characteristics of the main sample

Pseudonym	Age	Gender	Race	Ethnicity	Social class	Cognitive impairment	Social location
Joe Brown	75	Man	Black	African Canadian	Working/lower class	Mild-moderate	In-between
Jim Heather	74	Man	White	New Zealander	Professional/upper class	Mild-moderate	Multiply privileged
Ester Hernandez	76	Woman	Asian	Filipina	Working/lower class	Moderate-severe	Multiply marginalized
Gus Holden	73	Man	White	Anglo-Canadian	Professional /upper class	Mild	Multiply privileged
Angela Huggins	74	Woman	Mixed	Trinidadian	Middle class	Mild	Multiply marginalized
Bosse Knudsen	76	Woman	White	Danish	Middle class	Moderate	In-between
Nancy Matheson	87	Woman	White	Anglo-American	Professional/ upper class	Mild-moderate	Multiply privileged
Julianna Molnar	83	Woman	White	Hungarian Jewish	Middle class	Mild	In-between

the findings, or the findings should be used to inform research with a larger and even more diverse sample to establish generalizability.

Research Participants

The main research participants were eight community-dwelling older people with dementia who ranged from multiply marginalized to multiply privileged on the basis of their ethnicity, gender, class, and race. They were accessed through a hospital outreach program for older people in a large urban centre and an Alzheimer society in a small city, both in central Ontario. The participants were grouped based on the relative amounts of privilege and oppression to which they were likely to be subject due to the unique configurations of racialization, ethnicity, social class, and gender expression in their lives (see Hulko 2004). For example, though Nancy Matheson may appear to be the most privileged participant if one focuses largely on social class, her identity as a woman renders her subject to gender-based oppression, unlike the "dominant and privileged norm citizen: white, heterosexual, middle class, man" (Verloo 2006, 217). All the participants shared a non-normative status due to their disability (Alzheimer's disease or non-specified dementia) and age (the average was seventy-seven years), yet they differed from one another in terms of gender, class, ethnicity, and race. Table 10.1 lists their age, gender, race, ethnicity, social class, degree of cognitive impairment, and identifies each as either multiply marginalized (MM), in-between (IB), or multiply privileged (MP).

Experiencing Dementia: From "Not a Big Deal" to "a Nuisance" to "Hellish"

When I asked the participants what it is like to have this form of cognitive impairment, very few actually described it in the negative terms commonly found in the literature. There was more diversity of opinion, and more importantly, these varying views seemed to be connected to the social locations of the respondents. The more marginalized people dismissed the significance of dementia in their lives, and the more privileged ones confirmed the commonly held belief that dementia is a living hell, as illustrated by the following extract from the second interview with Jim Heather:

> *Interviewer:* Now how, what is it like to have Alzheimer's?
> *Jim Heather:* Hellish.
> *Interviewer:* Hellish?
> *Jim Heather:* Hmm.

For Jim Heather, the world "hellish" summed up his views on living with dementia (see Davis 1989; DeBaggio 2002). In contrast, for Joe Brown, forgetting things was not much of a problem:

Joe Brown: I forget things that I don't wanna remember.
Interviewer: Mm-hmm. But what's that like?
Joe Brown: Don't bother me.
Interviewer: Don't bother you? How come it doesn't bother you?
Joe Brown: I pay my bills, what else I gotta do. What, what else have
   I got to do, what other memory do I got to have?

Among participants who dismissed the significance of having dementia, some brushed it off as age related, and others focused on its lack of impact on their lives; this response was more common among the less privileged. For those who accorded dementia slightly more significance than did Joe Brown, several claimed that their memory problems were not particularly significant, as the things they tended to forget were not that important. For example, Angela Huggins noted that "I don't forget things I'm really interested in," and Nancy Matheson told me that "I always feel that if something's important, I'll remember it. I usually do." Others spoke in terms of a tolerable inconvenience. For example, Bosse Knudsen said, "Yeah, I'm forgetful ... and it's a nuisance."

The two most privileged participants, Jim Heather and Gus Holden, voiced the most pessimistic views of dementia. Heather, a former physician, remarked that it was "awkward knowing that in front of you lies the territory we've never experienced before and that it's getting worse uh, a slippery slope which is um, uh, either you don't know whether it's steep or going to be ... gradual." Gus Holden's views were not quite as negative as those of Jim Heather, yet he clearly identified dementia as a problem in his life: "You can fight it or try to overcome it or step around it, but it's there and it's not as if you can say that 'What a nuisance, I'll push it aside and carry on uh, my regular.' No, you can't, it's just a ... It is a different way of life." Holden claimed that Alzheimer's could not be referred to as a "nuisance," as it is much more significant than that, yet Bosse Knudsen used the word in describing her life with memory problems.

Clearly, real variability characterized participant experiences with dementia. These views were not static, however, as some people moderated them over time, others divulged more feelings as trust increased, and some learned to adapt to the limitations imposed by dementia. The reactions of and interactions with members of their social worlds proved to be important in understanding their subjective experiences of dementia, with all the participants being othered or marginalized to some degree (see Innes, Archibald, and Murphy 2004; The Group Members 2003) and social location affecting the degree to which this occurred, as is seen in the next section.

Othering Dementia: "She Has Dementia You Know"
The type of othering to which this research refers is derived from Simone

de Beauvoir's (1989, xxii) argument that "he is the subject, he is the absolute – she is the Other." To date, dementia studies have produced little discussion of this subject. An associated term – "marginalization" – has been used by both researchers (see Innes, Archibald, and Murphy 2004) and the people with dementia who belonged to an early stage support group (The Group Members 2003). In her taxonomy of the five faces of oppression, Iris Marion Young (1990, 53) explained that "marginalization is perhaps the most dangerous form of oppression [as] a whole category of people is expelled from useful participation in social life." The literature more commonly refers to "the other" and tends to restrict itself to descriptions of those who inhabit this category and what the experience is like for them, rather than explaining the process of othering – how and why one comes to be othered or to other those perceived as others. In this chapter, othering is the analytical lens through which the interactive components of participant experiences are best understood, as well as a material reality of living with dementia.

The silencing and social distancing to which people with dementia are subject occurred in most of the participant observation sessions. When I mentioned these incidents to the participants at follow-up interviews, I found that they were commonly unaware of this othering or actively denied that they had been treated any differently. A few, such as Jim Heather, did reflect on it. His first observation session took place at an airport hangar where his eldest son, Mike, manages one of the family businesses. During the subsequent interview, he acknowledged that he had noticed a change in his interactions with people at the hangar: in the past, they had been "much more free and easy in discussing things with [him] and that sort of thing." He believed that people with dementia should alert those with whom they spoke regarding their newly acquired deficits and disclose their "abnormality." This influenced his actions at the second observation session, which took place at a staff meeting in a clinic owned by Heather and his spouse, Patricia. As he used his position as chair of the meeting to talk about having "Alzheimer's-related problems and Parkinson's," I watched closely to see how staff would react. As can be seen in the notes below, neither the staff nor his spouse responded to his words, much less acknowledged the feelings behind his disclosure; instead, they silenced him and reproduced the othering I had witnessed at the first observation session:

> Jim Heather then talked of his interest in "this place"; about having been on the board for so long; how good it is for him to be "part of the team"; and how he would be upset if he was not able to "have a laugh with people" and "keep up with what people are doing." He ended by saying, with a smile on his face, "it's a sad time, but there you go." After his words, Elaine [staff person] raised the issue of the shredder again and a heated discussion ensued about this; there was neither an acknowledgement of Jim Heather's feelings

nor a response to his words by any of the people present. Jim Heather sat
and watched the action.

In discussing the reactions of the staff during our next interview, Heather
indicated that, having revealed his "abnormality," he could have been asked
to leave or end his involvement with the clinic, but that would have been
an extreme move on their part since he had been around for a long time
and there was no precedent for it.

Ester Hernandez had a much narrower social world than Jim Heather,
with few opportunities for engagement not in some way connected to her
dementia status. I rarely saw her treated as a person, in the sense described
by Tom Kitwood (1997), and not surprisingly, her acts of resistance tended
to be ignored as well. Although she was treated as excessively disabled, she
continually surprised me with her insightful comments, which often went
unheard or were misunderstood. Perhaps they were too unexpected from
an older person with dementia who was thought to lack both insight and
the ability to communicate, particularly in the English language. This was
evident during the "sunroom chatter" activity at the dementia day program
that she attended three days per week, the site of the first observation
session:

> The group leader asked if anyone knew what a "calling card" was and Ester
> said "yes, you give your card and I'll see you." The group leader did not seem
> to grasp the dual meaning of "calling card" so I explained that Ester was
> referring to how in the past you would present your calling card when you
> went to visit someone at their home or office. The group leader said "oh,
> that's a long time ago" in response and clarified this was a card used to make
> a telephone call.
>
> I was impressed by the speed with which Ester Hernandez came up with
> the answer to this question and how well she articulated her understanding
> of the purpose of a "calling card." The group leader was not visibly impressed
> herself, nor did she acknowledge Ester's skilful performance, an act which
> could have increased Ester's status and visibility in the group, yet also could
> have drawn attention to the group leader's own lack of knowledge.

An extreme example of how people with dementia are othered comes
from the second observation session with Bosse Knudsen at a seniors' group
at the Seventh Day Adventist Church to which she and her husband
belonged:

> While Bosse was meandering about, no one spoke to her; in fact they seemed
> to studiously ignore her. One woman came up to me ... and after we talked
> for a few minutes, I told her why I was there. When she noticed me talking

to Bosse, she pulled me aside, gave me a conspiratorial look and confided in me that "you can't talk to her – dementia – she has dementia you know."

Not only was this woman treating Bosse as the Other, but also she felt it her duty to instruct me in the techniques of othering so that I could conform to the practices of the group; my non-compliance disrupted her taken-for-granted assumptions about who should be othered and how this should be done. One other person disobeyed the group sanctions that day: the lay pastor came up to talk to Bosse Knudsen and placed a hand on her shoulder and, in that moment, Bosse Knudsen looked like the "people-person" she purported to be. I did not see anyone else treat Bosse Knudsen as a person (Kitwood 1997; see Baldwin and Capstick 2007) during the three hour session which included a presentation, discussion and lunch.

Angela Huggins was aware of the othering practices adopted by her daughter Ashley, which made her feel like "a decrepit old lady," particularly Ashley's newly adopted habit of referring to her as Gramma: "And – and now she calls me Gramma. And it aggravates me no end! In the store, 'Gramma!' And I don't answer. And everybody's looking, 'Where's Gramma?' You know? I mean, good God call me mommy!" When I asked if she had told Ashley how she felt about being called Gramma, Huggins said, "Several times but she forgets. I feel like a decrepit little old lady, with a little cane you know coming down the street. Good Lord!"

Many participants felt that the members of their self-identified communities did not treat them differently due to their memory problems, and for some this was indeed the case. As I accompanied Joe Brown on a typical walk around his neighbourhood, none of the people with whom he interacted treated him as a person with an abnormality. Being treated as the other did not figure strongly in the observation sessions with Julianna Molnar either. Angela Huggins and Ester Hernandez were not fully aware of being treated differently due to their dementia status but were both clearly aware of othering processes in relation to racialization, ethnicity, and age. Huggins called herself "just a beginning Alzheimer's patient ... not way back on the list," and she strenuously rejected the idea that she would be treated differently as her dementia progressed: "No, no, no ... no ... I'll be treated differently here [small city] because they think I'm a Black person, but as far as any other thing, no, no."

Othering occurred frequently in the participants' lives, though it was more often observed and captured in photographs than commented on by the participants. This section has presented only a small portion of the rich research data on othering, yet it is enough to show that the more privileged participants were othered to a greater extent than those who were marginalized in more than one domain, apart from dementia. It could be argued that the othering to which Bosse Knudsen and Ester Hernandez were subject was at least as pronounced as that accorded Jim Heather, as is the impression given by the data. However, these two women were the most cognitively impaired participants; therefore, one would expect them to be othered more often and to a greater extent, as marginalization or social exclusion is a feature of life with dementia (see Innes, Archibald, and Murphy 2004; The Group Members 2003; Wilkinson 2002).

The degree to which participants were subject to othering as a result of their dementia status varied by social location, in much the same way as experiencing dementia differed for this diverse group. This can be explained in part by the performance expectations of the participants' self-identified communities: the more privileged participants were pathologized for displaying any cognitive deficits whatsoever, no matter how minor, whereas their more marginalized counterparts seemed to be benefiting from a more expansive definition of "normal" within their communities and more tolerance for "slippage." This is related to the concept of resilience, as will be discussed below.

Theorizing Dementia: "Straight from the Horse's Mouth"

During my third and final interview with Angela Huggins, I tried to explain my rationale for talking directly to people with dementia. When I said, "So we need to find out what the experiences have been like," she finished my sentence with "straight from the horse's mouth." In explaining what was happening to them, the participants offered two theories regarding dementia – that it is a brain disease and that it is part of normal aging. Only the two most privileged participants – Gus Holden and Jim Heather – both of whom were white Western upper-class men, believed dementia to be a disease. Jim Heather referred to Alzheimer's as a "strange disease" and expressed a strong belief that "within probably two to five years, they'll uh, this will be a disease that, the Alzheimer part of it, will be, will be able to be conquered." Holden gave the following explanation for his Alzheimer's: "Well, uh, it's cancer of certain uh [intake of breath], systems in my body. That, that's not word for word but uh, that's what uh I was told." Although he used the language of cancer, rather than brain disease, he clearly saw dementia as a pathological state, not a normal part of aging. When I questioned Jim Heather about his use of the word "slipping" in reference to his awareness of the signs and symptoms of dementia, he explained that this was a euphemism for being on "a path of decline" and that he'd used it in the past when talking about his own patients: "For example, person with cancer and um, it, it's a euphemism I suppose to describe a patient's um, being on the slippery slope."

In contrast, every participant who was marginalized on at least one domain, whether race, ethnicity, class, or gender, invoked the "normal aging theory" – the belief that dementia is a natural part of the aging process – to explain the cause of their memory problems. This is exemplified by the following quote from Angela Huggins; during the first interview, when I asked her why this [Alzheimer's] was happening to her, she said, "I just think I'm getting older and, and I just, my memory isn't as good as it was 'cause my mother was just the same ... and nobody thought of putting her in an institution or anything like that."

She later noted, "It's not like I have cancer or something like that, you know. It's just, it's just uh, it's just, just a thing that happens when you're getting older." When I tried to ascertain whether she felt that dementia mattered in her life, she pointed out that "old age" posed more challenges than dementia: "It's not something I'm ashamed of or anything like that. I, I don't really think it matters ... It's more the old age that is bothering me because I can't keep up, I can't run, like I say I can't go dancing, you know, this type of thing." As noted above, racialization may have been a more significant factor in this participant's life, though certainly her disability, age, and gender could not be easily separated from each other, as seen in her earlier comment about feeling like "a decrepit old lady."

Nancy Matheson, who was the only multiply privileged woman in the sample and who usually chose to assert her individuality and incomparability, employed the normal aging theory to align herself with other older people. Doing so enabled her to assert her status as a "normal older person": "But it [dementia] doesn't bother me because I think it happens to everyone, you know." Joe Brown also felt that aging brought changes to which we need to adjust – "every dog has its day" – and that his age-related memory loss was not particularly significant, because, "I don't forget to pay my rent, to pay the hydro, etc. I eat, I sleep. Listen, dear, I'm 75 years old. Life's not the same when you're older."

Like Jim Heather, Julianna Molnar was a former physician, but whereas he subscribed to the pathological view of dementia – or brain disease theory – she referenced normal aging and drew on her medical credentials to legitimate her view of dementia as part of normal aging: "I know very well, I was a doctor. I know well that at a certain age, there are certain things that are forgotten and your brain [is] not working as it used to. For at a certain level, at a certain level, I think it's normal but I don't feel good about it."

As has been shown, only those two participants who were not marginalized due to their gender, race, class, or ethnicity held the view that dementia is a disease state or pathological. The others adhered to the idea that dementia was a normal aspect of aging, and there were indications that this constituted a tactic to decrease their marginalization as people with dementia. This section has also demonstrated that they were active meaning makers, who engaged in theorizing about dementia – what it is and why they had developed it. The next section discusses the insights gained from using an intersectionality and interlocking oppressions paradigm in research on dementia in later life.

The Dynamics of Privilege and Oppression

Social location clearly affects how one views dementia and how one lives with it. Although studies are emerging that focus on socio-culturally diverse older people with dementia and actually solicit their views rather than emphasizing those of caregivers or service providers, the tendency has been to isolate one identity factor, such as gender (Proctor 2001), sexual orientation (Price 2008; Ward et al. 2005), and race or ethnicity (see O'Connor et al. 2010). Power in relationships and feelings of powerlessness were central themes in Gillian Proctor's (2001) interviews with four older women with dementia in a day hospital, but it is unclear whether the power dynamics were related to their gender or their membership in a traditionally disempowered group.

My research revealed that the participants could not be essentialized or reduced to certain aspects of their identities in order to make sense of their varied perspectives on living with dementia, despite some suggestions of a gendered response to it. My tentative finding that men may attempt to control their dementia and be upfront about it, whereas women may be more likely to accept and mask it, is an area for future exploration. This would entail a sample with a greater proportion of men and would assess not only gender identity but also gender expression. However, separating gender from other aspects of identity would be inconsistent with an intersectionality approach, which was key to understanding the dynamics of privilege and oppression in the lives of this diverse group of older adults with dementia, rather than the specific identity categories to which they belonged. In other words, intersectionality was key to understanding the phenomenon of dementia and the ways in which it was subjectively experienced, not the specific identity categories themselves.

This study builds on Proctor's (2001) findings in that it shows the linkages across various forms of oppression and privilege, and how individuals' social location, which may be multiply marginalized, multiply privileged, or somewhere in between, can shape their experience of living with dementia. That is, the dynamics of privilege and oppression may be "structuring and destructuring the disease's developmental order" (Gubrium 1987, 20), as opposed to the particular identity category itself. Holding negative views of dementia may have more to do with how much privilege is afforded the particular social group(s) to which one belongs than with the fact that one is a man, or white, or majority ethnic, or upper middle class. The key factor is the power associated with these subject positions – in a particular time and place (see Hulko 2009b).

The concept of resilience also proved important in understanding why the more marginalized participants appeared to be the least frequently othered and did not see dementia as particularly problematic. In the literature on marginalized or oppressed peoples, "resilience" refers to an *acquired* rather than an *innate* survival mechanism that results from experiencing discrimination due to membership in a particular social group (see Brotman, Ryan, and Cormier 2003; Holstein and Minkler 2003; Kirmayer, Brass, and Tait 2000). Defined in this way, resilience captures the strengths and resources of marginalized communities that tend to be buried or overlooked in the multiple jeopardies tradition and other expressions of a "deficit-thinking mentality" (Minkler 1996), as numerous critical gerontologists have argued (see Calasanti 1996; Dressel 1991; Dressel, Minkler, and Yen 1997; Holstein and Minkler 2003; McMullin 2000; Minkler 1996).

It may well be that those who have experienced discrimination or disadvantage on the basis of racialization, gender identity, ethnic group membership, and/or socio-economic status are able to apply this resilience to their lives when they develop dementia. In this way, dementia becomes one more hurdle to overcome, just another thing to get on with, or "not a big deal." Unfortunately, family members and health care providers tend to interpret this response to dementia as indicating lack of insight or awareness, rather than an expression of resiliency in the face of adversity. It is possible, however, that resilience and lessons learned from comparable experiences of marginalization throughout the life course may be used to overcome marginalization due to dementia – strategically invoking normal aging to position oneself as a "normal" person.

Conclusions and Implications for Future Research
Several conclusions can be drawn from these findings. First, asking people about their experiences of living with a disabling condition such as dementia can generate rich data that not only challenge our existing knowledge base but also lead us toward a deeper and more complex understanding of the condition. It is possible and extremely valuable to undertake these sorts of investigations, both for the researchers and the researched, as has been argued convincingly (see Allan 2001; Dewing 2007; Hubbard, Downs, and Tester 2003; Reid, Ryan, and Enderby 2001; Wilkinson 2002). Moreover, it is possible to discuss complex and nebulous topics such as identity and social location with older people with dementia, and to yield significant insights. Although socio-culturally diverse older people with dementia may not use the language of intersectionality, their words and behaviours clearly indicate the relevance/applicability of this concept.

Second, the problematization of dementia occurs within a social and political context; it is not transmitted to and/or integrated into the "illness narratives" of all people with dementia in an identical fashion. The extent to which dementia is conceptualized as a problem varies; not all those who live with it view it as problematic, which appears to be related to the social location of the affected individual. This study suggests that the more privileged a person, the more likely she or he will be to view dementia in a negative light; and the more marginalized an individual, the more likely she or he will be to dismiss the significance of dementia and resist being viewed as the sum of her/his symptoms. Future research should aim to confirm these theoretical propositions through establishing transferability to other social contexts and/or generalizability based on a larger and more diverse sample.[2]

Lastly, the data clearly show that diversity makes a difference. When we expand the pool of respondents by factoring in "race," ethnicity, class, and gender, the resulting picture of life with dementia is bound to be more nuanced and complex, as it was in this research. Future research needs to consider these and other identity factors not addressed in this study, such as sexual orientation, age gradations (such as fifty to sixty-four years, sixty-five to seventy-nine years, and eighty to ninety-four years), (dis)ability, and faith, as these also form components of an intersectionality and interlocking oppressions paradigm, and are often overlooked (see Hulko 2009b). Intersectionality should be used as a theoretical lens and a metaphor for the interaction of complex and intertwined identity constructs; however, it should be introduced to research participants with caution, as it can be alienating to those whose life it is meant to capture.

Not only must we acknowledge that older people with dementia may conceptualize their experiences differently from one another, but we also need to consider the probability that their views and preoccupations will vary according to social location. Applying intersectionality to the context of their experiences draws attention to the differential amounts of privilege and oppression to which older persons with dementia are subject in their daily lives, irrespective of their shared identity as "persons with dementia," and challenges commonly held assumptions about life with a disabling condition such as this.

Notes

1   The family members included four opposite-sex spouses (two male, two female), three adult daughters, and one adult niece.

2   I recently completed grounded theory research on dementia with First Nation elders in British Columbia (Hulko et al. 2010) during which we assessed the transferability of this theory of dementia and intersectionality through the grounded theory method of "emergent fit" (Glaser 1978). We determined that this theory could not be used to explain the views of Secwepemc Nation elders on memory loss and memory care in later life, which underscores the unique nature of Indigenous knowledge and ways of life.

References

Allan, K. 2001. *Communication and consultation: Exploring ways for staff to involve people with dementia in developing services.* Bristol, UK: Policy Press.

Baldwin, C., and A. Capstick, eds. 2007. *Tom Kitwood on dementia: A reader and critical commentary.* Maidenhead, UK: Open University Press.

Bannerji, H. 1995. *Thinking through: Essays on feminism, Marxism, and anti-racism.* Toronto: Women's Press.

Becker, H. 1974. Photography and sociology. *Studies in the Anthropology of Visual Communication* 1(1): 1-19.

Brah, A., and A. Phoenix. 2004. Ain't I a woman?: Revisiting intersectionality. *Journal of International Women's Studies* 5(3): 75-86.

Brotman, S. 1998. The incidence of poverty among seniors in Canada: Exploring the impact of gender, ethnicity and race. *Canadian Journal on Aging* 17(2): 166-85.

Brotman, S., B. Ryan, and B. Cormier. 2003. The health and social service needs of gay and lesbian elders and their families in Canada. *Gerontologist* 43(2): 192-202.

Brown, L., and S. Strega, eds. 2005. *Research as resistance: Critical, indigenous and anti-oppressive approaches.* Toronto: Canadian Scholars' Press.

Calasanti, T. 1996. Incorporating diversity: Meaning, levels of research, and implications for theory. *Gerontologist* 36(2): 147-56.

Charmaz, K. 2000. Grounded theory: Objectivist and constructivist methods. In *Handbook of qualitative research.* 2nd ed., ed. N.K. Denzin and Y.S. Lincoln, 509-35. Thousand Oaks, CA: Sage.

—. 2002. Qualitative interviewing and grounded theory analysis. In *Handbook of interview research: Context and method,* ed. J.F. Gubrium and J.A. Holstein, 675-94. Thousand Oaks, CA: Sage.

—. 2006. *Constructing grounded theory: A practical guide through qualitative analysis.* Thousand Oaks, CA: Sage.

Collins, P.H. 2000. *Black feminist thought: Knowledge, consciousness and the politics of empowerment.* 2nd ed. New York: Routledge.

Combahee River Collective. 1983. The Combahee River Collective Statement. In *Home girls: A black feminist anthology,* ed. Barbara Smith, 264-74. New York: Kitchen Table: Women of Colour Press, 1977.

Crenshaw, K.W. 1989. Demarginalizing the intersection of race and sex: A black feminist critique of antidiscrimination doctrine, feminist theory and antiracist politics. University of Chicago Legal Forum, 139-67.

—. 1994. Mapping the margins: Intersectionality, identity politics, and violence against women of color. In *The public nature of private violence,* ed. M.A. Fineman and R. Mykitiuk, 93-118. New York: Routledge.

Davis, R. 1989. *My journey into Alzheimer's disease.* Bucks, IL: Scripture Press.

DeBaggio, T. 2002. *Losing my mind: An intimate look at life with Alzheimer's.* New York: Free Press.

De Beauvoir, S. 1989. *The second sex.* Trans. H.M. Parshley. London: Vintage.

De Vault, M.L. 1999. *Liberating method: Feminism and social research.* Philadelphia: Temple University Press.

Dewing, J. 2002. From ritual to relationship: A person-centred approach to consent in qualitative research with older people who have a dementia. *Dementia* 1(2): 57-171.

—. 2007. Participatory research: A method for process consent with persons who have dementia. *Dementia* 6(1): 11-25.

Downs, M. 1997. The emergence of the person in dementia research. *Ageing and Society* 17: 597-607.

Dressel, P. 1991. Gender, race and class: Beyond the feminization of poverty in later life. In *Critical perspectives on aging: The political and moral economy of growing old,* ed. M. Minkler and C. Estes, 245-52. Amityville, NY: Baywood.

Dressel, P., M. Minkler, and I. Yen. 1997. Gender, race, class, and aging: Advances and opportunities. *International Journal of Health Services* 27(4): 579-600.

Fine, M., L. Weis, S. Weseen, and L. Wong. 2000. For whom? Qualitative research, representations and social responsibilities. In *Handbook of qualitative research.* 2nd ed., ed. N.K. Denzin and Y.S. Lincoln, 107-31. Thousand Oaks, CA: Sage.

Glaser, B.G. 1978. *Theoretical sensitivity: Advances in the methodology of grounded theory.* Mill Valley, CA: Sociology Press.

Glaser, B.G., and A.L. Strauss. 1967. *The discovery of grounded theory: Strategies for qualitative research.* New York: Aldine.

Grady, J. 2001. Becoming a visual sociologist. *Sociological Imagination* 38(1-2): 83-119.

The Group Members. 2003. Reflections of an early stage memory loss support group for persons with Alzheimer's and their family members. *Alzheimer's Care Quarterly* 4(3): 185-88.

Gubrium, J. 1987. Structuring and destructuring the course of illness: The Alzheimer's disease experience. *Sociology of Health and Illness* 9(1): 1-24.

Hancock, A.-M. 2007. When multiplication doesn't equal quick addition: Examining intersectionality as a research paradigm. *Perspectives on Politics* 5(1): 63-79.

Harman, G., and L. Clare. 2006. Illness representations and lived experience in early-stage dementia. *Qualitative Health Research* 16(4): 484-502.

Harper, D. 2000. Reimagining visual materials: Galileo to Neuromancer. In *Handbook of qualitative research.* 2nd ed., ed. N.K. Denzin and Y.S. Lincoln, 717-32. Thousand Oaks, CA: Sage.

Hockey, J., and A. James. 1993. *Growing up and growing old: Aging and dependency in the life course.* London: Sage.

Holstein, M.B., and M. Minkler. 2003. Self, society and the "new gerontology." *Gerontologist* 43(6): 787-96.

Hopkins, P., and R. Pain. 2007. Geographies of age: Thinking relationally. *Area* 39(3): 287-94.

Hubbard, G., A. Cook, S. Tester, and M. Downs. 2002. Beyond words: Older people with dementia using and interpreting nonverbal behaviour. *Journal of Aging Studies* 16: 155-67.

Hubbard, G., M. Downs, and S. Tester. 2003. Including people with dementia in research: Challenges and strategies. *Aging and Mental Health* 7(5): 351-62.

Hulko, W. 2002. Making the links: Social theories, experiences of people with dementia, and intersectionality. In *The diversity of Alzheimer's disease: Different approaches and contexts,* ed. A. Leibing and L. Scheinkman, 231-64. Rio de Janeiro: CUCA-IPUB.

–. 2004. Social science perspectives on dementia research: Intersectionality. In *Dementia and social inclusion: Marginalised groups and marginalised areas of care in dementia research, policy and practice,* ed. A. Innes, C. Archibald, and C. Murphy, 237-54. London: Jessica Kingsley.

–. 2009a. From "not a big deal" to "hellish": Experiences of older people with dementia. *Journal of Aging Studies* 23(3): 131-44.

–. 2009b. The time- and context-contingent nature of intersectionality and interlocking oppressions. *Affilia: Journal of Women and Social Work* 24(1): 44-55.

Hulko, W., E. Camille, E. Antifeau, M. Arnouse, N. Bachynksi, and D. Taylor. 2010. Views of First Nation elders on memory loss and memory care in later life. *Journal of Cross Cultural Gerontology* 25: 317-42. Online First, 1 July 2010.

Innes, A., C. Archibald, and C. Murphy, eds. 2004. *Dementia and social inclusion: Marginalised groups and marginalised areas of dementia research, care and practice.* London: Jessica Kingsley.

Kirby, S., L. Greaves, and C. Reid. 2006. Experience, research, social change: Methods beyond the mainstream. 2nd ed. Peterborough: Broadview Press.

Kirmayer, L.J., G.M. Brass, and C.L. Tait. 2000. The mental health of Aboriginal people: Transformation of identity and community. *Canadian Journal of Psychiatry* 45(7): 607-16.

Kitwood, T. 1997. *Dementia reconsidered: The person comes first.* Buckingham, UK: Open University Press.

Kleinman, A. 1988. *The illness narratives: Suffering, healing and the human condition.* New York: Basic Books.

Krekula, C. 2007. The intersection of age and gender: Reworking gender theory and social gerontology. *Current Sociology* 55(2): 155-71.

Lambert, H., and C. McKevitt. 2002. Anthropology in health research: From qualitative methods to multidisciplinarity. *British Medical Journal* 325: 210-13.

Lather, P. 1991. *Getting smart: Feminist research and pedagogy with/in the postmodern.* New York: Routledge.

Lorde, A. 2007. Age, race, class and sex: Women redefining difference. In A. Lorde, *Sister outsider: Essays and speeches by Audre Lorde,* 114-23. Berkeley: Crossing Press, 1984.

Mama, A. 1995. Researching subjectivity. In A. Mama, *Beyond the masks: Race, gender and subjectivity,* 65-88. London: Routledge.

Marshall, M., and M.-A. Tibbs. 2006. *Social work and people with dementia: Partnerships, practice and persistence.* 2nd ed. Bristol, UK: Policy Press.

McMullin, J. 2000. Diversity and the state of sociological aging theory. *Gerontologist* 40(5): 517-30.

Minkler, M. 1996. Critical perspectives on ageing: New challenges for gerontology. *Ageing and Society* 16: 467-87.

O'Connor, D., S.-M. Chan, W. Hulko, L. Stern, and M. Yan. 2010. Contextualizing dementia: Conceptualizing culture. Manuscript under revision for *Journal of Aging Studies*.

O'Connor, D., A. Phinney, and W. Hulko. 2010. Dementia at the intersections: A unique case study exploring social location. *Journal of Aging Studies* 24(1): 30-39.

O'Connor, D., A. Phinney, A. Smith, J. Small, B. Purves, J. Perry, E. Drance, M. Donnelly, H. Chaudhury, and L. Beattie. 2007. Personhood in dementia care: Developing a research agenda for broadening the vision. *Dementia* 6(1): 121-42.

Price, E. 2008. Pride or prejudice? Gay men, lesbians and dementia. *British Journal of Social Work* 38(7): 1337-52.

Proctor, G. 2001. Listening to older women with dementia: Relationships, voices and power. *Disability and Society* 16(3): 361-76.

Prosser, J., and D. Schwartz. 1998. Photographs within the sociological research process. In *Image based research,* ed. J. Prosser, 115-30. London: Falmer Press.

Reid, D., T. Ryan, and P. Enderby. 2001. What does it mean to include people with dementia? *Disability and Society* 16(3): 377-92.

Seman, D. 2002. Meaningful communication throughout the journey: Clinical observations. In *The person with Alzheimer's disease: Pathways to understanding the experience,* ed. P. Braudy Harris, 134-49. Baltimore: Johns Hopkins University Press.

Steeman, E., B. Dierckx de Casterlé, J. Godderis, and M. Grypdonck. 2006. Living with early stage dementia: A review of qualitative studies. *Journal of Advanced Nursing* 54(6): 722-38.

Verloo, M. 2006. Multiple inequalities, intersectionality and the European Union. *European Journal of Women's Studies* 13(3): 211-28.

Ward, R., A. Vass, N. Aggarwal, C. Garfield, and C. Beau. 2005. A kiss is still a kiss? The construction of sexuality in dementia care. *Dementia* 4(1): 49-72.

Wenger, C. 2002. Interviewing older people. In *Handbook of interview research: Context and method,* ed., J.F. Gubrium and J.A. Holstein, 259-78. Thousand Oaks, CA: Sage.

Wilkinson, H., ed. 2002. *The perspectives of people with dementia: Research methods and motivations.* London: Jessica Kingsley.

Young, I.M. 1990. Five faces of oppression. In I.M. Young, *Justice and the politics of difference,* 39-65. Princeton: Princeton University Press.

Part 3
Social Context, Policy, and Health
Edited by Bilkis Vissandjée and Olena Hankivsky

11

An Intersectional Lens on Various Facets of Violence: Access to Health and Social Services for Women with Precarious Immigration Status

Jacqueline Oxman-Martinez and Jill Hanley

In this chapter, we shall explore the use of the concepts of systemic and structural violence in developing an intersectional understanding of health inequities for women of precarious immigration status. Our theoretical reflections, and the feminization of migration with precarious status, lead us to focus our essay on women as a heterogeneous group from a migration policy perspective. Health system inequities arise from the intersection of, on the one hand, unequal power relations between women with and without permanent immigration status (who also have varying social statuses based on age, gender, race, and so on), and, on the other hand, the different legal frameworks that govern the health systems in Canada's provinces and territories.[1] Obstacles that hinder access to the health system constitute facets of what we would argue is "systemic violence," a violence that is rooted within the public health and social service system, and that victimizes women with precarious immigration status. We define "structural violence" as the physical and psychological harm inflicted on these women by the socioeconomic inequalities intrinsic to Western capitalist economic and political structures. The links between processes of migration and the risk of violence and exploitation faced by immigrant women of precarious status are well established (Hanley and Shragge 2009; Hughes et al. 2007; Spitzer et al. 2004-8). In this analysis, the violence that is exercised by the state when there is a lack of access to health and social services for these women is deemed inadvertent because we assume it is not part of the legislative rationale.

This chapter is developed as follows. A first section discusses the feminization of international migration and, more specifically, the health and social service experiences of women migrants to Canada. We explore the policy framework shaping these experiences, the academic research on the topic, and the NGO perspectives on access to health and social services. Building on this, we propose a theoretical framework that weaves the concepts of systemic and structural violence into a macro and global approach to intersectionality. In conclusion, we argue that an intersectional approach will reveal how precarious immigration status intersects with systemic and socio-structural factors to result in the forms of violence studied and propose some new orientations to policies, practice, and research related to precarious status women migrants' access to health and social services.

Context of Women's Migration to Canada

In recent decades, armed conflicts, religious persecutions, and the ideological construction of the "security-terrorism" binary – reinforced around the world by the 11 September 2001 attacks (Measuring Security Measures Tour 2005) – have contributed to an increase of migrants who have fled their countries of origin and now find themselves part of the diverse Canadian reality yet hold a wide range of immigration statuses. Canada has also seen a feminization of migration, particularly in its more precarious immigration statuses, under which, for example, women are far more often classified as "dependants" than are men. This current Canadian reality creates situations that were not taken into account when health and social service policies and programs were originally conceived; these include the presence of refugees, trafficked human beings, temporary workers, and sponsored family members from various cultural backgrounds and with complex needs. As noted by Aarti Iyer, Gita Sen, and Piroska Östlin (2008), in general, and Halime Celik et al. (2008, 65), in particular, "current healthcare practices are structured in ways that support the neutral approach and keep dimensions of diversity invisible and hidden." Through the configuration of its socio-political and economic framework, Canada creates variations in access (not only to health and social services, but also to housing and stable jobs) according to gender, sex, language ability, ethnicity, religion, social location in the family, and other variables.[2]

Precariousness, meaning the lack of permanent residency and/or dependency on a third person for status (most often a family member or employer), is experienced differently depending on gender, age, race, ethnicity, religion, language, social location, and the health and/or migration path used (Oxman-Martinez and Lapierre Vincent 2002). Federal immigration policies foster the development of specific programs to fill low-paid, low-skilled jobs rejected by Canadians. Recent longitudinal studies have shown that, in terms of socio-economic integration, those who migrated to Canada since approximately 1990 have fared less well than those who came earlier (Statistics Canada 2006), a fact that has added to concerns about the Canadian immigration system. We must ask, therefore, if those whose status is secure have fared poorly in the last two decades, what of those with less than secure status? To be clear, we seek not to examine their economic success but merely their access to those services that are their basic human rights: health and social services.[3]

A significant number of immigration categories can be considered "precarious" in that they fail to confer the permanent right to remain in Canada and/or they are dependent on a third party such as a spouse or employer. These include refugee claimants, refugee claimants whose claims have been accepted but whose work permits and other Canadian documents have not yet been issued, temporary workers, sponsored family members, victims of human trafficking, and undocumented persons (those whose papers have expired or who entered Canada illegally).[4]

We observe an increasing proportion of precarious status migrants versus those with permanent status (permanent residents). According to Citizenship and Immigration Canada data (CIC 2007b), 236,758 permanent residents were admitted to Canada in 2007 (122,779 women and 113,979 men) versus 797,932 temporary residents (355,169 women and 442,763 men). This perhaps surprising difference is linked to the growth and implementation of sizable temporary work programs as well as restrictive migratory policies that reduce the length of stay in Canada and promote differential access to services (DeVoretz 2008). These figures are provided to indicate the size of the problem. Whereas 122,415 women in the temporary resident group are in Canada legally as temporary workers, most are asylum seekers, under a humanitarian order, foreign students, and others. Moreover, 4 percent of permanent residents (through regular migration) are dependent on a third party, which means that they too have a form of precarious status (CIC 2007b).[5] In general, the insecurity and dependence of these statuses make migrant women more vulnerable to violence than Canadian women with permanent status (Oxman-Martinez and Krane 2005; Krane, Oxman-Martinez, and Ducey 2001).

Exclusion of this vulnerable population from health and social services is currently framed by laws, policies, and programs at the federal and provincial levels of government. We have reviewed the Canadian scientific journals and grey literature on the immigration policies that place women under the broad umbrella of this precariousness. Many authors concur that specific immigration programs such as the Live-In Caregiver Program (LCP), the Seasonal Agricultural Workers Program (SAWP), the Low Skill Pilot Project (LSPP), family sponsorship programs, and the refugee protection system place women under this umbrella (Choudry et al. 2009; Hanley et al. 2006).

Access to Health and Social Services
The literature, including our own work, highlights the necessity of understanding how precarious immigration status intersects with systemic and socio-structural factors to result in systemic and structural violence, exacerbating the exclusion and social isolation of immigrant women in Canadian society. Although authors sometimes cite other areas of rights in their analysis, their focus remains on health and social services because of their

impact on individuals' general state of well-being. Previous research findings (Oxman-Martinez et al. 2005) concluded that precariousness has a differential impact on health according to gender, age, class, and ethnicity. Canadian work on the topic is expanding, and research in other countries has established a relationship between immigration status and access to and/or use of health services (Carmel 2001; Meyerowitz et al. 2000; Sudha and Mutran 2001).

As Margaret Whitehead (1991, 219) points out, national health policies, which are thought to serve the whole population, generally do not address the concerns of vulnerable sections of society. Migrants with precarious status are exposed "to unhealthy, stressful living and working conditions" yet experience difficulties in accessing essential health and other public services. Whitehead's (ibid., 221) definition of "equity" indicates that "equal access to available care for equal need implies equal entitlement to the available services for everyone." This definition extends equity to all temporary foreign workers, who are contributing to the growth of the country. Yet, in all the geographic areas where they live and work, these population segments face systemic barriers to accessing health services. Lack of access and the inability to use health and social services are related to precarious migratory status and intersecting underlying factors such as income, race, gender, dependency on a third person, age, or religion (Oxman-Martinez and Hanley 2007; Oxman-Martinez et al. 2005).

These health differentials are avoidable through a better and more universal health system, as stated by the World Health Organization (2007, 1).[6] In general, if one conceives of health as a key human rights issue, lack of access to it is a form of systemic violence. Governments have a responsibility regarding their people's health that can be fulfilled by the provision of adequate health and social measures: accessibility is among the five fundamental principles of Canada's health care system (Justice Canada 2003). Although Canada ranks among the top nations in the world in terms of health standards, these are not shared equally by all sectors of Canadian society (Bowen 2001).

NGO Perspectives

Canadian NGOs and community groups have taken positions on immigration and social policy issues, often directly related to specific programs that affect migrants of precarious status. Their reports and publications examine social policy according to its consequences in the lives of asylum seekers, victims of trafficking, seasonal agricultural workers, and live-in caregivers.[7] Though these reports do not analyze their information through the lens of systemic violence, they do highlight the negative and cumulative effects of public policy and practice on migrants' well-being.

In its submission to the Standing Committee on Human Resources, Social Development and the Status of Persons with Disabilities, KAIROS (2006) outlines the impact of the SAWP and the LCP on migrant workers. Due to the provisions of the SAWP, the government cannot enforce the labour laws that affect SAWP workers; nor can the workers collectively demand improvements in their working conditions. These problems are created by program regulations that allow the workers to be employed only by the employer mentioned on their visa and that force them to live on the employer's property. Workers are subject to abuse without recourse, as they can be fired and deported by their employer without review. Similarly, the LCP is critiqued for placing women in environments that foster exploitation (ibid.; Oxman-Martinez, Hanley, and Cheung 2004).

The Future Group (2006) argues that current legislation on human trafficking in Canada negatively affects trafficked persons in various ways, documenting that they are routinely detained and often deported from Canada. Their condition as victims of trafficking does not make them automatically eligible for refugee status, and until recently, they were not provided with any government-funded medical, psychological, or counselling support. It is important to note that since June and September 2007, they were eligible to obtain protection for periods of 120 and 180 days respectively under a temporary resident permit (CIC 2007a, 2008). Bill S-218, submitted by Senator Gerald Phelan, proposes a modification of the Immigration and Refugee Protection Act (IRPA) that would allow victims to stay in the country for three years, after which, under certain conditions, they may become permanent residents. In "Coming to Dance" (LACEV 2002), Mujer's coalition studied migrant "exotic" dancers and found that their working conditions and emotional well-being depended on, and dramatically changed according to, their immigration status and recruitment procedures. Women with temporary working visas experienced physical, sexual, and psychological abuse, as well as human rights violations.[8]

In "The Role of NGOs in Health Care Services for Immigrants and Refugees," the CCR (Canadian Council for Refugees) and the City of Toronto Public Health Department (1999) summarized their presentations at the fourth International Metropolis Conference. These proceedings point to a number of factors of isolation and exclusion suffered by migrants vis-à-vis the health care system, including lack of confidence in accessing health care and high rates of diagnosis of mental health problems. Women migrants with precarious status have not been studied extensively in relation to domestic violence, although the Latin American Coalition to End Violence against Women and Children (LACEV 2000) demonstrates how women of dependent status who must rely on their spouse or another family member suffer greatly from it, particularly as their experience is compounded by the isolation and exclusion occasioned by the migratory experience and by the precariousness of their status.

The CCR has documented a series of policy failures that negatively affect and socially exclude precarious status migrants (see, for example, CCR 2005, 2006a). The CCR (2006a) has also denounced the fact that processing fees for permanent resident applications have a discriminatory impact on certain groups on the basis of property and social status. The CCR indicates that persons without permanent resident status in Canada suffer from systemic discrimination in three fundamental areas: the right to family reunification (see also CCR 2004), the right to non-discrimination in the provision of government benefits and services, and the right of workers to organize and bargain collectively. Through case studies, the CCR reports the social effects of such exclusion and critiques the Canadian government policy regarding persons from moratorium countries (CCR 2006b).[9]

The following three excerpts, drawn from the fifty-one interviews conducted with former live-in caregivers as part of a 2004-8 study, illustrate the links between migration programs and risks of violence as well as exploitation (Spitzer et al. 2004-8). Live-in caregivers experience diverse forms of systemic and structural violence as well as painful sequels to them. Furthermore, the inherent violence of the system and the direct violence of employers are highlighted. Ultimately, we observe the prejudice that caused the physical and psychological isolation described by these female workers. Participant 2, a woman from Singapore who looked after three children in Beaconsfield, said, "I arrived here at March; in June I fall down the stairs and hit the top of my head. After that, they give me the receipt and I have to wait for my Medicare card. There's no way initially to get access to services because I didn't have my Medicare yet and I had to pay for that. It was a hundred sixty-eight."

Participant 4, who was from the Philippines and who worked in the outskirts of Montreal, spoke about her employer's behaviour when she herself became ill: "In my case, she doesn't allow me to get sick. She said that 'you're not allowed to get sick.' And so even though you're not feeling well, you still have to do that, you still have to work." She added, "You are sick and you are all alone, you can do whatever you want, like crying the whole day. It is really depressing but now whenever it happens, I tell myself, 'Hey, hey, stop it; you are doing it again; you have to think about something else.'"

These excerpts offer an overview of the reality facing women of precarious immigration status in trying to access Canadian health and social services. Awareness and knowledge around this issue are growing, as is the desire to address it in practice. In terms of research, however, we argue that it is necessary to propose a theoretical framework that intertwines the traditionally analyzed variables of this important issue with the concepts of systemic and structural violence.

Theoretical Framework of Intersectionality in Health Research and Policy

Intersectional theory has revealed the differing experiences of oppression by individuals within a group. Here we discuss how the intersectional approach to oppression is useful from a group perspective, adding the argument that a consideration of macro processes and the global economic framework is essential in understanding migrant experiences. As well, the concepts of systemic and structural violence are put forth as useful to the analysis of access to health and social services by women of precarious status.

Contemporary Canadian literature offers several theoretical approaches to migration. Theories relevant to this chapter include systemic and structural violence examined through the lens of an intersectional approach of oppression. Nira Yuval-Davis (2006, 195) states that "intersecting social divisions are used for political, legal and policy purposes at the different analytic levels in which intersectionality is located." She makes a case against the so-called triple oppression approach, affirming that there is no such thing as suffering from oppression "as Black," "as a woman," and "as a working-class person," arguing that each social division has a different ontological basis, which is irreducible to other social divisions. This matter transcends ontological queries in relation to the existing social divisions, and the ways they are dealt with, regarding specific forms of discrimination. It is relevant to note the presence of an amalgamation between vectors of discrimination as well as differences in identity groupings (ibid., 203).

The differential power relationships experienced by various identity groups in specific historical contexts remain largely unexamined. This issue has affected attempts to construct a methodological approach to intersectionality in development and human rights fieldwork, as pursued by the Charlotte Bunch Center for Women's Global Leadership (ibid., 203-4). According to Ange-Marie Hancock (2007, 67), there is an interaction and a relationship among relevant categories and the way in which ethnicity and gender play a role in the shaping of political institutions and the respective actors involved. Hancock identifies the mainstream ideology, the structural basis of social institutions, their bureaucratic hierarchies, and their practices, as well as the interpersonal interactions among individuals that are rooted in or affected by the categories of race, gender, and class.

Here we examine the intersectionality of oppression in the context of the impact of cross-cutting oppressions on immigrant women's health access, and we cite studies that demonstrate how Canadian federal policy creates a framework that shapes their health experiences. Jacqueline Oxman-Martinez et al. (2005) examine how women fall primarily into the "dependent" categories of immigration, consequently experiencing barriers in accessing health services. They argue that direct policy barriers and their unintended secondary effects intersect with each other and with socio-cultural barriers arising from the migrant's socio-economic and ethnocultural background to undermine equitable access to health. For example, "socio-cultural barriers may arise from a woman's cultural and ethnic background, her lack of knowledge of the host-country language, her level of social isolation, and her experiences with authorities both in her country of origin and in Canada" (ibid., 255). Sepali Guruge and Nazilla Khanlou (2004) support this through a critical approach derived from a post-colonial feminist perspective. B. Singh Bolaria and Rosemary Bolaria (1994) conclude that immigrants are more exposed than native-born Canadians to numerous workplace health hazards and observe that immigrant women are exposed to even more hazardous working environments. Various qualitative studies point to barriers for immigrant women in accessing health and social services (Stewart et al. 2008; Hyman et al. 2006; Whitley, Kirmayer, and Groleau 2006). In relation to the gendered dimension of migration, Evangelina Tastsoglou, Valery Preston, and Brian Ray (2005) assert that gender has not been sufficiently addressed in migration studies. They challenge researchers to go beyond adding in sex as a variable – to consider gender as embedded in cultural institutions and norms, through negotiated and historically constructed social practice. They point out that gender decisively shapes identity and interpersonal and social relationships, and that it determines access to resources during migration, settlement, and integration. Vijay Agnew (2007) has also examined and identified the inherently "racialized," gendered, and temporary nature ascribed to migrant women. Although these analyses of the oppression of migrant women are enlightening and well developed, they generally leave aside the macro processes and global economic framework that lie at the root of most migrants' decision to leave home.

Macro Processes and Global Economic Framework

In this section, we examine the ideological character of macro-level social processes through a political economy framework and how they are reinforced by a global perspective. Certain Canadian sociological approaches have analyzed the ideological character of state social practices. For example, Nandita Sharma (2001, 2002) illustrates how state practice itself organizes social differences and how social relations make possible certain state practices. Using institutional ethnography and Foucault's analysis of "governmentality," Dorothy Smith (2005) demonstrates how the recruitment of migrant workers is part of globalization and argues that state practices create the category of "foreign" for certain workers within the Canadian labour market. She reveals how presenting migrants as "problems" results not only in their physical exclusion but also in differentiation between them and other Canadians in ways that are both ideological in origin and material in outcome. In a comparable vein, Jacqueline Oxman-Martinez and Jill Hanley

(2007) analyze the concept of the otherness of migrants with precarious status, reinforcing the construct of exclusion.

Audrey Macklin (1999) argues that the purpose of institutional long-term migrant labour programs is to create the circumstances that enable employers to subject workers to wages and conditions that Canadian citizens and permanent residents will not accept. She analyzes the gendered nature of migrant work, arguing that as the female migrant's role moves away from the "public" into the "private sphere," Canadian law becomes increasingly silent. Analyzing Chinese migration, Guida Man (2004) concludes that Chinese women are being deskilled by Canadian policy and practice, and that this deskilling is complicated by the processes of globalization and economic restructuring, highlighting the polarizing effects of differentiation along gender, race, ethnicity, class, and citizenship lines. Habiba Zaman (2004) also approaches her study of the LCP from a political economy perspective. She examines race, class, and gender dynamics in transnational migration and states that the processes involved in the commodifying of migrant women workers in Canada turn them into "indentured labourers," a conclusion that is reinforced by the findings of Abigail Bakan and Daiva K. Stasiulis (1994).

Gender, age, and rural provenance render some women invisible in class terms. Similar processes occurred in Britain, where young Chinese and East European workers provided temporary labour in the agricultural and food-processing sector (McDowell 2008), and have also occurred across Canada, as studied by Oxman-Martinez et al. (2005). As Patricia Fernández-Kelly (2006, 6) indicates, in some areas of the world, young female migrants are "merely the providers of cheap and replaceable labour" rather than permanent members of the working class and so are excluded from access to benefits associated with permanent residence and citizenship.

Linda McDowell (2008, 505, 491) analyzes the possibility of bringing together constructs on labour segmentation and feminist scholarship related to intersectionality in order to capture the multiple relationships between the dimensions of identity that constitute complex social locations. We agree that state, political, and institutional practices and daily social engagements continue to produce and reinforce the categories of class, gender, race/ethnicity, and sexuality that negatively affect women's lives and well-being. The impact of globalization and the division of labour, as well as the international flows of capital and human beings, create a spatial dislocation for millions of migrant workers according to their class position, gender division, and skin colour, facilitating through migration the reconstruction of "racialized" and national stereotypes. This maintains the division between those who are labelled the deserving and the undeserving migrants, the first having a permanent resident status and the second a precarious migration status.

Systemic and Structural Violence under an Intersectional Lens

The intersection of a number of key variables with systemic and structural forms of violence has been underanalyzed. The theoretical underpinning of structural violence is the consideration of subtle or latent aspects of violence in women's lives (Farmer 1997, 2004; Galtung 1969). Our working definition, as stated above, considers systemic violence to be induced by the Canadian socio-political framework and expressed by laws, policies, and practices that structure migrants' personal experiences within our society (Oxman-Martinez et al. 2007). The concept of systemic violence implicates public policy, government practice, and the educational, social, and health systems, as well as the justice system. The consequences of this form of violence, exploitation, and abuse take diverse shapes in individual lives (ibid.). These symptoms manifest themselves in an increased level of vulnerability, depression, and mental distress, and are often associated with feelings of social exclusion and isolation.

Structural violence reflects pre-existing social and economic drawbacks in Canadian society, whereby dominant social policy and practice act to exclude, and therefore grant unequal opportunities to, different groups and categories of persons within Canada. Policy and practice hinder the transformation of aspirations into reality for a segment of the population. Great differences exist between persons' potential and their lived realities. As a respondent in our study on access to services for refugee claimants described it, "issues of abuse and power are not easy to deal with. The dynamics are complicated. People might be suffering from the Stockholm syndrome. These are complicated dynamics since there is the need to be socially recognized and loved. People who encourage exploitation are generally fairly knowledgeable and skilled in using the weaknesses of people who are emotionally fragile ... or who could be made so. The victims are isolated and misinformed individuals" (Oxman-Martinez, Lacroix, and Hanley 2005, 8-9).

Social inequalities become inherent in social structures and are manifested in asymmetrical power relations, as well as in the limitations of rights and services for certain persons. Discriminatory practices intersect with dominant culture, disadvantageous laws, and policies, thus ultimately transforming themselves into multiple forms of violence (Eckermann 1998; Braud 2003). Structural violence is therefore expressed in a deprivation of rights, individual alienation, and the inability to meet fundamental material needs (James et al. 2003). Physical manifestations of this violence are expressed in a person's state of health, whereas psychological violence may be reflected in alienation and abuse (Oxman-Martinez et al. 2007; Braud 2003; Farmer 1997, 2004; Dunn and Dyck 2000; Langevin and Belleau 2000).

Structural violence leads to the erosion of dignity and self-esteem in response to particular social situations, including the relationships of dependence on the employer. Though systemic and structural violence emanates from social organizations and institutions, it becomes apparent at the individual and interpersonal levels (Braud 2003; Farmer 1997, 2004; Dunn and Dyck 2000; Langevin and Belleau 2000). The theory of systemic violence has not been widely applied to migration issues. Its applicability is illustrated by a small number of Canadian studies. Yasmin Jiwani (2005) indirectly uses this theory to understand young migrant women's lives, emphasizing the impacts of violence at the intersections of race, class, gender, and age. She concludes that young women from racialized immigrant communities in Western Canada suffer from heightened vulnerability to systemic and institutional forms of violence.

Canadian migration policy thus dictates parallel yet contradictory paths: on the one hand, Canada chooses women with precarious status as potentially permanent immigrants, but on the other hand, they live a trial period, sometimes indefinitely, with this status as temporary workers or dependants. This apparatus of regulatory control, through policy and enforcement, invokes the notion of biopower developed by Michel Foucault (2004). The entirety of mechanisms, procedures, and control through power and the legal system is exercised on a territory and population in order to manage and organize the population-wealth relations. This strategy of power touches a variety of procedures that render individuals apt to function "well" in society.

Analyzing the mechanisms of systemic and structural violence in certain Canadian immigration policies and programs permits us to identify their detrimental outputs. Recent studies examine the consequences of these policies in the lives of precarious-status migrants. They exemplify how state policy can inflict violence on their lives, with the SAWP and the LCP receiving heavy attention (Grez 2005; Preibisch 2005; Barber 2000; Basok 1999, 2000; Satzewich 1988) and the LCP (Zaman 2004; Velasco 2002; Cohen 2000; Langevin and Belleau 2000; Pratt 1999; Grandea and Kerr 1998). We must conclude that the systemic and structural violence experienced by caregivers is in part predetermined and the result of political and judicial social constructs. The trafficking of women illustrates one of the worst forms of violence, in which the intersections of age, gender, race, ethnic origin, poverty, lack of resources, and other factors highlight the junction of the most severe case of social exclusion and exploitation. An important number of migrant women workers testify to the existence of this systemic and structural violence within their workplaces (Oxman-Martinez and Hanley 2007). The following example shows how systemic violence provoked by the LCP itself intersects in a woman's experience, creating a series of multiple oppressions that affect her physical and mental health, her working conditions, and her life stability: she is dependent on a third party (her employer), her migration status is temporary, and she faces the threat of deportation. She states, "I'm worried already, crazy, crying, asking to everyone if they know an employer that's going to be willing to sponsor me and calling every time to take me, saying this is my condition" (Oxman-Martinez et al. 2007); this is echoed in Denise Spitzer et al. (2004-8). The integration of migrant workers as a social group into broader Canadian society is thus seen to be characterized by differing levels of vulnerability and even social exclusion (Preibisch 2004).

Conclusion

As stated above, this chapter aims to respond to health inequities that arise from multiple unequal power relations within the health and social systems as well as from migration policies emerging from existing Canadian legal frameworks, and to do so through an intersectional lens. As Hancock (2007, 74) points out, the intersectional approach emphasizes the dynamic inter-action between individual and institutional actors, which reproduces and reinforces inequalities throughout the system. These inequities and inequalities inadvertently create multiple facets of violence such as the systemic and structural violence that affects the heterogeneous groups of women with various forms of precarious migration status. Research based on intersectional analysis in regard to this issue permits us to disclose the systems of oppression and exclusion that hinder access to and equity in health and social services, and to highlight the disparities among the diverse needs of these segments of the population. Celik et al. (2008, 69) and Aarti Iyer, Gita Sen, and Piroska Östlin (2008) found in their research that effective attention to diversity dimensions in health care practices is impeded by various barriers, as stated by Oxman-Martinez et al. (2005). These barriers are explained by lack of awareness and knowledge, shortcomings in information and communication, lack of cultural sensitivity, and mostly by organizational constraints, among other factors.

Women with precarious immigration status are particularly exposed to forms of vulnerability and even violence because of their lack of autonomy and their dependence on the primary applicant, often rooted in immigration policies and their eligibility criteria for social and health programs that are considered basic. They are frequently victims of socio-structural violence, previously defined as the physical and psychological harm provoked by the socio-economic inequalities intrinsic to the division of labour. Our working definition of systemic violence asserts that this violence is aggravated by the Canadian laws, policies, and practices that structure migrants' personal experiences of vulnerability within our society (Oxman-Martinez et al. 2007).

Migration programs and health and social practices, examined together, reveal tensions and contradictions that affect the health and well-being of women with precarious migration status. If they are to attain access and equity in health care, it is necessary to create solid foundations that will take solidarity and social justice into account, avoiding the gaps and barriers existing in the legal framework, including its policies, programs, and practice.

The full implementation of the law, and an authentic political will respectful of workers' rights, should diminish the possibilities of abuse and exploitation.

It is also crucial to support alliances with the women affected by the various cross-cutting systems of oppression and exclusion, and with the various political and social actors. As stated by most authors of the relevant theoretical and grey literature we analyzed, women in their various dimensions and categories constitute very heterogeneous groups and are thus characterized by their diversity in connection with race, ethnicity, age, ability or disability, socio-economic status, education, and sexual orientation.

Intersectional lenses are required in training at diverse levels and in various milieux. In academia, for example, medical, social work, nursing, public health, and management schools, among many others, should look at introducing or strengthening a cross-cultural approach that takes into account the increasing diversity of patients and personnel. At a community level, practitioners need to look at diversity and violence from a different and more innovative angle, and to change traditional ways of practice. From a feminist perspective, differing currents (autonomist, NGOs, participants) must adopt a unified strategy toward achieving the common goal of equity and access to health and social services for women with precarious immigration status.

The authors also propose the need to increase the dialogue with young people and to work on representations tied to violence in order to eliminate constructions that, in their minds, link "feminism" to outdated theoretical frameworks and thinking. It is necessary to find and build on solid bases for research that will provide an irrefutable rationale for equal rights for all (women and men) in the country, at home, and in bed as added later to the Chilean feminist slogan (Vargas 2003, 3, author's translation). This constitutes a key challenge that, once met, might facilitate the inclusion of the variables that distinguish the forms of oppression, exclusion, and violence in contextualizing the issues in question. The intersectional approach that facilitates the assembly of missing elements in the various layers of our society will thus contribute to building a fairer and more equitable one.

We intend to promote this intersectional analysis within and beyond the academic community and to contribute to a vast dialogue on differential access to social and health services among the actors implicated – policy makers, NGO representatives, academics, and students – emphasizing the role of systemic and structural violence. The relevance of the subject, studied within the Canadian migration context, and the lack of analysis on the links between access to health and social services, precarious immigration status, and violence emphasize its importance and its contribution to academic scrutiny, sound Canadian social policy, and useful information for programs or intervention in community organizations.

Finally, we firmly argue that government must submit legislation that takes into account the differences articulated above, in order to establish the same access to health and social services and their related rights for all workers in Canada. This legislation should be implemented in such a way as to respect all workers' rights independent of their current migration status and to eliminate critical existing gaps in service at federal, provincial, and municipal levels.

Notes

1 Each province has its own health system according to the Canada Health Act, yet provinces use the federal Immigration and Refugee Protection Act (IRPA) to define eligibility for coverage.

2 As Health Canada (2000, 14) explains, "*Gender* refers to the array of socially constructed roles and relationships, personality traits, attitudes, behaviours, values, relative power and influence that society ascribes to two sexes on a differential basis. Gender is relational – gender roles and characteristics do not exist in isolation, but are defined in relation to one another." Health Canada (2000, 8) also notes that "*sex* refers to the biological characteristics such as anatomy (e.g., body size and shape) and physiology (e.g., hormonal activity or functioning of organs) that distinguish males and females."

3 By "human rights," we mean the right of all individuals to have access to similar health and social services, regardless of their immigration status (Oxman-Martinez et al. 2005), as suggested in various human rights charters, from the United Nations' Universal Declaration of Human Rights to the Quebec Charter of Rights and Freedoms.

4 It is important to note that for the purpose of this chapter, we will not debate the issue of illegal migrants.

5 Migrants' status is considered to be "dependent on a third party" when their right to remain in Canada and/or their economic security relies on another person's actions. Examples include temporary workers whose visas are linked to a specific employer or permanent residents who are economically tied to their sponsoring family member. This dependence often translates to a lack of autonomy due to fear (sometimes unfounded) of deportation, bureaucratic constraints, limited knowledge about rights in the host country, language, and cultural barriers.

6 Health is "a state of complete physical, mental and social well-being and not merely the absence of disease or infirmity. The enjoyment of the highest attainable standard of health is one of the fundamental rights of every human being without distinction of race, religion and/or political belief, economic or social condition ... Governments have a responsibility for the health of their peoples which can be fulfilled only by the provision of adequate health and social measures" (World Health Organization 2007, 1).

7 The Seasonal Agricultural Workers Program (SAWP) allows for the entry of agricultural workers to assist in harvesting Canadian crops (HRSDC 2009). The Live-In Caregiver Program (LCP) is a temporary work program that recruits migrants to care for children, elderly people, or persons with disabilities in private homes without supervision. They must live in the home where they work. They may apply for permanent resident status after they have lived and worked in Canada for twenty-four months over a four-year period (CIC 2010).

8 Although the automatic approval of temporary work visas for exotic dancers has been ended following the media scandal surrounding the practice, "entertainers" and other categories of workers can still apply for and receive them. They are no longer automatically granted, but if the work described is legal and the employer shows a lack of available Canadian labour, there is no reason to refuse them.

9 Canada has imposed a moratorium on removals to eight countries – Afghanistan, Burundi, the Democratic Republic of Congo, Haiti, Iraq, Liberia, Rwanda, and Zimbabwe – because of conflict and/or other forms of insecurity there.

References

Agnew, V. 2007. The conundrum of inclusion: Race in public policy reports. In *Interrogating race and racism,* ed. V. Agnew, 325-51. Toronto: University of Toronto Press.

Bakan, A.B., and D.K. Stasiulis. 1994. Foreign domestic worker policy in Canada and the social boundaries of modern citizenship. *Science and Society* 58(1): 7-33.

Barber, P.G. 2000. Agency in Philippine women's labour migration and provisional diaspora. *Women's Studies International Forum* 23(4): 399-411.

Basok, T. 1999. Free to be unfree: Mexican guest workers in Canada. *Labour, Capital and Society* 32(2): 192-221.

–. 2000. He came, he saw, he ... stayed: Guest workers programs and the issue of non-return. *International Migration* 38(2): 215-38.

Bolaria, B.S., and R. Bolaria. 1994. Immigrant status and health status: Women and racial minority immigrant workers. In *Racial minorities, medicine and health,* ed. B.S. Bolaria and R. Bolaria, 149-68. Halifax: Fernwood.

Bowen, S. 2001. Access to health services for underserved populations in Canada. In *Certain circumstances: Equity in and responsiveness of the health care system to the needs of minority and marginalized populations: A collection of papers and reports prepared for Health Canada,* 1-60. Ottawa: Health Canada.

Braud, P. 2003. Violence symbolique et mal-être identitaire. *Raisons politiques* 99: 33-47.

Carmel, S. 2001. Subjective evaluation of health in old age: The role of immigration status and social environment. *International Journal of Aging and Human Development* 53(2): 91-105.

CCR. 2004. More than a nightmare: Delays in refugee family reunification. Canadian Council for Refugees. http://www.ccrweb.ca/nightmare.pdf.

–. 2005. Annual status report 2005. http://www.ccrweb.ca/status05.pdf.

–. 2006a. Annual status report 2006. http://www.ccrweb.ca/ASR2006en.pdf.

–. 2006b. Lives on hold: Nationals of moratoria countries living in limbo. http://www.ccrweb.ca.

CCR, and the City of Toronto Public Health Department. 1999. The role of NGOs in health care services for immigrants and refugees. Proceedings of the International Metropolis Conference Workshop, Washington, DC, 7-11 December. http://www.international.metropolis.net.

Celik, H., A. Tineke, G.A. Widdershoven, F.C.B. van Wijmen, and I. Klinge. 2008. Implementation of diversity in healthcare practices: Barriers and opportunities. *Patient Education and Counseling* 71(1): 65-71.

Choudry, A., J. Hanley, S. Jordan, E. Shragge, and M. Stiegman. 2009. *Fight back: Workplace justice for immigrants.* Halifax: Fernwood.

CIC (Citizenship and Immigration Canada). 2007a. Canada's new government strengthens protection for victims of human trafficking. News release, 19 June. http://www.cic.gc.ca.

–. 2007b. *Facts and figures 2007: Immigration overview, permanent and temporary residents.* Ottawa: Minister of Public Works and Government Services Canada. http://www.cic.gc.ca/english/pdf/pub/facts2007.pdf.

–. 2008. Assistance for victims of human trafficking. http://www.cic.gc.ca.

–. 2010. Working temporarily in Canada: The Live-In Caregiver Program. http://www.cic.gc.ca.

Cohen, R. 2000. "Mom is a stranger": The negative impact of immigration policies on the family life of Filipina domestic workers. *Canadian Ethnic Studies/Études ethniques au Canada* 32(32): 76-88.

DeVoretz, D. 2008. An action model of Canadian temporary immigration for the twenty-first century. *International Migration* 46(1): 3-17.

Dunn, J., and I. Dyck. 2000. Social determinants of health in Canada's immigrant population: Results from the National Population Health Survey. *Social Science and Medicine* 51(11): 1573-93.

Eckermann, A.K. 1998. The economics of Aboriginal education. *International Journal of Social Economics* 25(2-3-4): 302-13.

Farmer, P. 1997. On suffering and structural violence: A view from below. In *Social suffering*, ed. A. Kleinman, V. Das, and M. Lock, 261-83. Berkeley: University of California Press.

–. 2004. An anthropology of structural violence. *Current Anthropology* 45(3): 305-25.

Fernández-Kelly, P. 2006. *The global assembly line in the new millennium*. Working Paper 335. Princeton: Center for Migration and Development, Princeton University.

Foucault, M. 2004. *Sécurité, territoire, population: cours au Collège de France, 1977-1978*, ed. Michel Senelart, François Ewald, and Alessandro Fontana. Paris: Seuil Gallimard.

The Future Group. 2006. *Falling short of the mark: An international study on the treatment of human trafficking victims*. Calgary: The Future Group. http://www.thefuturegroup.org/TFGhumantraffickingvictimsstudy.pdf.

Galtung, J. 1969. Violence, peace and peace research. *Journal of Peace Research* 6(3): 167-91.

Gastaldo, D., J. Lima, F. Chakir, N. Bendris, and B. Vissandjée. 1998. Reproductive and sexual care for Arab Muslim women living in Quebec (Canada): Looking at religion, gender and immigration to have a better understanding of health. Final research report, Centre of Excellence on Women's Health, University of Montreal Consortium.

Grandea, N., and J. Kerr. 1998. "Frustrated and displaced": Filipina domestic workers in Canada. *Gender and Development* 6(1): 7-12.

Grez, E.E. 2005. Harvesting seeds of justice: The plight of migrant farm workers in Ontario. *Women and Environments International Magazine* 68-69: 16-19.

Guruge, S., and N. Khanlou. 2004. Intersectionalities of influence: Researching the health of immigrant and refugee women. *Canadian Journal of Nursing Research* 36(3): 32-47.

Hancock, A.-M. 2007. When multiplication doesn't equal quick addition: Examining intersectionality as a research paradigm. *Perspectives on Politics* 5(1): 63-79.

Hanley, J., J. Oxman-Martinez, M. Lacroix, and S. Gal. 2006. The "deserving" undocumented? Government and community response to human trafficking as a labour phenomenon. In Gender, Migration and Trafficking, ed. D. Chew. Special issue, *Labour, Capital and Society* 39(2): 78-103.

Hanley, J., and E. Shragge. 2009. Economic security for women: Organizing around immigration status and work. In *Public policy for women: The state, income security, and labour market issues*, ed. M. Griffin Cohen and J. Pulkingham, 353-73. Toronto: University of Toronto Press.

Health Canada. 2000. *Health Canada's gender-based analysis policy*. Ottawa: Minister of Public Works and Government Services Canada.

HRSDC (Human Resources and Skills Development Canada). 2009. Seasonal agricultural worker program. http://www.hrsdc.gc.ca.

Hughes, K.D., D. Spitzer, J. Oxman-Martinez, and J. Hanley. 2007. TFWs and caregiving: Canada's Live-In Caregiver Program (LCP). Paper presented at "Finding a Home in the Global Economy: Temporary Foreign Workers in Alberta," Work and Learning Network Symposium, University of Alberta, Edmonton, 6 December.

Hyman, I., T. Forte, J.D. Mont, S. Romans, and M.M. Cohen. 2006. Help-seeking rates for intimate partner violence (IPV) among Canadian immigrant women. *Health Care for Women International* 27(8): 682-94.

Iyer, A., G. Sen, and P. Östlin. 2008. The intersections of gender and class in health status and health care. *Global Public Health* 3(Suppl. 1): 13-24.

James, S.E., J. Johnson, C. Raghavan, T. Lemos, M. Barakett, and D. Woolis. 2003. The violence matrix: A study of structural, interpersonal and intrapersonal violence among a sample of poor women. *American Journal of Community Psychology* 31(1-2): 129-41.

Jiwani, Y. 2005. Walking a tightrope: The many faces of violence in the lives of racialized immigrant girls and young women. *Violence against Women* 11(7): 846-75.

Justice Canada. 2003. *Canada health act*. http://laws.justice.gc.ca.

KAIROS: Canadian Ecumenical Justice Initiatives. 2006. Joint submission to the Standing Committee on Human Resources, Social Development and the Status of Persons with Disabilities. http://www.kairoscanada.org/.../JointSubmission_HUMA_MigrantWorkers_6Sept06.pdf.

Krane, J., J. Oxman-Martinez, and K. Ducey. 2001. Violence against women and ethno-racial minority women: Examining assumptions about ethnicity and "race." *Canadian Ethnic Studies* 32(3): 1-18.

LACEV (Latin American Coalition to End Violence against Women and Children). 2000. No (wo)man's land research project. http://www.mujer.ca.

–. 2002. Coming to dance, striving to survive: A study on Latin American migrant exotic dancers. Research report. http://www.mujer.ca.

Langevin, L., and M.C. Belleau. 2000. *Trafficking in women in Canada: A critical analysis of the legal framework governing Immigrant live-in caregivers and mail order brides.* Ottawa: Status of Women Canada.

Macklin, A. 1999. Women as migrants: Members in national and global communities. *Canadian Woman Studies* 19(3): 24-31.

Man, G. 2004. Gender, work and migration: Deskilling Chinese immigrant women in Canada. *Women's Studies International Forum* 27(2): 135-48.

McDowell, L. 2008. Thinking through work: Complex inequalities, constructions of difference and trans-national migrants. *Progress in Human Geography* 32(4): 491-507.

Measuring Security Measures Tour. 2005. *Yasmin Jiwani: security or terrorism?* Video. http://citizen.nfb.ca.

Meyerowitz, B.E., S.C. Formenti, K.O. Ell, and B. Leedham. 2000. Depression among Latina cervical cancer patients. *Journal of Social and Clinical Psychology* 19(3): 352-71.

Oxman-Martinez, J., and J. Hanley. 2007. L'identité assignée du statut d'immigration précaire et l'accès aux services de santé: la construction sociale de l'exclusion. In *Éthique de l'altérité*, ed. Marguerite Cognet and Catherine Montgomery, 119-35. Quebec City: Presses de l'Université Laval.

Oxman-Martinez, J., J. Hanley, and L. Cheung. 2004. *Another look at the Live-In-Caregivers Program.* Working Paper 24. Montreal: Centre d'Excellence Immigration et Métropoles.

Oxman-Martinez, J., J. Hanley, L. Lach, N. Khanlou, S. Weerasinghe, and V. Agnew. 2005. Intersection of Canadian policy parameters affecting women with precarious immigration status: A baseline for understanding barriers to health. *Journal of Immigrant Health* 7(4): 247-58.

Oxman-Martinez, J., E. Jimenez, J. Hanley, and I. Bohard. 2007. La dynamique triangulaire dans le processus d'incorporation des demandeurs d'asile, les politiques migratoires et le rôle des organismes communautaires. *Refuge* 24(2): 76-85.

Oxman-Martinez, J., and J. Krane. 2005. Un décalage entre théorie et pratique? Violence conjugale et femmes issues des minorités ethniques. Special issue, *Journal international de victimologie* 3: 1-10.

Oxman-Martinez, J., M. Lacroix, and J. Hanley. 2005. *Victims of trafficking in persons: Perspectives from the Canadian community sector.* Ottawa: Department of Justice Canada, Research and Statistics.

Oxman-Martinez, J., and N. Lapierre Vincent, eds. 2002. *Precarious immigration status, dependency and women's vulnerability to violence: Impacts on their health.* Conference proceedings. Montreal: Centre for Applied Family Studies, McGill University, and Immigration and Metropolis (Domain 4).

Pratt, G. 1999. Is this Canada? Domestic workers' experiences in Vancouver, B.C. In *Gender, migration and domestic service,* ed. J.H. Momsen, 23-42. New York: Routledge.

Preibisch, K.L. 2004. Migrant agricultural workers and processes of social inclusion in rural Canada: Encuentros y desencuentros. *Canadian Journal of Latin American and Caribbean Studies* 29(57-58): 203-39.

–. 2005. One woman's grain of sand: The struggle for the dignified treatment of Canada's foreign agricultural workers. *Canadian Woman Studies* 24(4): 98-101.

Satzewich, V. 1988. The Canadian state and the racialization of Caribbean migrant farm labour 1947-1966. *Ethnic and Racial Studies* 11(3): 282-304.

Sharma, N. 2001. On being not Canadian: The social organization of "migrant workers" in Canada. *La revue canadienne de sociologie et d'anthropologie/Canadian Review of Sociology and Anthropology* 38(4): 415-39.

–. 2002. Immigrant and migrant workers in Canada: Labour movements, racism and the expansion of globalization. *Canadian Woman Studies* 21-22(4-1): 18-25.

Smith, D.E. 2005. *Institutional ethnography: A sociology for people.* Toronto: AltaMira Press.

Spitzer, D., K. Hughes, J. Oxman-Martinez, and J. Hanley. 2004-8. The land of milk and honey: After the Live-in-Caregiver Program. Research project.

Statistics Canada. 2006. Survey of labour and income dynamics (SLID): Preliminary, labour and income interview questionnaire for reference year 2006. http://www.statcan.ca.

Stewart, M., J. Anderson, M. Beiser, E. Mwakarimba, A. Neufeld, L. Simich, and D. Spitzer. 2008. Multicultural meanings of social support among immigrants and refugees. *International Migration* 46(3): 123-59.

Sudha, S., and E.J. Mutran. 2001. Race and ethnicity, nativity, and issues of health care. *Research on Aging* 23(1): 3-13.

Tastsoglou, E., V. Preston, and B. Ray. 2005. Gender and migration intersections. *Canadian Issues* (Spring): 91-93.

Vargas, V. 2003. Los procesos feministas latinoamericanos en el nuevo milenio: Identidades descentradas en lo nacional y lo global. In *Emergencia de los movimientos sociales en la Región Andina*, 1-8. http://hdl.handle.net.

Velasco, P. 2002. Filipino migrant workers amidst globalization. *Canadian Woman Studies* 21-22 (4-1): 131-35.

Whitehead, M. 1991. The concepts and principles of equity and health. *Health Promotion International* 6(3): 217-28.

Whitley, R., L.J. Kirmayer, and D. Groleau. 2006. Understanding immigrants' reluctance to use mental health services: A qualitative study from Montreal. *Canadian Journal of Psychiatry/Revue canadienne de psychiatrie* 51(4): 205-9.

World Health Organization. 2007. Constitution of the World Health Organization. http://www.who.int.

Yuval-Davis, N. 2006. Intersectionality and feminist politics. *European Journal of Women's Studies* 13(3): 193-209.

Zaman, H. 2004. Trans-national migration and the commodification of immigrant female labourers in Canada. *International Journal of Canadian Studies/Revue internationale d'études canadiennes* 29: 41-61.

12

Place, Health, and Home: Gender and Migration in the Constitution of Healthy Space

Parin Dossa and Isabel Dyck

This chapter considers the health practices of immigrant and refugee women living in Vancouver, British Columbia. Specifically, it explores how these women's everyday health-promoting and healing activities are implicated in the production of "healthy space" in a large culturally diverse city. It intends to contribute to literature in health geography and medical anthropology that is framed by recent work that seeks to investigate the role of everyday activity in producing meanings and experiences of space as "healthy" or its converse (Gesler 2005; Smyth 2005) but always in connection with wider social relations and political economies. Such works show differentials in the experience of places as healthy or unhealthy and link with the larger problematic of the interconnections between place, culture, and health (Gesler and Kearns 2001). The interesting tension between agency and structure is an ongoing theme – although in reworked frameworks following the well-rehearsed dismantling of a "macro" and "micro" distinction initially prompted by Anthony Giddens's structuration theory (Dyck and Kearns 2005). Our focus is on the possibilities for agency as revealed through the practice of health "in place" that takes into account the political economy of health informed by the paradigm of intersectionality.

Our comparison of two groups of women, South Asian Sikhs from Punjab and Afghan Muslim refugees, serves to build an understanding of how their respective relationships to place inform and circumscribe their health practices. The women are of varying educational and social backgrounds, left their home countries under differing circumstances, and enjoy different levels of financial and personal security in Canada. The comparison acknowledges the effects of such differences on the specificity of their health practices, but there are notable commonalities related to their *particular* political and social positioning in Canada as ethnic minorities entering through the "humanitarian" family reunification and refugee categories of Canadian immigration policy. In the chapter, we draw on insights from health geography and medical anthropology to unravel how such features of their lives inflect the ways they seek viable space for raising healthy families.

We explore the tension between the political economy framing of the materialities of the women's lives and their everyday carving out of room for agency as they attempt to create healthy homes in diaspora space. Although their projects of health and home are constrained and shaped by the effects of structural processes in the form of local material and social conditions, the women rework these felt effects in their day-to-day health practices. However, such practices are not best understood as simply local, but as intricately interwoven with material resources and/or cultural knowledge located and constructed within a context of transnational connections and memories of home. The production of healthy space, then – with the domestic sphere as a core site – situates the women as transnational subjects with a complex relationship to place.

The chapter begins with a brief discussion of the literature that informs its conceptual approach. A description of the study methods follows. The major sections of the chapter draw on data from in-depth individual and group interviews and focus on three areas of everyday health practice: food purchasing, preparation, and consumption; home-based or traditional medicine; and religious observance. We use the contrast between the two groups of women to emphasize the embeddedness of their material and ideational projects of home and health in the interlocking of immigrant status, local materialities, and a transnational sense of belonging. We also bring home the importance of taking into account the aspect of agency alongside the political economy of health. As it stands, the intersectionality paradigm has highlighted only the structural dimensions – multiple relations of power. The women's ability to negotiate these complex relations has been largely muted. We conclude with a comment on the contribution of our analysis to theorizing the production of healthy space.

Political Economy of Health and Intersectionality

During the last decade, the body of literature on two critical and interrelated paradigms – political economy of health and the framework of intersectionality – has grown. This work has increasingly focused on women's health. The emphasis on women, more specifically on gender relations, has brought home fresh insights on the complex ways in which gender is embedded in social, political, and economic relations. The framework of intersectionality is complicated by the additional factors of race, nationality, migration, and displacement. Due to global and national patriarchal systems, women experience health inequalities on a larger scale than do men. With its focus on the macro-level workings of the system, the political economy of health has further highlighted class and gender differences in context-specific ways

(Lock 2001; Navarro 2002). Furthermore, it has shown how political and economic systems inform what is otherwise considered as neutral and objective medical practice. Political economy of health and the framework of intersectionality locate women's health experiences within broader structures of power, affecting an important shift from the individual body to the political body (Baer 2008; Donahue and McGuire 1995; Nettleton 1996; Tsalikis 1989; Hart 2006).

However, less sustained attention is accorded to how these macro-level structures affect the everyday realities of women. What are perceived as mundane and less important activities (food preparation, catching a bus, shopping) hold promise to reveal the fault lines of the system while showing how people from the margins of society remake their worlds in relation to wider socio-political and economic relations (political economy). In foregrounding women's agency, this chapter reconfigures the framework of intersectionality to show its workings from the bottom up. Through their everyday practices, women engage in complex relationships addressing the ambiguities of being othered and how their otherness is worked on and transformed. They too draw on the framework of intersectionality (local and transnational, displacement and settlement, material and symbolic) to create healthy spaces embedded in larger structures of power. Thus, the transformative potential of the intersectionality paradigm, as emphasized by Rita Dhamoon and Olena Hankivsky in Chapter 1 of this volume, is revealed in its emphasis on process, agency, and fluidity of socially constructed boundaries. An emphasis on agency helps to deconstruct reified and essentialized constructs (Baer 2008; Close 1995; Brodwin 2007).

Situating Migrant Women's Health Practices

Following the lead of Wil Gesler's (1992) interest in the association between healing processes and particular places, geographers have examined the use and experience of places of healing in a variety of settings (Williams 1999). Particular landscapes are neither intrinsically healthy nor unhealthy: rather, they may be used, experienced, and perceived differently by different people (Conradson 2005; Gesler 2005; Wakefield and McMullan 2005). Following work on the role of everyday activity in the cultural production of landscapes as material, symbolic, and lived cultural phenomena (Cresswell 2003), some scholars have eschewed an exclusive focus on "exotic" healing places, preferring to examine the productive capacity of daily activity in the construction and experience of healthy spaces. A variety of spaces that are conducive to health and well-being are being explored (Smyth 2005) in relation to multiple locations that women occupy in the process of migration and resettlement. The gendering of the productive action in constructing healthy space, however, has received little attention, and migrants have been rendered socially invisible in the cartography of healthy spaces.

Nevertheless, work in the therapeutic landscape tradition of health geography provides a potentially useful perspective in studying migrant health practices through its recent emphasis on process and diversity. Early recognition of the tension between local action and wider processes in producing spaces of well-being, and the acknowledgment that different groups may experience landscapes differently, suggests that the everyday actions of migrants need situating within the imbrications of local and global processes in their lives. Anthropology also has a long engagement with the tricky explication of tensions between structural forces and agency, revitalized through work on gender and diaspora within the context of contemporary globalization. "Diaspora" refers to the intricate ties that migrant communities maintain with their homeland; as Rebecca Elmhirst (2000, 487) states, it "provides a useful way of framing identities" that challenges a static view of "an ahistorical indigenous identity" where women are conceptualized as a unitary category. Diasporas, as cultural and political terrains, are shown to be gendered, with myth, memory, history, and travel as media through which home is reconstituted in the country of destination (see Brah 1996; Yeoh and Willis 1999). Women are seen to reconstruct and rework hegemonic scripts of identity through everyday practices that blur public and private space (Mankekar 2002: Yeoh and Willis 1999) and by constructing transnational identities (Panagakos 2004). A crucial area that remains unexplored, however, is that of women's work in constituting healthy homes in diaspora, with home understood in the sense of a transnational domain.

The promise of a focus on everyday practices in revealing the workings of human agency is particularly emphasized in feminist work, which insists that it is in local materialities, linked to the wider world through reciprocal processes, that we can see women's cultural and place-making work (Massey 1994; Ong 1999; Staeheli 2003). This point needs elaboration in light of an orientation where the global is "macro-political economic and the local is situated, culturally creative and resistant" (Ong 1999, 4). To forestall analytical confinement of the local to the cultural, Aihwa Ong (ibid.) suggests that we "analyze people's everyday actions as a form of cultural politics embedded in specific power contexts." Narrative accounts from marginalized subjects are particularly valuable in such excavation (Lawson 2000).

Studies in health geography and medical anthropology take up such a focus and methodology, looking at the *particular* location of certain minority groups within the power relations surrounding flows of migrants to Western nations. For example, Caroline Kerner et al. (2001) discuss the impact of temporary protected status on the health and health care behaviour of Salvadoran women in the US, and Natalie Grove and Anthony Zwi (2006) note the "knock-on" effects of social marginalization on the health of forced migrants. Parin Dossa (2004) similarly points to the significance of immigration processes in shaping how Iranian women reconstruct place in Canada, and Lenore Manderson and Pascale Allotey (2003) further show the complexity of such processes as a context for health behaviour in the Australian context. Studies such as these echo Ong's work (1995, 1999), which considers the biopolitical construction of Cambodian refugees in California as "a particular kind of American minority" within dominant ideas of "healthy and culturally correct subjects" (Ong 1995, 1246), a status that defines them as other.

It is in this stream of work, which indicates the intertwining of social, economic, and political processes at various spatial scales, that we see immigrants and refugees as creative agents in negotiating their otherness as they seek to construct healthy lives. Their narrative informs both our analysis and our use of qualitative methods in seeking insight into the negotiation of healthy space from marginalized locations in society.

Study Methods and Participants

In this ethnographic study, women were recruited through settlement agencies. Individual semi-structured interviews were conducted with ten South Asian women and ten Afghan women. Six additional South Asian women and four Afghan women then participated in four sequential group interviews. South Asian and Afghan research assistants conducted the interviews in the women's first language. They were invited to talk about their experiences of immigration and various aspects of living in Canada, including their mothering work, household organization, paid work, and ways of managing health and illness. All the interviews addressed the same topics, but the group interviews promoted an interactive storytelling mode of communication that allowed the women to discuss them in some depth. The group interviews promoted an interactive storytelling mode of communication and allowed the women to discuss the same issues in some depth. Although the fieldworkers used one interview guide throughout and pursued similar topics in the group and individual interviews, they followed an established principle of qualitative research, in that questions were not presented in the same order every time, and the women could raise subjects of particular concern to them (Hammersley and Atkinson 2005). However, close collaboration with the fieldworkers ensured uniformity in topics covered. Close reading of transcripts and comparison across both types of interviews and groups involved discussion among researchers of emerging substantive and theoretical themes.

The South Asian women, all Sikhs from Punjab, lived in various low- to middle-income city and suburban neighbourhoods of Vancouver, where there are concentrations of immigrants from India, principally from Punjab. Most lived in well-maintained single-family dwellings, and all but one were married. All but two – one with teenaged children and one who was a single parent – lived in nuclear or extended households with children of elementary school age. They had been in Canada for between two and twenty years, and had low education levels (high school) relative to the Canadian-born population. Like their husbands, all except two (one cared for her grand-children during the day) worked in low or semi-skilled sectors of the labour market. They worked in food-processing plants, farming, a flower nursery, restaurants, or as cashiers. Some were training for similar jobs. None had worked for pay in India.

The Afghan women, all Muslims, had been in Canada for two to fifteen years. All had children and four headed single-parent households, having lost their husbands through war. All but two entered Canada as UN Con-vention refugees via other countries, including India, Pakistan, and Iran. They were placed by settlement agencies in a low-income housing area in a culturally diverse inner suburb that is part of the urban sprawl of Vancouver, and most lived in apartment blocks. Unlike that of the South Asian women, their educational level ranged from high school to university. Prior to com-ing to Canada, like their husbands, most had worked in skilled occupations. Their previous jobs included teaching and research laboratory work, and one had been a seamstress. They had experienced deskilling in Canada, with most holding part-time jobs in service occupations, such as cashier and casual retail work, child care, and housecleaning. One was a store manager in a family business. All, however, described themselves as homemakers.

Negotiating Healthy Homes from a Migrant Location

In the following discussion, we consider aspects of immigration and settle-ment experience that frame the ideational and material projects of healthy homes and healthy bodies, which underpin the women's construction of healthy spaces. We focus on three specific domains of health practice and their spatiality that were prominent in the women's narratives: preparing nutritious meals, managing illness episodes, and prayer. Their accounts bring home that, for them, keeping healthy is not an atomized activity but one bound up with their experiences of migration and settlement where health inequalities are informed by class, "race," and nationality. We see their health work filling in gaps in biomedical practice, using traditional remedies as a valued system in its own right, and the performance of cultural work in the constitution of healthy identities in the context of diaspora. How health practices were interpreted and enacted indicate the linking of mode of entry into Canada, the subsequent material, social, and economic conditions of the women's day-to-day lives, and past cultural practices relating to a re-membered home.

Gender and Migration

Migrant women's experiences of particular places will vary according to whether gender identities are reaffirmed or challenged through migration

(Boyle 2002). In our study, there were marked differences in the circumstances of migration, with the forced migration and refugee status of the Afghan women contrasting with the planned migration of the South Asian women who entered Canada as family class immigrants. However, despite the considerable difference in the women's migration and settlement experience and in the human capital that they embody – in terms of educational qualifications and job skills – normative constructions of gender, associating women with the domestic realm, were reinscribed by state policy through migration. For the South Asian women, migration patterns in which family reunification has been central, with women entering as dependants, serve to reaffirm their primary responsibility for health and care work. For the Afghan women, identification with the home and children's futures takes on particular significance in the context of ruptured families, lost homes, and the absence of labour market participation appropriate to their qualifications.

Whereas the South Asian women had joined husbands, other relatives, or fiancés in a well-established Sikh community and continued to enjoy connections with India through, for example, the exchange of goods, visiting between the two countries, and ongoing migration from the same region of India, the Afghan women's accounts depicted severing of ties and loss. All had been affected by the conflict in Afghanistan, and none anticipated return; as one woman commented, "War in our home country has left us with broken families." The differing modes of entry into Canada for the two groups of women spilled over into the material and social conditions underpinning their health practices. The thinly resourced landscape of the Afghan women, who relied on social services, newly made acquaintances, and poorly paid work or welfare payments, contrasted with the South Asian women's often rich family life, familiar goods and services, and dense social networks of the Sikh community. The South Asian women commented that it was easy "to make a lot of 'aunties,'" an affectionate term for other Sikhs with whom they could engage in social life and enlist support, whereas the Afghan women were more likely to speak of loneliness. Shirin, for example, spoke of her isolation from her extended family: "At times, I just sit and cry for hours."

There was contrast, too, in the groups' economic standing and financial security. Although the South Asian women worked in low-paid jobs, as their husbands often did, two incomes and a variety of in-kind support – such as help with job finding, house maintenance, child care, and housework – gave them some financial stability, secure housing, and a sense of belonging in their neighbourhoods. As one participant commented, "I didn't have much of a problem coming over because I was coming into my own family ... I didn't have a problem finding employment because my brother worked there [a flower nursery] already." On the other hand, regardless of whether they were lone parents or married, the Afghan women spoke of their precarious financial situation and considerable uncertainty about their future prospects in Canada. Like their husbands, none had been able to translate their past educational and professional skills into the labour market, and they were re-evaluating the priorities in their lives. Nargis, for example, whose husband was killed in Afghanistan, came to Canada with her four children after being in Iran for seven years. Financially dependent on the state for three years and living in overcrowded conditions in a two-bedroom apartment, she saw her children as her priority in Canada: "I have a big responsibility on my shoulder ... [The children] have been homeless for a long time ... They have suffered a lot. They need help." Similarly, Shirin experienced a reduced material life and financial insecurity. She had reworked her priorities around her children's needs and their futures, commenting that "mothers have the responsibility of making sure that kids grow up to be good citizens" and that children "should be happy and healthy."

Both sets of women interpret meanings of healthy homes and healthy bodies under the conditions of migration and attempt to translate such meanings into everyday health practices, as we discuss below. When they talked about food, dealing with illness, and religious practice, therefore, their relationship to place framed their experiences and actions. This not only related to home and neighbourhood space in Canada but also to their countries of origin, which remained an anchor point in their discussions of healthy homes and healthy bodies.

Food, Health, and Cultural Negotiation

Both groups of women combined long-standing knowledge about healthy food from their countries of origin with knowledge gained in Canada through a variety of sources, such as doctors, their children's schools, television, and print media. They included both indigenous cuisine and Canadian foods in the repertoire of their household consumption patterns. Although the choice of food products differed from home to home, both groups sought to meet the needs of children growing up as Canadian citizens. Like the Bengali American families in Krishnendu Ray's (2004) study, the women can be seen to be navigating from home the "public" institutions signifying modernity and the "ethnic" spaces of community life, holding in tension the cultural knowledge of home with that of dominant narratives of Canadian belonging. To be an "appropriate citizen" indicates notions of appropriate food consumption, so that food practices are not neutral but set within relations of power and exclusions of national cultural imaginaries (Gunew 2002; Probyn 1998). Furthermore, to be a "good citizen" is to take responsibility for healthy eating; certainly, a plethora of public health messages about nutrition and food consumption appearing in a variety of media complicate the relationship between food and health (King and Watson 2005).

This complex meaning of food showed in the women's accounts, re-affirming the notion that food signifies and presences social and geographical worlds (Bell and Valentine 1997). However, though there were commonalities in their provisioning strategies, their different migration histories framed their specific practices and the way in which a personal politics of food interwove with the notion of the home as healthy space.

The institutional depth of the Sikh community and the fact that they lived where Sikhs were clustered meant that the South Asian women had ready access to the stores and markets of the locally known Little Indias. As one woman said, "you can get everything here" to create traditional dishes, and like others, she noted the freshness of local produce that was considered central to producing a healthy meal. Cooking and eating Indian food, primarily vegetarian, was common, and emphasis was laid on cooking from scratch. Although home preparation of meals was time consuming, and several of the women were in paid employment, it was part of all the women's household routines. The ready availability of inexpensive ingredients and often help with cooking from family members, such as a grandmother or sister-in-law, facilitated the inclusion of well-known recipes and ways of cooking in what the women considered a healthy lifestyle. Nevertheless, ideas about healthy food were not static. Children were purveyors of nutritional information acquired at school, which women heeded. Surbjeet, for example, said, "Now when [my son] tells me that his teacher said they should eat certain things, I buy those things." The women spoke of how they tried to avoid "risky" food that they learned about through schools, the media, or their local social networks; the spicy, fatty, salty, high-sugar-content food they had been accustomed to in India was sometimes modified.

The Afghan women also emphasized the importance of fresh ingredients, and they cooked familiar dishes, but finding appropriate ingredients was a more difficult and time-consuming task than for their South Asian counterparts. They found some spices locally but travelled several kilometres across the city to specialist outlets to buy other foodstuffs necessary for indigenous recipes. Like the South Asian women, they were conscious of health messages about food ingredients and had learnt from the media about hidden salt and sugar in canned and packaged foods. They modified traditional recipes to consume less salt and fat, one noted that "the meat that we buy here comes with a lot of fat but this was not the case in Afghanistan," and some talked of screening out oily food or ingredients grown with pesticides. They worked hard to serve balanced meals that included vegetables, rice, meat, fruits, and milk. Often living on a precarious income, they spent extra time shopping for affordable foods, wanting to avoid cheap fast food for health and cultural reasons. All felt that Afghan cuisine was important from the point of view of reconstructing a disrupted life and ensuring the children did not lose the "taste" of Afghanistan. As Shirin put it, "Our children must not forget what it is to be a Muslim and what it is to be an Afghan."

Nevertheless, though traditional fare was the mainstay of food served in the home, both groups of women recognised that raising children in Canada also meant that Canadian foods needed to be part of the household's food-scape. Some of the South Asian women spoke of accommodating the desire of husbands, too, to incorporate Canadian foods, including meat, into the weekly round of dishes. Fast foods such as pizza, pasta, and hamburgers, eaten out, were used as a treat for children or to reward their success at school. The women considered "outside" food as inferior to home-cooked food but felt that children should participate in the food culture of Canada if they were to be successful in Canadian society. Like the South Asian women, they wanted to raise children true to their cultural heritage but also wished them to succeed in Canadian society. They responded to children's desires to eat foods representing Canadian popular culture and tastes, usually preparing these at home, modifying ingredients.

Food, then, was not simply a nutritional issue but one of negotiation of cultural belonging in multiple and reconfigured contexts of social, economic, and political relations. The home was a "safe" site for the production of healthy food, admitting Canadian tastes as well as adhering to valued cultural food practices. In the case of the Afghan women, there was also evidence of a more direct politics of food. For example, one spoke of the "multicultural days" at her children's school (when parents brought in ethnic foods) as a site for such cultural negotiation and claiming validity for an Afghan identity. She used such events as an opportunity to tell politicized stories of life in Afghanistan to teachers and non-Afghan parents, thus adding to the variety of narratives of belonging in Canada. Jo-Anne Lee and Linda Cardinal (1998, 230) suggest that mothers' transmission of cultural knowledge provides "other" bases for identity formation for children that have the potential to destabilize the "hegemonic core of Canadian nationalism." Yet, in their food work, the women in our study were creating a balance between Canadian belonging (through acceptance of Canadian popular food) and cuisine that provided a transnational sense of home. Children, too, negotiate their cultural identities as they bring consumer culture, tastes, and Canadian public health knowledge to the family table. The home in these ways is constructed as healthy space, fostering healthy bodies and ways of appropriate cultural belonging.

Healing Knowledge and Spaces

The association of food with a migrant identity and a remembered distant home was particularly sharp in discussions of the use of herb- and spice-based traditional and home remedies in illness management. Here too the significance of social networks in settlement experience is apparent (Bauder 2005; Hagan 1998). Literature on immigrant use of traditional healing methods tends to focus on a debate between their use as cultural conservatism or as efficient consumerism (Chabot 1999). The examples from the women of our study suggest this debate must take account of the larger context of the negotiation of this health work. Difference in use of traditional remedies cannot be simply associated with different educational levels and debate over the value of "modern" medicine versus traditional knowledge. The women's accounts indicate how their experiences of the dislocation of home, together with current experiences of diaspora space, situate their negotiation of competing health care knowledge.

Women from both groups showed a rich knowledge of alternative healing practices, transmitted over generations, but their use was much more common among the South Asian women. They regarded such *desi* medicines (home remedies) as "part of our culture" and as safer than prescription medicines. They found them cheap and easy to use; many ingredients were readily accessible in local shops and markets. A typical approach was "we see what the problem is and give the appropriate treatment," considering both home remedies and the biomedical health care system in responding to illness. They favoured a preventative approach to illness: "Desi meds may not have benefit but they don't have a side effect either ... But you don't give a person with a heart attack desi meds and keep them at home. For this type of thing, you need to go to the doctor." Women were able to purchase most ingredients for desi medicines locally, and they incorporated medicinal ingredients into daily routines. As one woman described, "We make *sund* once per week and we have ginger and garlic in there with *paneer* [cheese] so the kids will eat it. If we do this once per week, it helps alleviate certain issues like stomach problems."

A variety of traditional healing remedies were taken for granted as an appropriate approach to well-known conditions, and social networks were important in the exchange of information and in supporting women in their quest for good health. The following excerpt from a group interview indicates valued collective cultural knowledge and the familial links in problem solving around health issues, in this case stomach complaints: "Doctors can't diagnose *thurn* here, but we know what it does; you get an upset stomach, food doesn't digest properly, hands and feet hurt ... And there is another one called *gund*. And if you have both thurn and gund – well, then doctors here will keep you in the hospital and not get rid of it. But our elders know what it is and how to deal with it ... My niece comes here from Comox and gets it [gund] taken out because doctors don't know about it, but us Punjabis know about it."

Women commonly share knowledge of remedies with friends and acquaintances, and knowledge of traditional healing approaches is widespread in the community. Women spoke of gaining healing information from a number of sources; for example, Haminder commented, "[I hear from] the Punjabi papers or through an elder – like an auntie or uncle. If we tell someone what problem we have – they tell us what desi medicine to use." Transnational networks also figured in their accounts, with women speaking of relatives who sent medicines from India and family members who consulted a traditional healer when on visits back to India.

This operationalization of a collective knowledge through networks spanning Canada and India contrasted with the Afghan women's experience. The political history of Afghanistan figured prominently in their accounts of managing health issues. They talked of Afghanistan as an unstable, shifting landscape of care. Its virtues as a source of herbal remedies and modern medicine were now in question, but it continued to be a source of knowledge, as well as a yardstick in assessing quality of health care in Canada. In nostalgic accounts, the women spoke of the violence inflicted on a landscape of healing. One stated that the remedies they used in Afghanistan were now beyond their reach: "Instead of herbs, the country is filled with landmines." Others noted the deterioration of the health care system through regime changes and foreign intervention: "Before the Mujahedeen and the Taliban we had a great medical system. We had very nice hospitals and very smart and well-educated doctors ... These hospitals were very modern ... Today we have nothing, but back then we had everything. We were a modern country."

The women stressed this situation, aware that the West has looked on Afghanistan as inferior, or in Edward Said's (1978) terms, through the discourse of Orientalism in which an uncivilized and barbaric "they" is contrasted with the civilized and progressive "we." Women went out of their way to explain that in peaceful times (before the Soviet invasion), Afghanistan had a viable system of health care that included both biomedicine and alternative healing, and people judged which would work best for them. They talked of foreign occupation undermining this system with the result that healing and tending of the sick had become a home affair administered by women. They spoke of using traditional remedies for "minor things, like chest pain, ear aches and colds," and they had combined biomedical and traditional remedies. One woman gave the example of her father-in-law, who had high blood pressure; she described a powdered substance made from cherry seeds that "we would put in a bottle for him to take" and spoke of giving him the water from boiled *sinjeat* and *lekat* leaves to keep his blood pressure normal. Few, however, used home remedies in Canada. Some consider their usage as part of a practice embedded in female-centred networks, which are now lost to them. They also noted that the younger generation lacked interest in home remedies. As one woman said, "The new generation looks for modern-day new things ... They want to look to the future and not the past."

Ray's (2004) suggestion – that food practices of migrant cuisine slowly assert a reorientation of hegemonic conceptions of place – can be applied to home healing practices. In our study, use of traditional healing practices by the South Asian women served to claim space for alternative conceptions and modes of healing that contest dominant biomedical constructions. As in food production, remedies made and administered at home are created by the women as a component of home as healthy space. Such healthy space, however, is not confined to the local but incorporates material and symbolic aspects of a distant home of origin, both in terms of living cultural knowledge and material health-giving substances. The Afghan women, who have lost connection with such home-based healing expertise, seek care primarily through the Canadian health system embedded in unequal relations of "race," gender, class, and space.

Prayer, Health, and Place

Prayer is our last example of women's constitutive activities of healthy space, and here we look at how and where they use prayer in their daily lives. Religious observance has received little attention in literature on migrant health, or even in the burgeoning field of intersectionality and the policy prescriptions that stem from it (Urbanek 2009; see also Reimer-Kirkham and Sharma, Chapter 5 this volume). For the women, it was part of a bundle of health-promoting activity; it also provided both groups with moments of repose and a way of coping with worries as they took on the multiple responsibilities of work in the domestic sphere, often in conjunction with participation in the labour market.

Like food provisioning and illness management, the practice of prayer spans home, neighbourhood, and institutional space. Although some South Asian women regularly attended an established *gurdwara* (temple), and Afghan women attended Friday prayers at a makeshift mosque in a neighbourhood school, the home remained the core site for prayer. Prayer was spoken of as everyday practice, usually seamlessly integrated into the temporality and spatiality of daily chores. Prayers might be used throughout the day, but all noted prayer at the start of the day as a firm routine. A South Asian woman's description of the beginning of her daily routine as "I put on tea and start prayers" was typical. An Afghan woman similarly included prayer along with her mothering practices as she described her busy schedule: "I get up early in the morning and I say my prayers. I make sure all my sons wash up and wear proper clothes for school. I also make breakfast for them." Prayers were said at other times of the day, too, either at home or as women went about their chores.

For the South Asian women, prayer was a taken-for-granted practice, part of belonging to the Sikh community. There is a known repertoire of prayers of different lengths, with specific requirements as to when they should be said. However, the women displayed flexibility in how and when prayer could be used, as illustrated in one exchange:

> *Woman 1:* In the morning I do Sukhmani Sahib [a prayer that can be said at any time] and the five *bharnees* and in the evening I do Rheas Sahib.
> *Interviewer:* Sukhmani Sahib is a long one, how long does it take you?
> *Woman 1:* It just seems really long in the beginning but it only takes thirty-five minutes.
> *Woman 2:* If you can't do it in the morning, you can do it in the afternoon or at night or before you go to sleep.

The Afghan Muslim women also spoke of the flexibility in how they practised prayer in Canada and the modifications they made, including the use of public space. One noted, "The important thing is that we pray. This does not mean that we can always pray five times a day or that we always have the time to put on [special prayer outfit]." Women used strategic moments to say a few minutes of prayer in a sitting position, wherever they might be, with their head covered and facing Mecca when possible. An exchange with Nargis, who had asked for a few minutes to pray during the interview, illustrates this slotting of prayer into the spaces of her daily routine:

> *Interviewer:* Do you often pray in public?
> *Nargis:* Whenever I get the opportunity. Lunchtime is a good time, but any time is fine.
> *Interviewer:* Do other people [non-Muslims] make any comments?
> *Nargis:* Sometimes they ask me questions. Other times they say nothing. They carry on with whatever they are doing.

For the Afghan women, prayer was a central feature in their day-to-day lives, and they spoke of its particular significance for them as they struggled with their current situations. Shirin explained that prayer and faith in Allah helped her and other Afghan women to cope with the loss of family members in Afghanistan, as well as with their new life in Canada. Some women read *Quran-e Sharif* when they felt depressed or sad. Prayer was also key to their identity as Afghan Muslims, and they encouraged children or grandchildren to pray as part of maintaining traditions and culture.

Although the Sikh community's religious faith is visible on the landscape through the substantial gurdwaras that echo the style of those in India, the Afghan women had no direct equivalent. Instead, the visibility of the temporal and spatial dimensions of their faith in everyday public spaces is created through their embodied practices. The integration of home, prayer, health, and healing suggests, however, that the daily rituals of prayer comprise a project beyond that of religious observance and everyday coping. Lila Abu-Lughod (1998, 3) observes that, "in the post modern world women [their bodies] have become potent symbols of identity and visions of society and the nation," a script that is not denuded of agency. It is through the temporality and spatiality of prayer, embodied in women's practices, that we see women reinscribing the landscape – extending the healing practices of a healthy home into public space. As they offer prayers in times of crisis, sadness, or sickness in homes and neighbourhood space, they further build the home and neighbourhood as healthy space – in material, social, and symbolic dimensions.

Conclusion

This chapter set out to consider women's agency in producing healthy space in a major immigrant destination city in Canada. Our analysis has focused on the embeddedness of their health practices in place, bringing to bear a conception of place that dismisses a notion of boundedness. Rather, we attempt to examine the intertwining of the local social and material conditions that frame women's health practices with ongoing transnational attachments and processes of settlement experience shaped by migration patterns and policy. Healthy space is not simply locally constituted but involves relationships and materialities stretched over space (Massey 1994). Despite the differences in their dislocation and settlement experiences, the narrative accounts of the women express a collective experience of positioning in Canadian society as other. In the course of their day-to-day practices – obtaining and preparing nutritious food, dealing with illness, and prayer – the women actively seek to create their homes as healthy spaces within the ambiguities of a migrant identity discursively constructed as marginal to national economic goals. Although differences in forced and planned migration were substantial, the home country remained an anchor point in the women's interpretation and practice of health (see also Sherrell and Hyndman 2004).

It is within the various constitutive spaces of home, the material, social, and symbolic qualities of which span their adopted country and home of origin, that women interpret health and its management. To be healthy involves not only the physical body but also the ability to participate in Canadian society as an "appropriate" cultural body. For both groups, access to social and material resources, including housing, work, and social networks, frames the specificity of their health practices. For the women from Afghanistan, the difficulties of rebuilding a life are formidable. Their reflections on personal losses were interwoven with the violence inflicted on their home country, a violence that spills over to long-held health and healing knowledge and religious faith. Women struggled to make space for these in

Canada. The South Asian women entered Canada with living connections with India, through marriages, the exchange of goods, and ongoing migration flows. Yet both groups negotiated fields of knowledge and health practices in ways that provided their children with opportunities to be "flexible citizens" (Ong 1999) who would be connected to a remembered symbolic homeland as well as citizens of Canada.

We have emphasized the home as the primary site from which women orchestrate and construct their health practices, although these also spill over into neighbourhood space. Taking place in the nooks and crannies of everyday life, their endeavours are not easily discernible. Yet, as noted in feminist work, it is within such hidden spaces that women contribute to place making, although as Nancy Scheper-Hughes (1992) warns us, the conditions under which women forge their lives can be severely constraining. In conceptualizing the women's health practices as constitutive of healthy space within the multicultural landscape of this major city, we suggest that their actions, though constrained, indicate the productive capacity of reproductive work. As the women seek to construct healthy lives, we see their agency both located within and constitutive of a complex spatiality of home space and belonging. The key challenge for such analyses is to bridge the divide between political economy of health and agency in the context of intersectionality. This paradigm helps us to see that women and other marginalized populations can occupy multiple social locations to advance their own cause for justice.

Acknowledgments
We are indebted to the women who participated in the study, to the interviewers Jas Gill, Gulalai Habib, Bindy Kang, and Poran Poregbal, and to NGOs for recruiting the women. The research was funded by RIIM, the Vancouver Centre of Excellence in Research on Immigration and Integration in the Metropolis (www.riim.metropolis.net).

References
Abu-Lughod, L. 1998. Feminist longings and postcolonial conditions. In *Remaking women, feminism and modernity in the Middle East,* ed. L. Abu-Lughod, 1-27. Princeton: Princeton University Press.

Baer, H.A. 2008. The Australian dominative medical system: A reflection of social relations in the larger society. *Australian Journal of Anthropology* 19(3): 253-71.

Bauder, H. 2005. Habitus, rules of the labour market and employment strategies of immigrants in Vancouver, Canada. *Social and Cultural Geography* 6: 81-97.

Bell, D., and G. Valentine. 1997. *Consuming geographies: We are where we eat.* London: Routledge.

Boyle, P. 2002. Population geography: Transnational women on the move. *Progress in Human Geography* 26: 531-43.

Brah, A. 1996. *Cartographies of diaspora: Contesting identities.* London: Routledge.

Brodwin, P. 2007. Mediations of power in contemporary medical anthropology. *Anthropology in Action* 14(3): 1-5.

Chabot, C. 1999. Immigrant health care issues and the use of alternative health systems in Canada: An examination of recent literature. Unpublished paper, Department of Sociology and Anthropology, Simon Fraser University, Burnaby, BC.

Close, E.L. 1995. A political economy perspective on home care labor. *Dissertation Abstracts International, A: The Humanities and Social Sciences* 56(1): 361-A.

Conradson, D. 2005. Landscape, care and the relational self: Therapeutic encounters in rural England. *Health and Place* 11: 337-48.

Cresswell, T. 2003. Landscape and the obliteration of practice. In *Handbook of cultural geography*, ed. K. Anderson, M. Domosh, S. Pile, and N. Thrift, 269-81. London: Sage.

Donahue, J.M., and M.B. McGuire. 1995. The political economy of responsibility in health and illness. *Social Science and Medicine* 40(1): 47-53.

Dossa, P. 2004. *Politics and poetics of migration: Narratives of Iranian women from the diaspora.* Toronto: Canadian Scholars' Press.

Dyck, I., and R.A. Kearns. 2005. Structuration theory: Structure and agency in everyday life. In *Key approaches in human geography: Philosophies, people and practices,* ed. S. Aitken and G. Valentine, 86-97. London: Sage.

Elmhirst, R. 2000. A Javanese diaspora? Gender and identity politics in Indonesia's trans-migration resettlement programme. *Women's Studies International Forum* 23: 487-500.

Gesler, W.M. 1992. Therapeutic landscapes: Medical issues in light of the new cultural geography. *Social Science and Medicine* 34(7): 735-46.

–. 2005. Therapeutic landscapes: An evolving theme. *Health and Place* 11: 295-97.

Gesler, W.M., and R.A. Kearns. 2001. *Culture/place/health.* London: Routledge.

Grove, N.J., and A.B. Zwi. 2006. Our health and theirs: Forced migration, othering, and public health. *Social Science and Medicine* 62(8): 1931-42.

Gunew, S. 2002. Introduction: Multicultural translations of food, bodies, language. *Journal of Intercultural Studies* 21: 227-37.

Hagan, J. 1998. Social networks, gender and immigrant incorporation: Resources and constraints. *American Sociological Review* 63: 55-67.

Hammersley, M., and P. Atkinson. 2005. *Ethnography: Principles in practice.* 2nd ed. London: Routledge.

Hart, J.T. 2006. *The political economy of health care: A clinical perspective.* Bristol, UK: Policy Press.

Kerner, C., A.J. Bailey, A. Mountz, I. Miyares, and R.A. Wright. 2001. "Thank God she's not sick": Health and disciplinary practice among Salvadoran women in northern New Jersey. In *Geographies of women's health,* ed. I. Dyck, N.D. Lewis, and S. McLafferty, 127-42. London: Routledge.

King, M., and K. Watson, eds. 2005. *Representing health: Discourses of health and illness in the media.* Basingstoke, UK: Palgrave Macmillan.

Lawson, V.A. 2000. Arguments within geographies of movement: The theoretical potential of migrants' stories. *Progress in Human Geography* 24: 173-89.

Lee, J.-A., and L. Cardinal. 1998. Hegemonic nationalism and the politics of feminism and multiculturalism in Canada. In *Painting the maple: "Race," gender and the construction of Canada,* ed. V. Strong-Boag, S. Grace, A. Eisenberg, and J. Anderson, 215-41. Vancouver: UBC Press.

Lock, M. 2001. Medicalization: Cultural concerns. In *International encyclopaedia of the social and behavioral sciences,* ed. Neil J. Smelser and Paul B. Baltes, 9534-39. Oxford: Pergamon.

Manderson, L., and P. Allotey. 2003. Story-telling, marginality, and community in Australia: How immigrants position their difference in health care settings. *Medical Anthropology* 21: 1-21.

Mankekar, P. 2002. India shopping: Indian grocery stores and transnational configurations of belonging. *Ethnos* 67: 75-98.

Massey, D. 1994. A global sense of place. In *Space, place and gender,* ed. D. Massey, 146-56. Manchester: Manchester University Press.

Navarro, V. 2002. A historical review (1965-1997) of studies on class, health, and quality of life: A personal account. In *The political economy of social inequalities: Consequences for health and quality of life,* ed. V. Navarro, 13-30. Amityville, NY: Baywood.

Nettleton, S. 1996. What makes women sick: Gender and the political economy of health. *Sociology of Health and Illness* 18(3): 423-25.

Ong, A. 1995. Making the biopolitical subject: Cambodian immigrants, refugee medicine and cultural citizenship in California. *Social Science and Medicine* 40(9): 1243-57.

–. 1999. *Flexible citizenship: The cultural logics of transnationality.* Durham, NC: Duke University Press.

Panagakos, A.N. 2004. Recycled odyssey: Creating transnational families in the Greek diaspora. *Global Networks* 4: 299-311.

Probyn, E. 1998. Mc-identities: Food and the familial citizen. *Theory, Culture and Society* 15: 155-73.

Ray, K. 2004. *The migrant's table: Meals and memories in Bengali-American households.* Philadelphia: Temple University Press.

Said E. 1978. *Orientalism.* New York: Vintage Books.

Scheper-Hughes, N. 1992. *Death without weeping: The violence of everyday life in Brazil.* Berkeley: University of California Press.

Sherrell, K., and J. Hyndman. 2004. *Global minds, local bodies: Kosovar transnational connections beyond British Columbia.* RIIM Working Paper Series 04-10. Vancouver: Research on Immigration and Integration in the Metropolis.

Smyth, F. 2005. Medical geography: Therapeutic places, spaces and networks. *Progress in Human Geography* 29: 488-95.

Staeheli, L. 2003. Women and the work of community. *Environment and Planning* 35: 771-77.

Tsalikis, G. 1989. The political economy of decentralization of health and social services in Canada. *International Journal of Health Planning and Management* 4(4): 293-309.

Urbanek, D. 2009. Towards a processual intersectional policy analysis. Project proposal for QUING (quality in gender and equality policies). http://www.quing.eu.

Wakefield, S., and C. McMullan. 2005. Healing places of decline: (Re)imagining everyday landscapes in Hamilton, Ontario. *Health and Place* 11: 299-312.

Williams, A., ed. 1999. *Therapeutic landscapes: The dynamic between wellness and place.* Lanham, MD: University Press of America.

Yeoh, B.S.A., and K. Willis. 1999. "Heart" and "wing," nation and diaspora: Gendered discourses in Singapore's regionalisation process. *Gender, Place and Culture* 6: 355-72.

13

Preventing and Managing Diabetes: At the Intersection of Gender, Ethnicity, and Migration

Bilkis Vissandjée and Ilene Hyman

Over the last century, global population mobility has exposed immigrant families to a broad range of contextual stressors that have contributed to increasing both their vulnerability to adverse health events and their resilience and capacities (Newbold 2009; Hyman 2007; DesMeules et al. 2005; Ng et al. 2005; Vissandjée et al. 2004; Hyman 2001; Anand et al. 2000; Razum, Zeeb, and Rohrman 2000; Vissandjée et al. 2000). A number of chapters in this volume illustrate the importance of accounting for contextual factors as differences in health status and beyond biology. Global forces, such as cultural, political, and ecological change, have been shown to exert a powerful effect on health, providing a backdrop for a complex set of factors that operate at the individual and community levels: transition experiences, education, health literacy, income, social status, type of housing, employment, health services, personal health practices, and physical environment. These factors shape immigrant lives in multi-faceted ways so that being an immigrant not only constitutes a legal status but also encompasses a set of complex realities and experiences (Commission on Social Determinants of Health 2008).

Though studies on the development of chronic diseases and mortality differentials support the healthy-immigrant effect and its loss over time, more work is required toward integrated research on determinants of health, chronic diseases, and mortality in consideration of the intersections of gender, ethnicity, and migration (Hankivsky and Christoffersen 2008; Hyman 2007; Johnson, Greaves, and Repta 2007; Vissandjée et al. 2007; Ng et al. 2005; Pérez 2002; Hyman 2001; Dunn and Dyck 2000). Research also suggests that recent immigrant women are less likely than their Canadian-born counterparts to report chronic conditions but that they have a greater likelihood than immigrant men of developing a chronic disease over time. These findings point to the necessity of examining the intersections between global, community, and individual determinants of health. The influence of socio-economic position on health and illness experiences has been well established. However, as James Nazroo (2003) stresses, socio-economic in-equalities cannot fully explain ethnic inequalities in health. As a number of chapters in this volume indicate, discrimination figures prominently as a direct and indirect determinant of health. The argument has also been made that women's and men's socio-cultural context, including their cultural and migratory experiences, shapes their exposure to health-damaging agents and determines what their individual resources for promoting health may be. Although studies have indicated that the process of acculturation or progressive integration produces changes in health, it has also been suggested that different dimensions of the process may be associated with different types of outcomes. Moreover, the literature attests to the importance of cultural beliefs and migration experience in perceptions of health and of what makes one ill or healthy.

The heterogeneity of experience among immigrant women and men calls for analyses of intersecting determinants, such as country of birth, country of origin (if different), countries in the migratory trajectory prior to arrival in the destination host society, and experiences of migration as they relate to health. This heterogeneity also affects immigrant integration and may result in an inequality of access to social networks mediated by gendered processes (Johnson, Greaves, and Repta 2007; Reid, Pederson, and Dupéré 2007; Spitzer 2005). The process of acculturation or progressive integration produces changes in health and may be associated with differing types of outcomes. However, few studies that take account of number of years since arrival in the host country as a contributing determinant have investigated health status or chronic conditions as perceived by diverse populations. In this regard, it has been demonstrated that capacities for handling the stress of diabetes and subsequent diabetes-coping strategies vary in relation to interdependent determinants such as quality of poverty, housing, know-ledge of the right food, and accessing it when needed (Oldroyd et al. 2005; Gafvels and Wändell 2005; Sarkadi and Rosenqvist 2002).

Type 2 diabetes is most commonly diagnosed in women and men over forty years of age; however, with the rapid rise in obesity, a risk factor that affects immigrant women and men differentially, much younger women and men are increasingly presenting with this chronic condition. Women and men from certain countries in South Asia are at higher risk of obesity because their nutritional requirements may not be adequately met, their physical activity may be limited, and they face high levels of stress (Gucciardi et al. 2007). Significant differences in the prevalence of obesity between immigrants of different ethnic origins have also been observed (Misra and Ganda 2007). These studies demonstrate that there is a non-negligible risk of developing obesity, thereby increasing the risk of diabetes, with length of stay in a host society. The importance of gene-socio-environmental inter-action needs to be given further attention.

To better understand the importance of an intersectional analysis in the development, implementation, and evaluation of programs for the prevention and management of diabetes, this chapter begins with a review of certain social determinants of health as they affect health status, access to health care, and the development of chronic diseases. Relevant risk factors and successful interventions for preventing and managing diabetes among immigrant populations are discussed, and at the end of the chapter, the issue is considered through the lens of intersectionality. At the centre of our reflections are the evolving social contexts of women experiencing migration, and more specifically, the notion that women exposed to numerous risk factors during their integration are also vulnerable to chronic diseases. The aim in using intersectional discourse to understand these "moving" contexts as they relate to diabetes prevention and management is to identify factors for vulnerability so that better interventions may be developed for a condition. In addition, this chapter underscores the importance of keeping up a constant search for the protective and resilience factors of immigrant women, even though they may not be allowed to exercise their capacities fully. A number of best practices for preventing and managing diabetes in immigrant populations and certain ethnic groups are then presented, and outcomes in terms of controlling diabetes and related conditions among women are discussed.

Determinants of Immigrant Health: New Approaches or Old Ways Revamped?

The term "determinants of health" was adopted by Health Canada in 1994 to describe factors that influence population health; these include income and social status, social-support networks, education, employment and working conditions, physical environment, social environment, personal health practices, healthy child development, health services, gender, and culture (Health Canada 1994). The term "social determinants of health" has emerged to reflect the fact that health is largely influenced by a wide range of social and economic factors, and that health promotion and policy must consequently not be limited to biomedical- and behavioural-risk-factor approaches (Raphael 2007; Wilkinson and Marmot 2003). The social determinants of immigrant health include socio-economic status, country of origin, length of stay in the host country, lifestyle, language proficiency, social support, degree of social exclusion, recognition of professional credentials, job security, education in early life, family role, and perceived stressful events (Abate and Chandalia 2007; Hyman 2007; Misra and Ganda 2007; Vissandjée, Abdool, and Dupéré 2005).

Any examination of the determinants of immigrant health has to consider complex issues of interdependence, the dynamic interplay between different levels of determinants, the life course perspective, and the context of migration (Hyman and Jackson 2011; Vissandjée and Battaglini 2010; Raphael 2007). Determinants of health may be conceptualized as operating on macro, community, family, and individual levels. Women and men are nested within their families, which are layered through and within multiple communities and are ultimately moulded in a broader societal context, in which there is a dynamic interplay of factors operating at multiple levels (Bierman, Ahmad, and Mawani 2009). This complex interplay may give rise to chronic diseases as a product of the dynamic interaction between the determinants of health associated with each of the levels.

Like sex, gender – however elusively defined in terms of social norms and power relations – has been identified as a factor in potential disparities in access to quality health care services (Kunti, Kumar, and Brodie, 2009; Llácer et al., 2007; Vissandjée, Abdool, and Dupéré 2005; Hyman 2001). Such complexity demands a place for a perspective that recognizes ongoing exposures to risks and to protective factors from gestation through childhood, youth, mid-life, later life, and across generations. A life course perspective makes it possible to shed light on the way in which certain conditions (such as stroke and stomach cancer) relate to gendered childhood circumstances, whereas others (such as lung cancer and onset of type 2 diabetes) depend more on one's roles as an adult woman or man, and still others depend on cumulative exposures over a lifetime (WHO 2007). With respect to immigrant health, a life course approach highlights the critical importance of considering trajectories from premigration through to resettlement. Age at migration and its impact on settlement experiences, including education and labour market experiences, are among the determinants of changes in a person's "vulnerable" status (Schaafsma and Sweetman 2001).

Since social determinants of health may be distributed differently and affect varying population subgroups differentially, the need to consider intersectionality is critical (Newbold 2009; Pittaway and Bartolomei 2002). Intersectionality is an approach that seeks to examine the ways in which a number of socially and culturally constructed categories – such as race/ethnicity, belonging to a specific community, social roles and power relations, social class, sexual orientation, geography, age, disability/ability, migration status, and religion – are viewed as dynamic parameters of social identity, which itself emerges at intersecting levels within multiple levels of power to result in sustained inequalities (racism, classism, sexism, ableism, homophobia) (Hankivsky 2005).

Critical Intersections: Sex, Gender, Ethnicity, and Migration Experience

Building on the dynamic definition of gender presented in many chapters in this volume, and as we disentangle the risk and protective factors associated with diabetes prevention and management among immigrant women, we must focus on the complexity of gender and how it relates to other intersecting determinants in order to prevent inequalities. Colleen Reid et al. illustrate the point very well in Chapter 4 of this volume; they argue for the importance of an intersectional analysis that pays particular attention to the internal dynamics of social identities and locations as they evolve and interact to affect immigrant women's health opportunities and risks.

Some risk factors are related to structural elements that stem from particular immigration policies: notably, labour-force opportunities, which may contribute to dietary and lifestyle changes that are not entirely under a recent immigrant woman's control. However, depending on her access to and uptake of resources for improving quality of life, her capacity for control should evolve. There is a growing literature on the effects of insecure legal status on health, notably for the increasing number of refugees who live in legal limbo (Caulford and Vali 2006; Oxman-Martinez et al. 2005). Qualitative evidence suggests that immigration policies that deny rights and privileges to refugees and promote geographic dispersal and delays in family reunification such events have negative health effects (Arcury et al. 2004; Ashton et al. 2003). Of particular concern is the finding that an immigrant's need for social support often leads to a secondary migration away from areas of economic opportunity (Simich, Beiser, and Mawani 2003). Settlement policies typically focus on the early stages of the transition and overlook intermediate and long-term integration needs such as access to language, health and legal literacy, and training in specific skills for women, which are some of the best examples of invisible social exclusion processes. The three-month waiting period for coverage under provincial health plans in several provinces does nothing to lower already compromised health care access barriers. Such situations are quite dramatic for immigrant women (Simich, Wu, and Nerad, 2007; Im and Yang, 2006; Gagnon, Tuck, and Barkun, 2004). Income insecurity and poverty are significant negative stressors on anyone's physical and mental health (Raphael 2007). Poverty affects access to basic needs (nutritious food and safe shelter) and thus limits the ability to fully participate in the host society.

Applying the concept of social inequalities to the field of public health helps clarify a number of salient questions, including the following: If racial categories are a social product rather than a biological fact, how can one explain the differences in health outcomes observed among some ethnic groups? Observed health disparities between different groups thus come to be understood as dynamic biological expressions of race relations rather than as reflections of underlying static differences in biology (Krieger 2003; Subramanian and Kawachi 2004). Whereas trauma, stress reactions, lowered self-esteem, and similar effects may have a direct impact on health, racism affects it indirectly through differential exposure to determinants of health – for example, by restricting socio-economic mobility and thus contributing to differential access to resources (Harris et al. 2006; Brondolo et al. 2003). The multi-faceted relationship (which requires intersectional analysis) between perceptions of discrimination and socio-economic status is complex, for the consequences restrict those who feel discriminated against to a certain socio-economic position whereas the "risk factor" of ethnicity remains a constant antecedent.

Nancy Krieger (2003) documented multi-level intersecting pathways linking racism to health outcomes across the life course of racialized families. She identified complex linkages between economic and social deprivation, exposure to toxic substances and hazardous social conditions, peer-inflicted trauma, targeted marketing of inadequate commodities, and limited access to health care and counter-racism strategies, especially among women. Similar results have been documented in Canada (Hyman 2007; Kazemipur and Halli 2000).

Migration and Diabetes: Epidemiology and Risk Factors
The global prevalence of diabetes has been estimated at around 2.8 percent for all age groups. Type 2 diabetes accounts for at least 90 percent of the disease worldwide (Wild et al. 2004). Rates for the disease among certain "ethnic" groups in countries such as Canada and the United States have been shown to increase with length of stay. Rates among Asian Americans, South Asians, and women and men from islands such as Haiti appear to be rising more quickly than in other ethnic groups (Désilets et al. 2007; Barnett et al. 2006; Public Health Agency of Canada 2005; Hux and Tang 2003).

In Canada, the disease affects more than 2 million people, a disproportionate number of them members of vulnerable communities, and its prevalence is rising (Raphael 2003). South Asians and West Asians in Ontario comprise 12 percent of the diabetes population but account for less than 4 percent of the general population.

Diabetes is not only more prevalent among certain ethnic groups but also varies in appearance and progression across and between groups of women and men depending on genetic-environmental interactions. Since the genes that regulate enzymatic function and other lipid-metabolism structural components vary across gene pools, certain genetically linked ethnic groups are more subject than others to adiposity, particularly abdominal obesity, a significant indicator of diabetes risk (Scheuner 2008; Misra and Ganda 2007; Raphael et al. 2003). For instance, women and men from some South Asian countries are thought to be particularly susceptible to abdominal obesity, which results from increased levels of central fat distribution and ultimately affects the type of diabetes (Abate and Chandalia 2007; Oldroyd et al. 2005). A greater susceptibility to dyslipidemia and hypertension among people from these countries also plays a role in the onset of the disease. In addition, those from countries in Southeast Asia, Latin America, and Africa have a three- to four-times greater risk of contracting type 2 diabetes than their Canadian-born counterparts (Kumar and Houlden 2005; Oldroyd et al. 2005).

The transition to Western dietary habits, particularly the intake of less fibre, more saturated fats, and an increased simple-sugar load in high-calorie foods, often combined with a more sedentary urban lifestyle, facilitates phenotypic expression that catalyzes the development of diabetes (Jaber et al. 2003; Misra and Ganda 2007). The gradient tracing the risk of obesity and the onset of type 2 diabetes in certain ethnic groups has been correlated with rising community affluence and urbanization resulting from progressive integration into a society. Investigations have thus revealed differences between and within ethnic groups in terms of their predisposition to biological factors that contribute to the onset of type 2 diabetes (Hosler and Spence 2004). Also deemed to be at greatest risk were immigrant women, recipients of Medicaid in the US, urban residents, and people with less than high school education. Most women refugees and elderly migrants are characterized by limited access to adequate diet, lack of health and legal literacy, socio-economic disadvantage, language barriers, and unstable networks. Gender intersects with these diabetes risk factors since women must often juggle complex demands in their domestic work but have limited access to resources, such as the classes they should attend to find decent employment (Pittaway and Bartolomei 2002). What is more, depression and anxiety have been associated with poor-diet behaviours leading to the diabetes precursor of abdominal obesity (Désilets et al. 2007; Oldroyd et al. 2005).

Adequate nutrition therapy is crucial to diabetes prevention and management among immigrants. Such therapy has been incorporated into diabetes self-management education and has been efficacious and cost-effective in improving blood pressure, serum lipids, and glycemic control (Gucciardi et al. 2007). From an intersectional perspective, issues of access to diabetes self-management resources, low diabetes literacy and low participation and retention rates in educational sessions are among the obvious risk factors for lack of proper management (Rothman et al. 2004; Gilmer, Philis-Tsimikas, and Walker 2005; Strine et al. 2005; Gilmer and O'Connor 2010). The intersecting social determinants of health that emerge along a woman's migration trajectory may explain these issues. In turn, lack of access and comprehension leads to non-compliance and poor clinical outcomes in a context of economic disadvantage (Cooper 2002; Raphael et al. 2003). These illustrations highlight the importance of considering intersections between migration-related variables, such as migration status (category of entry), country of birth, source country, and length of stay, on the one hand, and biological determinants of health (such as age and sex), post-migration stresses, gender roles that modulate access to health care, and other determinants of chronic-disease development, on the other.

Need for New Approaches: The Contribution of Intersectional Analysis

In public health practice, the demand for evidence-based approaches and interventions founded on best practices has increased. Indeed, these are crucial, for they integrate the best available evidence, the health care provider's expertise, and the patient's individual or cultural values. Viewing health care through an intersectional lens reveals that best practices must fully consider the intersecting demands that women and men experience differentially in daily life. In this regard, Lawrence Green (2006) recommends synthesizing various types of research in addition to randomized controlled trials in order to take into account the influence of place, setting, and culture. It is critical, he suggests, to focus on processes as well as practices, so that interventions can be combined, adapted, and tailored to the needs of specific groups, especially the most vulnerable (see also Arskey and O'Malley 2005; Murray et al. 2003; Hyman and Guruge 2002). In Green's (2006, 25) view, the greatest mistake in best-practice research is that "it seeks a magic bullet, a package to put on a shelf in any community where professionals can pull it off and apply it." If health professionals apply best practices and processes rooted in an intersectional perspective, they could help empower the community rather than focus unduly and exclusively on the individual, who may already be under great stress.

In Chapter 1 of this volume, Rita Dhamoon and Olena Hankivsky's compelling argument for applying an intersectional perspective to disease management follows along the same lines in seeking "sensitive approaches to empowerment." From an intersectional perspective, individual-level strategies, which focus exclusively on medical and lifestyle risk factors, cannot be labelled "best practices," because they tend to overlook the processes by which both micro- and macro-structural factors shape the experience and outcomes of cardiovascular and other diseases (Dhamoon and Hankivsky, Chapter 1 this volume). The application of intersectional analysis to best practices remains unclear, largely misunderstood, and dauntingly complex. However, it may be the most efficient way to respond to the numerous critical risk factors that lead to the sustained social and health inequalities experienced by women, men, and communities who are often at the crossing point of two or more marginalized identities (Hankivsky and Christoffersen 2008).

The next section of this chapter will present an analysis of interventions aimed at preventing or managing type 2 diabetes. Some have demonstrated their effectiveness; some have proven only partially effective. The intersectional analysis is rarely explicit; some interventions applied it successfully without acknowledging it. However, deconstruction of the "success factors" points directly to an awareness of the influence of intersecting determinants.

Preventing and Managing Diabetes: Selected Success Stories

Macro-level programs and policies are generally designed to eliminate structural barriers and so enable immigrants to participate fully in Canadian society by providing them adequate income, labour-force opportunities, housing, and community social structures. In seeking to best improve the health of vulnerable women and men, policies and programs need to reconsider exclusionary terms and conditions to take into account risk factors for the development of diabetes and chronic diseases (as discussed earlier). For instance, in Canada, the interpretation of the Canada Health Act varies from province to province, resulting in inconsistent health-coverage eligibility for economically insecure recent immigrants (Oxman-Martinez et al. 2005). Those who have the means can purchase health insurance for the waiting period, but the cost is prohibitive for many. Furthermore, even for people who can afford it, insurance provides a response only to emergency health issues and does not cover preventive care or advice. Given that the healthy immigrant effect ends with the immigrants' loss of their original above-average health status, sensitive prevention and management measures are imperative, for the immigrants may end up in a worse socio-economic situation than in their country of origin (Gravel et al. 2008; Midiema, Hamilton, and Easley 2008).

In diabetes prevention and management, literacy regarding the disease and its health-altering ramifications is crucial to the attainment of positive diabetes-management health outcomes (Gucciardi et al. 2007; Bruce et al. 2003). Best diabetes-treatment practices and processes must focus on such factors from an intersectional perspective in order to develop and implement comprehensively sensitive interventions: that is, interventions that are sensitive at both the individual and the community level and that systematically involve lay partners so as to move beyond a simple summing of individual "oppressions" and social identities (Hankivsky and Christoffersen 2008). In this regard, family and social networks may act either as risk or protective factors. The management of chronic illness takes time, resources, access to resources, effort, and motivation, requirements that may not always be evident, for example, to some of the immigrant women whose life context was discussed above (Midiema, Hamilton, and Easley 2008). What is more, it has been well illustrated that the context of vulnerability is not fixed in time. Rather, very successful interventions should enable vulnerable women suffering from type 2 diabetes to manage their disease and so escape some dimensions of their vulnerability. An immigrant woman may thus learn to free herself from imposed cultural expectations of her body, gain control over it, and adjust nutrition and physical therapies in accordance with her needs and her understanding of her health status.

The guidelines presented by the Canadian Diabetes Association in 2008 indicated that best practices should be based on an annual assessment of demographic and clinical criteria. Women and men should be screened for diabetes every three years with a fasting plasma-glucose test. The interval should be reduced to two years for vulnerable populations: people with first-degree diabetic relatives and members of high-risk groups such as Aboriginal community members, those known as Hispanics, and immigrant women and men from countries in Asia, South Asia, and Africa.

RE-AIM (reach, efficacy, adoption, implementation, maintenance) is an approach that has been applied to identify successful diabetes-management interventions. With this approach, an intervention is deemed successful if it satisfies a majority of the elements of the acronym: it has reached out to the targeted vulnerable community, efficiently delivered knowledge of the intervention, evaluated adoption of the intervention, ensured full implementation of a self-management program as part of a daily routine, and monitored maintenance of the intervention (Eakin et al. 2002). Although it provides a useful tool for assessing the efficacy of diabetes-management practices, RE-AIM does not explicitly acknowledge intersectionality or the use of a gendered lens.

Project Dulce is an intervention that satisfied several of the RE-AIM components over a one-year period. It is described as a stepped-care diabetes nurse case management program and culturally oriented peer-led self-empowerment training program targeting an ethnically diverse group (Gilmer 2005). The clinical components included diabetes counselling by nurses and certified diabetes educators, bilingual medical assistance, and classes taught in the native language with a health care worker who was an "ethnic match." Interactive story-sharing meetings were held, during which personal beliefs about and experiences of diabetes were discussed; the purpose was to empower low-income, ethnically diverse women and men who perceived diabetes management as a major burden. Intersecting identities were revealed in a comfortable, safe space. Cultural misunderstandings about the disease were cleared up. Diabetes literacy was improved, and hemoglobin, blood pressure, and cholesterol levels all decreased, as did hospital expenditures (Gilmer 2005).

An action-research framework for a four-year project involving clinicians, project managers, and diabetic women and men was proposed for some ethnic groups in an impoverished district of London, England (Greenhalgh,

Collard, and Begum 2005). Story-telling sessions were held in the presence of bilingual health advocates from the participants' communities. An account of the intersections of the multiple realities experienced by diabetic women and men was sought. Much of the discussion focused on diagnosis, diet, exercise, checkups, and tips on healthier eating with "ethnically" familiar ingredients. Success was measured against the capacity participants acquired in negotiating the significance of becoming progressively more "diabetically" literate. Indeed, literacy and knowledge of resources and how to access them are essential ingredients to fight "vulnerability," thereby being able to move upwards in the "health ladder" along with the challenges of negotiating the stresses associated with migration experiences. Focuses on culturally and gender sensitive information as well as on technical skills required for diabetes prevention and management will contribute to the fabric of empowerment that is built progressively along with the integration process (Hjelm et al. 2005; Clar et al. 2010; Spallek, Zeeb, and Razum 2010).

Studies that examined patient accounts for non-compliance with diabetes self-care regimens along with physician compliance-gaining response noted the inconsistency of value associated with ethnic and sex matching. However, greater confidence and a decrease in unhealthy behaviours were among the positive outcomes. This sense of confidence had to be rooted in the positive perspective required to enable disadvantaged immigrant women to extricate themselves from certain dimensions of the label of vulnerability. Meanwhile, it was noted, spiritual barriers were encountered because of the lack of involvement by family members in the implementation of interventions. Such barriers are quite difficult to manage in relation not only to diabetes but to women's independence per se (Helme and Harrington 2004; Hosler and Spence 2004).

Although selected interventions yielded improvements in some health outcomes behaviours, future studies should consider culturally based beliefs and norms specific to the community being monitored to ensure maximum efficiency of outcomes. Further to a study that monitored the lipid content and blood pressure of fifty-five type 2 Russian immigrants before and after information-exchange sessions included a Russian-speaking intern. While 90 percent of women and men adopted the lipid-control medications and the angiotensin converting enzyme, the study failed to present an intersectional analysis of structural (macro) and community-level facilitators in this success rate. Yet, the need to maximize language and cultural convergence was discussed at length, giving way to the fact that a more systematic gender and cultural sensitive approach would have allowed a proper understanding of what worked and why for each group (Mehler et al. 2004).

Further to in-depth interviews about physician practice with thirty immigrant men and women of Greek, Indian, Chinese, and Pacific Island cultural backgrounds, language concordance and ethnic matching were assessed to be important determinants (Mehler et al. 2004). However, the analysis of the strategy failed to go a step further and include sensitivity to immigrant women's life trajectories; this is needed to go beyond basic understanding of diabetes management and allow a proper gender-sensitive uptake and compliance to the challenges of the maintenance of a healthy lifestyle. There is a greater chance that women with more knowledge might also be empowered and so change their label as vulnerable actors. The authors might have gone still further to discuss the value of a prismatic panoramic view of the pros and cons while disentangling intersecting oppressions. Perceived gender roles and the power of health care professionals certainly play a role at the intersection of the various determinants of health and risk factors for type 2 diabetes (Kokanovic and Manderson 2007; Sulaiman et al. 2007; Wallin, Lofvander, and Ahlstrom 2007).

A study in which facility-based care was offered in the form of women's support groups to indigenous female Mayan populations in Guatemala clearly highlighted that the decision to participate was clearly associated with feelings of high self-worth, self-esteem, and some confidence that they would be in a safe and culturally appropriate program in familiar compounds. Building affiliations among community advocates, members, and health care providers was another key aspect of this success story. Trust and reputation accounted for a large part of the health care services attendance quotient in the community, providing insight into the personal values of the indigenous women (Llácer et al. 2007; Schooley et al. 2007; Vissandjée, Apale, and Wieringa, 2009).

Moving Forward

Trust and reputation are directly associated with women's participation in most programs. They are also ingredients of autonomy that become intertwined in the social contexts of immigrant women the longer they stay in the host society. Cultural and gender sensitivity, participatory methods, a call for sensitivity on the part of health care professionals, and recognition of diverse intersecting identities and social conditions would allow for the progressive construction of a dense network that incorporates a number of intersecting sensitivities to develop successful interventions.

Although structural approaches to the prevention and management of diabetes, such as anti-poverty campaigns, social inclusion, employment, and housing equity programs have not been systematically implemented nor evaluated for their effects, a number of community and individual level actions, such as the examples presented, have yielded improvements in health status and diabetes control. These actions converge to the importance of an intersectional analysis in order to address the evolving nature of vulnerability on the one hand and resilience on the other among a diversity of immigrant women.

This is a call to move beyond gender-sensitive health research. Too many interventions for immigrant women are unsuccessful because of a lack of attention to differences in pre- and post-migration social and cultural norms between groups of immigrant women. When they are, it is often unintentional. To properly understand and contribute to the adequate management of conditions such as type 2 diabetes among women experiencing migration, women's health research needs to incorporate the existence of intersecting determinants and clarify and substantiate them. It will thus be able to advance comprehension of the influence of social determinants of health and address social inequalities in health. In this regard, more thought is needed about the right approach. Identifying concrete practices remains a challenge; the key is to implement health programs and policies that take increasing account of intersecting determinants of health in ways that include and work with immigrant women (individual-level actions). To do so often requires contextual macro-level policy action as well as community-sensitive participation.

Acknowledgments

Sincere thanks to Brittany Wray for her sustained assistance with a number of versions of this chapter.

References

Abate, N., and M. Chandalia. 2007. Ethnicity, type 2 diabetes and migrant Asian Indians. *Indian Journal of Medical Research* 125: 251-58.

Anand, S., S. Yusuf, V. Vuksan, and S. Devanesen. 2000. Differences in risk factors, atherosclerosis, and cardiovascular disease between ethnic groups in Canada: The Study of Health Assessment and Risk in Ethnic groups (SHARE). *Lancet* 356: 279-84.

Arcury T.A., A.H. Skelly, W.M. Gesler, and M.C. Dougherty. 2004. Diabetes meanings among those without diabetes: Explanatory models of immigrant Latinos in rural North Carolina. *Social Science and Medicine* 59: 2183–93.

Arskey, H., and L. O'Malley. 2005. Scoping studies: Towards a methodological framework. *International Journal of Social Research Methodology* 8(1): 19-32.

Ashton, C.M., et al. 2003. Racial and ethnic disparities in the use of health services: Bias, preferences or poor communication? *Journal of General Internal Medicine* 18: 146–52.

Barnett, A.H., et al. 2006. Genetic or environmental effect? *British Heart Journal* 72(5): 413-21.

Bierman, A., F. Ahmad, and F. Mawani. 2009. Gender, migration and health. In *Racialized migrant women in Canada: Essays on health, violence, and equity,* ed. V. Agnew, 203-33. Toronto: University of Toronto Press.

Brondolo, E., R. Rieppi, K.P. Kelly, and W. Gerin. 2003. Perceived racism and blood pressure: A review of the literature and conceptual and methodological critique. *Annals of Behavioral Medicine* 25(1): 55-65.

Bruce, D.G., W.A. Davis, C.A. Cull, and T.M.E. Davis. 2003. Diabetes education and knowledge in patients with type 2 diabetes from the community: The Fremantle Diabetes Study. *Journal of Diabetes and Its Complications* 17(2): 82-89.

Canadian Diabetes Association. 2008. Clinical practice guidelines for the prevention and management of diabetes in Canada. *Canadian Journal of Diabetes* 32 (Suppl. 1).

Caulford, P., and Y. Vali. 2006. Providing health care to medically uninsured immigrants and refugees. *Canadian Medical Association Journal* 174(9): 1253-54.

Clar, C., et al. 2010. Self monitoring of blood glucose in type 2 diabetes: Systematic review. *Health Technology Assessment* 14(12): 1-140.

Commission on Social Determinants of Health. 2008. *Closing the gap in a generation: Health equity through action on the social determinants of health.* Final Report of the Commission on Social Determinants of Health. Geneva, World Health Organization.

Cooper, H. 2002. Investigating socio-economic explanations for gender and ethnic inequalities in health. *Social Science and Medicine* 54(5): 693-706.

Désilets, M.C., M. Rivard, B. Shatenstein, and H. Delisle. 2007. Dietary transition stages based on eating patterns and diet quality among Haitians of Montreal, Canada. *Public Health Nutrition* 10(5): 454-63.

DesMeules, M., J. Gold, Z. Cao, J. Payne, B. Lafrance, B. Vissandjée, E. Kliewer, and Y. Mao. 2005. Disparities in mortality patterns among Canadian immigrants and refugees, 1980-1998: Results of a national cohort study. *Journal of Immigrant Health* 7(4): 221-32.

Dunn, J.R., and I. Dyck. 2000. Social determinants of health in Canada's immigrant population: Results from the National Population Health Survey. *Social Sciences and Medicine* 51: 1573-93.

Eakin, E.G., S.S. Bull, R.E. Glasgow, and M. Mason. 2002. Reaching those most in need: A review of diabetes self-management interventions in disadvantaged populations. *Diabetes/Metabolism Research and Reviews* 18: 26-35.

Gafvels, C., and P.E. Wändell. 2005. Coping strategies in men and women with type 2 diabetes in Swedish primary care. *Diabetes Research and Clinical Practice* 71(3): 280-89.

Gagnon, A.J., J. Tuck, and L.A. Barkun. 2004. Systematic review of measurement strategies for refugee women's health. *Health Care for Women International* 25: 111-49.

Gilmer, T.P., and P.J. O'Connor. 2010. The growing importance of diabetes screening. *Diabetes Care* 33(7): 1695-97.

Gilmer, T.P., A. Philis-Tsimikas, and C. Walker. 2005. Outcomes of Project Dulce: A culturally specific diabetes management program. *Annals of Pharmacotherapy* 39(5): 817-22.

Gravel, S., J-M. Brodeur, B. Vissandjée, F. Champagne, and K. Lippel. 2008. Incompréhension par les travailleurs immigrants victimes de lésions professionnelles de leurs difficultés d'accès à l'indemnisation. *Migrations et Santé* 131: 12-37.

Green, L.W. 2006. From research to "best practices" in other settings and populations. *American Journal of Health Behavior* 25(3): 165-78.

Greenhalgh, T., A. Collard, and N. Begum. 2005. Sharing studies of complex intervention for diabetes education in minority ethnic groups who do not speak English. *British Medical Journal* 330: 628-31.

Greenhalgh, T., A. Collard, D. Campbell-Richards, S. Vijayaraghavan, F. Malik, J. Morris, and A. Claydon. 2011. Storylines of self-management: Narratives of people with diabetes from a multiethnic inner city population. *Journal of Health Services Policy* 16: 37-43.

Gucciardi, E., M. DeMelo, R. Lee, and S. Grace. 2007. Assessment of two culturally competent education methods: Individual versus individual plus group education in Canadian Portuguese adults with type 2 diabetes. *Ethnicity and Health* 12(2): 163-87.

Hankivsky, O. 2005. Gender mainstreaming vs. diversity Mainstreaming: A preliminary examination of the role and transformative potential of feminist theory. *Canadian Journal of Political Science* 38(4): 977-1001.

Hankivsky, O., and A. Christoffersen. 2008. Intersectionality and the determinants of health: A Canadian perspective. *Critical Public Health* 18(3): 1-23.

Harris, R., M. Tobias, M. Jeffreys, K. Waldegrave, S. Karlsen, and J. Nazroo. 2006. Effects of self-reported racial discrimination and deprivation on Maori health and inequalities in New Zealand: Cross-sectional study. *Lancet* 367(9527): 2005-9.

Health Canada. 1994. Strategies for population health: Investing in the health of Canadians. http://www.phac-aspc.gc.ca/ph-sp/pdf/strateg-eng.pdf.

Helme, D.W. and N.G. Harrington. 2004. Patient accounts for noncompliance with diabetes self-care regimens and physician compliance-gaining response. Patient Education and Counselling 55: 281-92.

Hjelm, K.G., et al. 2005. Beliefs about health and diabetes in men of different ethnic origin. *Journal of Advanced Nursing* 50: 47-59

Hosler, A.S., and M.M. Spence. 2004. Diabetes and its related risk factors among Russian-speaking immigrants in New York State. *Ethnicity and Disease* 14: 372-74.

Hux, J.E., and M. Tang. 2003. Patterns of prevalence and incidence of diabetes. In *Diabetes in Ontario*, ed. J. Hux, G. Booth, P. Slaughter, and A. Laupacis, Chapter 1. Toronto: Institute for Clinical Evaluative Sciences. http://www.ices.on.ca.

Hyman, I. 2001. *Immigration and health*. Health Policy Working Paper Series. Ottawa: Health Canada.

–. 2007. *Immigration and health: Reviewing evidence of the healthy immigrant effect in Canada*. CERIS Working Paper 55. Toronto: Joint Centre of Excellence for Research on Immigration and Settlement. http://ceris.metropolis.net.

Hyman, I., and S. Guruge. 2002. A review of theory and health promotion: Strategies for new immigrant women. *Canadian Journal of Public Health* 93(3): 183-87.

Hyman, I., and B. Jackson. Forthcoming 2011. The healthy immigrant effect: A temporary phenomenon? *Health Policy Research Bulletin* (January).

Im, E.O., and K. Yang (2002). Theories on immigrant women's health. *Health Care Women International* 27(8):666-81.

Jaber, L.A., M.B. Brown, A. Hammad, S.N. Nowak, Q. Zhu, A. Ghafoor, and W.H. Herman. 2003. Epidemiology of diabetes among Arab Americans. *Diabetes Care* 26(2): 308-13.

Johnson, J.L., L. Greaves, and R. Repta (2007). *Better science with sex and gender: A primer for health research*. Vancouver: Women's Health Research Network.

Kazemipur, A., and S. Halli. 2000. The invisible barrier. Neighbourhood poverty and integration of immigrants in Canada. *Journal of International Migration and Integration* 1(1): 85-100.

Kokanovic, R., and L. Manderson. 2007. Exploring doctor-patient communication in immigrant Australians with type 2 diabetes: A qualitative study. *Journal of General Internal Medicine* 22: 459-63.

Krieger, N. 2003. Does racism harm health? Did child abuse exist before 1962? On explicit questions, critical science, and current controversies: An ecosocial perspective. *American Journal of Public Health* 93(2): 194-99.

Kumar, S.S., and R. Houlden. 2005. Ethnocultural diversity and the diabetes epidemic in Canada: A call to action. *Canadian Journal of Diabetes* 29(2): 84-85.

Kuntie, K., S. Kumar, and J. Brodie. 2009. *Diabetes UK and South Asian Health Foundation recommendations on diabetes research priorities for British South Asians*. Diabetes UK.

Llácer A., M.V. Zunzunegui, J. del Amo, L. Mazarrasa, F. Bolumar. 2007. The contribution of a gender perspective to the understanding of migrants' health. *Journal of Epidemiology and Community Health* 61(Suppl. 2): ii-10.

McDonald, J.T., and S. Kennedy. 2005. Is migration to Canada associated with unhealthy weight gain? Overweight and obesity among Canada's immigrants. *Social Science and Medicine* 61(12): 2469-81.

Mehler, P., R. Lundgren, I. Pines, and K. Doll. 2004. A community study of language concordance in Russian patients with diabetes. *Ethnicity and Disease* 14: 584-88.

Midiema, B., R. Hamilton, and J. Easley. 2008. Climbing the walls: Structural barriers to accessing primary care for refugee newcomers in Canada. *Canadian Family Physician* 54(3): 335-36.

Misra, A., and O. Ganda. 2007. Migration and its impact on adiposity and type 2 diabetes. *Nutrition* 23(9): 696-708.

Murray, M., T. Bodenheimer, D. Rittenhouse, and K. Grumbach. 2003. Improving timely access to primary care: Case studies of the advanced access model. *Journal of the American Medical Association* 289: 1042-46.

Nazroo, J.Y. 2003. The structuring of ethnic inequalities in health: Economic position, racial discrimination and racism. *American Journal of Public Health* 93(2): 277-84.

Newbold, B. 2005. Health status and health care of immigrants in Canada: A longitudinal analysis. *Journal of Health Services Research Policy* 10(2): 77-83.

–. 2009. "The Short-Term Health of Canada's New Immigrant Arrivals: Evidence from the LSIC." *Ethnicity and Health* 14(3): 315-36.

Ng, E., R. Wilkins, F. Gendron, and J.M. Berthelot. 2005. The changing health of immigrants. *Canadian Social Trends* 78: 15-19.

Oldroyd, J., M. Banerjee, A. Heald, and K. Cruickshank. 2005. Diabetes and ethnic minorities. *British Medical Journal* 81: 486-90.

Oxman-Martinez, J., J. Hanley, L. Lach, N. Khanlou, S. Weerasinghe, and V. Agnew. 2005. Intersection of Canadian policy parameters affecting women with precarious immigration status: A baseline for understanding barriers to health. *Journal of Immigrant Health* 7(4): 247-58.

Pittaway, E., and L. Bartolomei. 2002. Refugees, race, and gender: The multiple discrimination against refugee women. *Dialogue* 19(6): 21-32.

Public Health Agency of Canada. 2005. Building a national diabetes strategy: Synthesis of research and collaborations. http://www.phac-aspc.gc.ca.

Raphael, D. 2003. The social determinants of the incidence and management of type 2 diabetes mellitus: Are we prepared to rethink our questions and redirect our research activities? *International Journal of Health Care Quality Assurance* 16(3): 10-20.

–. 2007. *Poverty and policy in Canada: Implications for health and quality of life.* Toronto: Canadian Scholars' Press.

Razum, O., H. Zeeb, and S. Rohrmann. 2000. The "healthy migrant effect"– Not merely a fallacy of inaccurate denominator figures. Letter to the editor. *International Journal of Epidemiology* 29: 191-92.

Reid, C., A. Pederson, and S. Dupéré. 2007. Addressing diversity in health promotion: Implications of women's health and the intersectional theory. In *Health promotion in Canada: Critical perspectives.* 2nd ed., ed. M. O'Neil, A. Pederson, S. Dupéré, and I. Rootman, 75-90. Toronto: Canadian Scholars' Press.

Rothman, R., D. DeWalk, R. Malone, B. Bryant, A. Shintani, B. Crigler, M. Weinberger, and M. Pignone. 2004. Influence of patient literacy on the effectiveness of a primary care-based diabetes disease management program. *Journal of the American Medical Association* 292(14): 1711-16.

Sarkadi, A., and U. Rosenqvist. 2002. Social network and role demands in women's type 2 diabetes: A model. *Health Care Women International* 23: 600-11.

Schaafsma, J., and A. Sweetman. 2001. Immigrant earnings: Age at immigration matters. *Canadian Journal of Economics* 34(4): 1066-99.

Scheuner, M.T. 2008. Delivery of genomic medicine for common chronic adult diseases: A systematic review. *Journal of the American Medical Association* 299(11): 1320-44.

Schooley, J., C. Mundt, P. Wagner, J. Fullerton, and M. O'Donnell. 2007. Factors influencing health care-seeking behaviours among Mayan women in Guatemala. *Midwifery* 7(11): 411-21.

Simich, L., M. Beiser, and F.N. Mawani. 2003. Social support and the significance of shared experience in refugee migration and resettlement. *Western Journal of Nursing Research* 25(7): 872-91.

Simich, L., F. Wu, and S. Nerad. 2007. Status and health security: An exploratory study of irregular immigrants in Toronto. *Canadian Journal of Public Health* 98(5): 369-73.

Spallek, J., H. Zeeb, and O. Razum. 2010. Prevention among immigrants: The example of Germany. *BMC Public Health* 10 (92): 191-92.

Spitzer, D.L. 2005. Engendering health disparities. *Canadian Journal of Public Health* 96 (supp 2): S78-96.

Strine, T., C. Okoro, D. Chapman, G. Beckles, L. Balluz, and A. Mokdad. 2005. The impact of formal diabetes education on the preventive health practices ad behaviors of persons with type 2 diabetes. *Preventive Medicine* 41(1): 79-84.

Subramanian, S.V., and I. Kawachi. 2004. Income inequality and health: What have we learned so far? *Epidemiologic Reviews* 26: 78-91.

Sulaiman, N.D., J.S. Furler, E.J. Hadj, H.M. Corbett, and D.Y. Young. 2007. Stress, culture and "home": Social context in Turkish and Arabic-speaking Australians' views of diabetes prevention. *Health Promotion Journal of Australia* 18(1): 63-68.

Vissandjée, B., S. Abdool, and S. Dupéré. 2005. Empowerment beyond numbers: Substantiating women's political participation. *Journal of International Women's Studies* 7(2): 123-41.

Vissandjée, B., A. Apale, and S. Wieringa. 2009. Exploring social capital among women in the context of migration: Engendering the public policy debate. In *Racialized migrant women in Canada: Essays on health, violence, and equity*, ed. V. Agnew, 187-203. Toronto: University of Toronto Press.

Vissandjée, B., and A. Battaglini. 2010. Santé des femmes: A la croisée des questions de genre, ethnicité et migration. In *Santé et services sociaux de première ligne en milieu plurieth-nique*. Éditions Rémi Saint Martin, Québec, 277 88.

Vissandjée, B., M. Desmeules, Z. Cao, S. Abdool, and A. Kazanjian. 2004. Integrating eth-nicity and migration as determinants of Canadian women's health. *BioMed Central Women's Health* 4(Suppl. 32).

Vissandjée, B., W. Thurston, A. Apale, and K. Nahar. 2007. Women's health at the intersec-tion of gender and the experience of international migration. In *Women's health in Canada: Critical perspectives on theory and policy*, ed. M. Morrow, O. Hankivsky, and C. Varcoe, 221-43. Toronto: University of Toronto Press.

Vissandjée, B., M. Weinfeld, M. Dupéré, and S. Abdool. 2000. Sex, gender, ethnicity and access to health care services: Research and policy challenges for immigrant women in Canada. *Journal of International Migration and Integration* 2(1): 55-75.

Wallin, A.M., M. Lofvander, and G. Ahlstrom. 2007. Diabetes: A cross-cultural interview study of immigrants from Somalia. *Journal of Nursing and Healthcare of Chronic Illness* 16(11c): 305-14.

Wild, S., et al. 2004. Global prevalence of diabetes: Estimates for the year 2000 and projec-tions for 2030. *Diabetes Care* 27: 1047-53.

Wilkinson, R., and M. Marmot, eds. 2003. *Social determinants of health: The solid facts*. 2nd ed. Geneva: World Health Organization.

World Health Organisation (2007). A conceptual framework for action on the social deter-minants of health. Discussion paper for the Commission on Social Determinants of Health. April, Geneva.

14

Intersectionality Model of Trauma and Post-Traumatic Stress Disorder

Joan Samuels-Dennis, Annette Bailey,
and Marilyn Ford-Gilboe

Since the official recognition of post-traumatic stress disorder (PTSD) in the third edition of the *Diagnostic and Statistical Manual of Mental Disorders* (DSM-III) (American Psychiatric Association 1980), extensive research has focused on identifying effective psychosocial and pharmaco-therapeutic treatments for it, as well as understanding the psychological, physiological, social, and ecological factors that cause this condition. Although psychiatry recognized the unique features of PTSD as early as the mid-nineteenth century, the impetus for the inclusion of PTSD in the DSM-III arose from the political actions of Vietnam veterans' advocacy groups and anti-war mental health workers who saw the need to move beyond multiple diagnoses such as phobias, depression, anxiety, and personality disorders toward a unique psychiatric profile for psychological symptoms exhibited by individuals who were exposed to single or multiple traumatic events (Herman 1997; McNally 2004).

The political agenda that facilitated the induction of PTSD into the DSM introduced an inherent gender bias in the conceptualization of PTSD-precipitating events, or Criterion A (see Table 14.1). Thus, Criterion A, as initially defined, legitimized the experiences of male war veterans as *outside the range of usual human experience* but failed to account for the traumatic experiences encountered by women and children (rape excluded) who also exhibited PTSD symptoms (American Psychiatric Association 1980). The next two decades would witness the evolution of Criterion A as feminist clinicians lobbied the DSM-PTSD committee to recognize violence against women and girls, including childhood abuse and intimate partner violence (IPV), as traumatic events that could cause PTSD (Burstow 2005; Herman 1997; Humphreys and Joseph 2004).

The goal of the feminist movement was to have clinicians and researchers alike appropriately assess and diagnose women's exposure to and reactions to assaultive traumas (Herman 1997). Such a shift on the part of mental health service providers and researchers would allow for the achievement

Table 14.1

Conceptualizing of Criterion A

DSM	Criterion A
DSM-III, 1980	The person has experienced a catastrophic stressor that is outside the range of usual human experience.
DSM-III-R, 1987	The person has experienced an event that is outside the range of usual human experience and that would be markedly distressing to almost anyone, e.g., serious threat to one's life or physical integrity; serious threat or harm to one's children, spouse, or other close relatives and friends; sudden destruction of one's home or community; or seeing another person who has been or is being, seriously injured or killed as the result of an accident or physical violence.
DSM-IV, 1994 DSM-IV-TR, 2000	The person has been exposed to a traumatic event in which both of the following were present: • The person experienced, witnessed, or was confronted with an event or events that involved actual or threatened death or serious injury, or a threat to the physical integrity of others; • The person's response involved intense fear, helplessness, or horror.

of three significant objectives. First, it would highlight the impact of gender-based violence on the mental health of women and girls. Second, emerging information on the effects of gender-based violence would facilitate a transition in mental health professionals' views of women's response to trauma and, consequently, absolve women of labels such as borderline personality disorder, histrionic personality, and dependent personality. Third, this shift would begin to unravel the social, political, and ideological systems that support and maintain violence against women and girls (Berg 2002; Herman 1992; Humphreys and Joseph 2004).

This move has led to the proliferation of theoretical and empirical literature addressing variations in women's exposure to violent traumas and the extent to which these traumas affect women's risk for developing PTSD (Andrews, Brewin, and Rose 2003; Breslau 2002; Gavranidou and Rosner 2003; Walker et al. 2004). Gender plays a significant role in the trauma-PTSD process, both in terms of the types of traumas men and women are likely to encounter over their lifetime and the unique ways in which women respond to traumatic events that are violent in nature (Breslau 2002; Herman 1997). However, a number of observations concerning the course of PTSD suggest that though the initial trauma exercises a central role in its development, the persistence of symptoms is associated with the presence or absence of specific personal and social resources that are not only determined by gender but also by women's multiple and intersecting social identities (Andrews, Brewin, and Rose 2003; Benight and Bandura 2004; Brewin, Andrews, and Valentine 2000). This suggests the need to move beyond examining gender as the primary structural factor that influences women's exposure to traumatic experiences and their psychological response to trauma. The use of frameworks that examine how the privilege and disadvantage implied by women's multiple and intersecting social statuses shape their experiences and their access to resources is crucial to understanding the development and persistence of PTSD.

Theorists and researchers espousing an intersectional perspective argue that social location – an individual's position within a social hierarchy conferred by multiple and interconnected social statuses (such as race/culture/ethnicity, gender, class, ability/disability) – shapes women's lived experiences and their differential or unequal access to resources, power, autonomy, and privilege (McMullin 2004; Symington 2004; Yuval-Davis 2006). Further, they argue that the social statuses that comprise social location are not mutually exclusive, static, or abstract; rather, they are interlocking systems of oppression that mutually support and define each other. Within this framework, trauma is not a monolithic phenomenon; instead, social location directly and indirectly influences the nature of trauma, the interpretation of the experience, the responses of others, and the personal and/or social resources available for responding to trauma.

Intersectionality Model of Trauma and PTSD

This chapter describes the intersectionality model of trauma and PTSD (IMT-PTSD), a framework that attempts to move researchers and clinicians beyond the traditional stress-response framework that guides much PTSD research toward a model that contextualizes women's physiological and psychological responses particularly to violent or assaultive traumas. The model (see Figure 14.1) situates PTSD within a social determinant of health perspective. It suggests that disparities in mental well-being reflect both the intersection between people's diverse experiences and the social context of their lives.

Unlike traditional frameworks, which focus on the individual's psychological and physiological response to trauma, the IMT-PTSD model addresses how structural opportunities and constraints facilitate or hinder health. Consistent with Susan Berg's (2002) position, we argue that the person-centred focus of the stress-response framework serves to decontextualize and depoliticize the experiences of women. Furthermore, the overwhelming use of such frameworks has resulted in a long-term introspective examination of women's personal vulnerabilities to trauma, rather than a collective appraisal of the social factors that both promote violence and limit women's

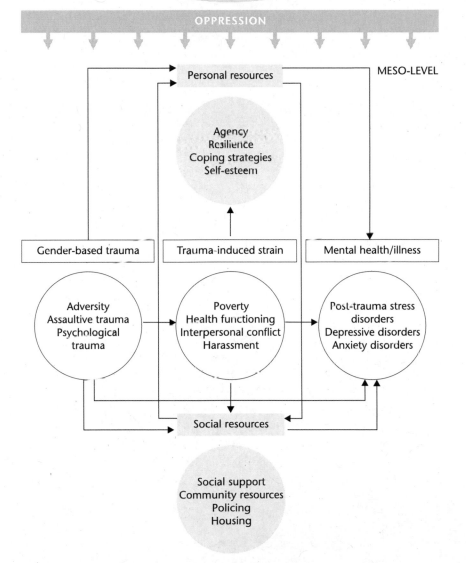

Figure 14.1 **Intersectionality model of trauma and PTSD**

ability to mobilize those personal, health, and social resources that facilitate the management of PTSD symptoms.

The IMT-PTSD model integrates current literature with principles of intersectionality (Crenshaw 1994) and the stress process model (Pearlin 1989, 1999) to provide a framework for conducting research that is sensitive to the nature of women's traumatic experiences and the ways in which intersectionality limits or supports access to the resources needed to promote mental health. The framework focuses on the structural and political context of women's lives with the explicit understanding that social status defines the conditions of life to which people are exposed. Assumptions of the IMT-PTSD include the following:

- Oppression operates naturally in various forms and levels (sexism, economic deprivation, racism/ethnocentrism, social exclusion) in modern society.
- A complex interaction between different forms of oppression determines individuals' power, resilience, and well-being.
- Political and structural characteristics uniquely affect people's mental health and well-being through socially created advantages and disadvantages in the distribution of social resources.
- The effects of trauma are proliferative in that exposure to one type of trauma gives rise to other negative and detrimental experiences, the effects of which surface and recede or function in combination with other life experiences to affect mental health.

As depicted in Figure 14.1, the IMT-PTSD model suggests that mental health is determined by macro-level factors (political and structural) that intersect to shape oppressive experiences – power inequalities, discriminating social relations, and the inequitable distribution of health and social resources. In turn, these intersecting factors facilitate a meso-level trauma-PTSD process, whereby gender-based traumas (primary stressor) directly and indirectly affect people's mental health through their influence on the availability of personal and social resources (mediating resources), and exposure to trauma-induced strain – chronic stressors and strains that arise as a direct consequences of the initial traumatic experience (secondary stressors).

Macro-Level Determinants of Mental Health

The stress process (Pearlin 1999) is a conceptual model and a general orienting framework used to guide research that seeks to emphasize the link between social and economic statuses, life circumstances, and the health and well-being of people. A fundamental assumption of the model is that people's hierarchical position in the stratified orders of social and economic class, gender, race, and ethnicity inherently entails inequalities in the possession of power, privilege, and prestige. Furthermore, these positions have the potential to affect well-being indirectly through their influence in shaping the context of people's lives, the stressors to which they are exposed, and the mediating resources they possess. The stress process model outlines six constructs with an emphasis placed on social and economic statuses as the central converging factor that influences all other constructs in the model. The model includes three forms of stressors: first are neighbourhood ambient stressors – the problems and threats encountered in everyday neighbourhood life. Second are primary stressors – an initial life event or the chronic strain that arise from an individual's life context (such as social status and roles) and social context (such as neighbourhood of residence). Third are secondary stressors, which develop as a direct consequence of exposure to the primary stressor. Each type of stressor has a direct and indirect impact on the individual's well-being, but their affect is hindered, prevented, and buffered by moderating and mediating resources (Pearlin 1999).

Stress mediators and moderators, including the individual's coping repertoires, level of social support, and level of mastery, represent the social and personal resources that individuals and families mobilize to contain, regulate, or otherwise ameliorate the effects of stressors (ibid.). Mediating and moderating resources helps us to understand why individuals exposed to the same stressors experience a wide array of differing outcomes. Mediating and moderating resources is thought to serve a protective function that can be exercised in three ways: by functioning proactively to prevent the occurrence of a stressor or the proliferation of a secondary stressor, by modifying or minimizing the harmful impact of stressful conditions, and by perceptually controlling the meaning of the stressor in ways that reduce its threat and potential painful consequences (Pearlin 1999).

In his overview of the stress process, Leonard Pearlin (1999) makes an argument for the normative reality of life hypothesis, suggesting that neighbourhoods are typically composed of individuals whose key statuses (such as race, age, socio-economic condition) are similar. He further suggests that people who share similar statuses experience similar hardships to which they respond in similar ways and with similar resources. Although Pearlin recognized the potential for neighbourhoods to affect people's health, a significant critique of the stress process framework is that it attends only to the individual-level effects of neighbourhoods in the form of ambient strain. In the model, ambient strain is reflected by risk of exposure to violence, poor physical state of the neighbourhood, high residential turnover rates resulting in lost social networks and reduced social cohesion, and the absence of social programs and services.

The stress process as outlined by Pearlin (ibid.) provides a foundation for understanding how neighbourhoods affect the everyday lives of individuals and the importance of social and economic status as central determinants of health. However, it falls short in highlighting how the intersection of

Structural intersectionality	Political intersectionality
→ Multiple and intersecting systems of domination	→ Process through which the political interests of women are denied
• Social oppression • Economic oppression • Representational oppression • Institutional oppression	• Political dialogue • Legal directives • Government policies

Figure 14.2   **Structural and political intersectionality**

these structures at the macro level influences various forms of oppression experienced by people. In developing the IMT-PTSD model, we build on this foundation by combining the individual-level components of the stress process (stress exposure, stress mediators/moderators, stress outcome) with the structural and political dimensions of the intersectionality perspective (see Figure 14.2). In doing so, we address not only the individual's experience but the ways in which these experiences intersect with neighbourhood structure and politics to perpetuate the varying forms of oppression women experience. Within this context, "oppression" refers to a process and an outcome whereby power exerted within political, social, environmental, and interpersonal relationships intersects to create advantages and disadvantages for psychological well-being. The model makes oppression visible as the key factor that links the arrangement of our socially structured world to the mental health and well-being of people.

Intersectionality is a critical social theory concerned with uncovering how structural and political factors (Figure 14.2) intersect to influence the health of individuals and groups (Crenshaw 1989, 1994). It was introduced as a philosophical critique of feminist theory and anti-racist discourses of the 1970s and 1980s, which granted primacy to gender or race as the most important sources of discrimination faced by women and minorities. Intersectionality places an emphasis on critically examining how various forms of oppression, such as racism, sexism, and classism, intersect to influence the multi-dimensionality of women's lived experiences and health.

The IMT-PTSD model incorporates Kimberly Crenshaw's (1994) distinction between structural and political intersectionality and places it within a neighbourhood context. Structural intersectionality refers to social, economic, representational, and institutional forms of oppression present in neighbourhoods that foster differential access to resources and exposure to trauma (ibid.). "Neighbourhood" in its broadest sense refers to geographic boundaries including countries, provinces/territories, cities, and regions.

Within neighbourhoods, structural intersectionality attends to co-relating systems of oppression that are supported by socially ascribed identities. In contrast, political intersectionality highlights how the political interests of various groups within neighbourhoods are obscured and sometimes jeopardized by political dialogue, legal directives, and government policies that ignore or suppress issues of oppression with implications for fairness/ unfairness, equity/inequity, and justice/injustice in society (Crenshaw 1994; Fernandes 2003).

The IMT-PTSD model suggests that neighbourhoods provide a geographic and social space whereby the structural and political profiles of neighbourhood supersede individual social and economic status in determining the types and sources of oppression to which residents are exposed as well as the resources available for coping with and managing trauma responses. Pearlin (1999) suggested that neighbourhoods comprise people with similar social and economic statuses, lived experiences, and resources. This argument begs the following question: Does the structural profile of neighbourhoods influence the traumatic life experiences of people, or do traumatized people move into neighbourhoods with particular profiles? Current literature does not support a social selection process whereby traumatized and mentally ill individuals settle into the most disadvantaged neighbourhoods. Rather, a myriad of studies support the hypothesis that neighbourhoods influence people's stressful and traumatic experiences. A growing body of research has demonstrated that disadvantaged neighbourhoods are characterized by increased exposure to violence (Burke, O'Campo, and Peak 2006; Cunradi et al. 2000; Miles-Doan 1998), resource deprivation (Allard, Rosen, and Tolman 2003), and mental health problems (Aneshensel and Sucoff 1996; Diez Roux 2001; Galea et al. 2006; Galea et al. 2007; Henderson et al. 2005; Leventhal and Brooks-Gunn 2003; Silver, Mulvey, and Swanson 2002). Thus, in keeping with current literature, we suggest that neighbourhood structure and politics may advantage or disadvantage individuals both in terms of exposure to a particular set of traumas and the accessibility of resources that regulate the impact of those events on people's well-being.

In Figure 14.3, we suggest that neighbourhood economic status as well as ethnic/racial and family structure distribution may unwittingly disadvantage women in their ability to access, for example, high-quality mental health care because the best practitioners may choose not to work in such neighbourhoods. Structurally related disadvantages may also intersect with political dialogue and policies that suppress the awareness of violence in the life of women and girls. For example, current and evolving privacy laws, although developed to protect the rights of individuals, may inadvertently and systematically silence women and girls regarding their exposure to violence. Additionally, such policies may result in the loss of critical information that

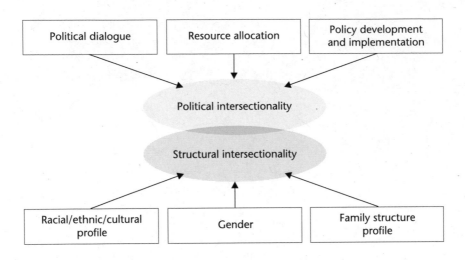

Figure 14.3   **Neighbourhood structural and political intersections**

would bring to the forefront the experiences of people living in specific neighbourhoods and consequently limit the development of community- or group-specific interventions.

In the IMT-PTSD model, as outlined in Figure 14.1, political intersectionality sits above structural intersectionality to illustrate the hierarchal dynamics of this relationship. Thus, though both have important contextual roles to play, neighbourhood policies and political dialogue relevant to trauma prevention have a much greater potential for creating environments that facilitate the perpetuation of violence against women and girls. There are several ways in which this may occur. First, policies that address the prevention of gender-based trauma may be absent. Second, policies may be developed that fail to acknowledge that structural intersectionality influences the types of trauma people experience. Thus, some policies are unsuccessful in purposefully and effectively targeting the prevention of traumas known to affect particular groups both within and across neighbourhoods. Third, political intersectionality may limit or enhance the availability of personal, health, and social resources resulting in differential access within and across neighbourhoods.

Meso-Level Determinants of Mental Health
The meso-level components of the IMT-PTSD model (Figure 14.1) depict the proposed relationship between five constructs: gender-based trauma, trauma-induced strain, personal resources, social resources, and mental health. The model acknowledges exposure to trauma as the central cause of PTSD.

However, the fact that not all individuals exposed to a traumatic event develop PTSD has led theorists and researchers to consider why, in the post-trauma period, some individuals do not develop PTSD, others experience it with recovery, and still others experience it without recovery. Employing Pearlin's stress process model, we argue that the severity of impact of any given trauma on women's mental health is mediated by interpersonal stressors and resources. Specifically, our review of current literature suggests that exposure to gender-based trauma will precipitate exposure to stressors/strains and deplete women's personal and social resources. In turn, each is proposed to affect PTSD symptom levels, such that women's personal and social resources are associated with less severe PTSD symptoms, whereas greater strain is associated with more severe PTSD symptoms. Additionally, this process is influenced by structural and political intersectionality.

Gender-Based Trauma

Gender-based trauma, as outlined in the model, refers to non-naturally occurring traumatic experiences that are motivated and supported by entrenched beliefs about the socially ascribed roles, responsibilities, and locations of individuals belonging to the male and female sex. Pearlin (1999) identified trauma as a type of life event that includes a wide range of severe situations such as loss through death, natural disasters, accidents, and rape, and are distinguished from other life events by their sudden occurrence, level of severity, and long-lasting impact. We suggest that this conceptualization does not adequately attend to the types of trauma that women encounter over their lifetime. A gender-sensitive conceptualization of trauma needs to account for those experiences, such as childhood abuse (physical, emotional, and sexual) and partner abuse (physical, emotional, and sexual), which, although not discrete or short-lived events, are nevertheless outside the range of usual human experience (American Psychiatric Association 2000).

In her documentation of the link between domestic captivity and complex PTSD, Judith Herman (1997) argued that the experiences and psychological responses of individuals exposed to political captivity (hostages, prisoners of war, concentration-camp survivors) and domestic captivity (survivors of domestic battering, childhood physical or sexual abuse, and organized sexual exploitation) are inherently similar. Although the context of captivity differs, tactics used by perpetrators, including force, intimidation, and manipulation to gain power and control over their victims, are almost identical. Recognizing the profound psychological alterations that occur among individuals exposed to prolonged periods (months to years) of violence, captivity, and total control by another, we offer a gender-sensitive conceptualization of trauma with the underlying assumption that, for many women, experiences of trauma are multiple, overlapping, and enduring (Kaysen, Resick, and Wise 2003).

Two types of gender-based trauma are particularly relevant to the IMT-PTSD model: assaultive traumas and psychological traumas. The former are discrete and/or enduring offensive physical and sexual encounters including childhood physical abuse, childhood sexual abuse, intimate partner violence (IPV), and non-intimate sexual assault that precipitate a state of intense fear, anxiety, and apprehension, loss of control, and powerlessness in the victim (Herman 1997). Psychological traumas are enduring, emotionally overwhelming, and personally uncontrollable life circumstances, such as childhood emotional abuse and witnessing parental IPV, that are often characterized by fear, intimidation, and manipulation, render individuals powerless, and profoundly alter their view of themselves, others, and the world (Goodman, Saxe, and Harvey 1991; Herman 1997).

This conceptualization of trauma is informed by the understanding that higher rates of PTSD among women do not reflect their greater vulnerability to mental illness, but rather differences in the nature and culmination of their traumatic experiences (Breslau, Chilcoat, Kessler, Peterson, and Lucia 1999; Follette et al. 1996; Schumm, Briggs-Phillips, and Hobfoll 2006). Over their lifetimes, women and girls are more likely than men and boys to experience assaultive and psychological traumas, which, in turn, increase their risk for developing PTSD. Results of one recent study (see Finkelhor et al. 2005; Turner, Finkelhor, and Ormrod 2006) revealed that, during childhood (two to nine years of age), rates of physical and sexual abuse against boys and girls are about equal. However, as children transition to adolescence, where socially ascribed beliefs concerning gender roles become entrenched, girls experience sexual abuse and sexually based dating violence more so than boys, whereas boys are more likely to experience physical abuse (Banyard, Cross, and Modecki 2006; Briere and Elliott 2003; Cyr, McDuff, and Wright 2006; Kilpatrick and Saunders 1997; Turner et al. 2006). Furthermore, as adolescents transition to adulthood (eighteen years and older), women experience more assaultive trauma, including rape and IPV, than their male counterparts, whereas men are at greater risk of non-sexualized assaultive violence such as physical assault by a stranger, being robbed, being threatened with a weapon, and combat (Astin et al. 1995; Breslau, Chilcoat, Kessler, and Davis 1999; Coker et al. 2005; Elliott, Mok, and Briere 2004; Resnick et al. 1993).

Although the model allows for the examination of how specific gender-based traumas influence mental health, we suggest that the *constellation* of women's lived experiences matters most to their well-being. Primacy granted to any one traumatic event denies the fact that all experiences shape the current context of women's lives and their mental well-being. Life adversities – discrete or short-lived non-violent events that are disruptive in nature because of their level of severity and sudden occurrence (Pearlin 1999) – must also be included in this constellation, as their effects on mental health have been demonstrated in previous studies (Avison, Ali, and Walters 2007; Avison et al. 2008; Breslau, Chilcoat, Kessler, and Davis 1999; Lloyd and Turner 2003). Understanding the complex relationship between trauma exposure and mental health problems also requires an examination of the interrelationship between intersectionality, trauma exposure, trauma-induced stressors/strains, and the availability of personal and social resources.

Personal Resources

Personal resources represent internal strengths or capacities that assist individuals in their daily life and in coping with the effects of stressful or traumatic experiences. They include but are not limited to coping styles, mastery, personal empowerment, self-esteem, and agency. Among all personal resources, the IMT-PTSD model grants primacy to agency, which refers to people's capacity for appraising and assigning meaning to their life circumstances, making meaningful choices, and engaging in activities that create personal, social, and political change (Bandura 2001; Benight and Bandura 2004; McMullin 2004). Agency represents both a process and an outcome. In the context of women's traumatic experiences, this process includes an evaluation of the potential harms or benefits of the traumatic event with respect to one's values, goals, commitments, and health, an assessment of activities that may be helpful in overcoming previous trauma or preventing future exposure, and the enhancement of one's sense of empowerment through engagement in the process of conscientization, or raised consciousness (Carr 2003; Finfgeld 2004; Ryles 1999). The IMT-PTSD model draws on empirical and theoretical literature, and identifies agency as a key factor that influences the development and persistence of PTSD symptoms.

Although a number of personal resources have been examined as mediators of the trauma-PTSD process, studies of self-efficacy may provide the most comparable insights regarding the protective influence of agency in the post-trauma period. Albert Bandura (2001) and Charles Benight and Albert Bandura (2004) suggest that, among the many mechanisms of human agency, none is more central than people's beliefs in their efficacy to manage their own functioning and to exercise control over events that affect their lives. The mediating role of self-efficacy in the trauma-PTSD process has been examined across a range of traumatic experiences including exposure to combat (Ginzburg et al. 2003), terrorist activities (Hobfoll, Canetti-Nisim, and Johnson 2006), physical injury caused by non-domestic violence (Johansen et al. 2007), and child abuse (Vranceanu, Hobfoll, and Johnson 2007). These studies have consistently shown that exposure to trauma diminishes levels of perceived self-efficacy, which, in turn, increases the risk for PTSD or elevated PTSD symptoms.

The importance of agency has also been noted in the pioneering work of researchers in the field of intimate partner violence (Ford-Gilboe, Wuest, and Merritt-Gray 2005; Wuest et al. 2003). The grounded theory study of Judith Wuest et al. (2003), describing the process through which women promote their health after leaving an abusive partner, speaks to the essence of agency as conceptualized here. The health promotion process, called "strengthening capacity to limit intrusion," addresses the ways in which women purposefully work toward establishing a predictable empowering environment that provides a foundation for strengthening their own and their children's health. This study identifies intrusion as the central problem that single mothers face after leaving an abusive partner. According to Wuest et al. (2003, 600) and Marilyn Ford-Gilboe, Judith Wuest, and Marilyn Merritt-Gray (2005), intrusion refers to "external control or interference that demands attention, diverts energy away from family priorities, and limits women's choices." It may include harassment/abuse by ex-partners, abuse-related health complications, stressors arising from seeking and obtaining support, and undesirable changes to patterns of living.

Although these authors did not use the term "agency," women's capacities as identified in their studies are consistent with the many elements of agency. This conceptualization of agency enables us to view women as reflective, reflexive, and possessing the capacity to engage in personal, social, and political change. Although the IMT-PTSD model argues that health is socially determined, the inclusion of agency in the model acknowledges that women are not static objects that are acted on. Rather, even after exposure to trauma, they have the capacity for making choices and behaving in meaningful ways that alter their social world.

Trauma-Induced Stressors/Strains

Trauma-induced strains arise as a direct consequence of exposure to gender-based traumas. They include but are not limited to functioning, disrupted social networks, poverty, and interpersonal conflict. Among all trauma-induced stressors/strains, the IMT-PTSD model grants primacy to social strain, which refers to the enduring conflicts and strains that women face in their daily lives that arise from their social networks and interpersonal relations. Specifically, it refers to the chronic absence of social support and/or consistent problematic interactions with members of their social network. In her conceptualization of complex PTSD, Judith Herman (1992) suggests that women subjected to prolonged and repeated trauma develop an insidious, progressive form of PTSD that is characterized by significant irrevocable interruptions in personality – most notably, disruption of identity and an inability to form close, trusting relationships with others. Such individuals are plagued with difficulties regulating emotions, variations in re-experiencing of trauma, alterations in self-perception, alterations in how they relate to others, loss of hope and faith, and preoccupation with the perpetrators of violence. Given these changes, the IMT-PTSD model posits that gender-based trauma gives rise to secondary stressors in the form of social strain, which develops as a direct consequence of the social network's response to women's experiences and women's own responses. The combination of these stressors leads to a social environment of heightened conflict and depleted supports, resulting in more complex and chronic symptomology.

Although social support has generally been conceptualized as a personal or social resource that mediates or moderates the relationship between stress and mental health problems, recent studies have identified the unavailability of social support and qualitatively poor interactions with one's social network as key determinants of the severity of PTSD symptoms (Andrews et al. 2003; Bradley, Schwartz, and Kaslow 2005; Brewin et al. 2000; Coker et al. 2002; Hyman, Gold, and Cott 2003; Ozer et al. 2003; Schumm, Hobfoll, and Keogh 2004; Schumm, Briggs-Phillips, and Hobfoll 2006). These studies suggest that when members of their social networks respond negatively to their traumatic experiences, women's PTSD symptoms are indirectly affected, influencing self-esteem, use of maladaptive coping strategies, and self-blame.

In their assessment of how the quantity (number of people) and quality (practical, emotional, and critical) of social support in women's social networks explain PTSD symptomology, Alytia Levendosky et al. (2004) found that criticism was the only significant predictor of PTSD symptoms. Andrews, Brewin, and Rose (2003) studied six qualitative dimensions of social support (availability of others, confiding in others, emotional support, practical support, negative responses, and satisfaction with support) and found that a negative response to women's assault experiences was the only significant predictor of PTSD symptoms, six months after physical or sexual assault. Further to this, Anne Coker et al. (2002) examined the relationship between received support versus absent or inconsistent support from friends, family, and a current non-abusive spouse and PTSD symptoms in a sample of women previously exposed to IPV. Like previous research, their study revealed that receiving consistent high levels of emotional support from any of the three sources reduced women's PTSD symptom levels, with emotional support from friends having the greatest effect.

Scott Hyman, Steven Gold, and Melissa Cott (2003) found that the type of social support received was related to PTSD symptom levels. Both self-esteem support (the perception that others value the abused individual) and appraisal support (the perception that one is able to obtain advice when coping with a problem) were related to women's PTSD symptom level: the higher the support, the less intense the symptoms, and vice versa.

Social Resources
Social resources refer to formal (community-based) and informal (familial, kin, friend) support that fosters the healthy development of individuals, families, and communities. Social resources foster a sense of safety and security,

and providing tangible resources to individuals in need. They encompass services and supports such as safe housing, symptom management, advocacy, and mediation. Given that women's mental health is influenced by structural and political factors that are largely beyond their control (Crenshaw 1994; Wuest et al. 2006), public policies ascribed to neighbourhood and communities affect their mental health through the development of mental health promotion strategies and the availability and/or accessibility of formal supports and resources across multiple sectors. Gender-based trauma is a complex health and social problem that is best addressed by interventions that cut across multiple sectors and have the mutual goal of reducing stress/ trauma exposure and improving women's access to personal, social, and economic resources. We suggest that access to social supports and resources may influence PTSD symptomology in multiple ways including enhancing safety, symptom resolution, and re-establishing social network and family routines. Although the published literature has not evaluated the efficacy of such social programs, the IMT-PTSD model acknowledges the particular health benefits of safety-promoting services/resources, religious or spiritual support, counselling and legal services, stable, secure, and affordable housing services, income assistance services, and mental health services.

Conclusion

In North America, women and girls are victimized because the laws, policies, and social mores of the society in which they live continue to support the oppression of women, children, ethnic groups, and the poor. As trauma researchers, we know that important work remains to be done in identifying how we help those exposed to trauma, but it is even more essential to look upstream at the intersection of systems that perpetuate the victimization of women. The IMT-PTSD model offers a framework for examining the social mechanisms that contribute to PTSD among women. The model makes explicit the need to examine how neighbourhood structural and political intersectionality influences exposure to gender-based trauma, the response of self and others to violence, and access to community and institutional supports that facilitate recovery from PTSD. Although the model has yet to be tested, its use may help to contextualize and politicize violence against women, resulting in research that clearly and collectively highlights the complex interplay of social factors that lead to violence against women and subsequent PTSD.

References

Allard, S.W., D. Rosen, and R.M. Tolman. 2003. Access to mental health and substance abuse services among women receiving welfare in Detroit. *Urban Affairs Review* 38(6): 787-807.

American Psychiatric Association, ed. 1980. *Diagnostic and statistical manual of mental disorders*. 3rd ed. Washington, DC: American Psychiatric Association.

American Psychiatric Association. 2000. 309.81 Posttraumatic stress disorder. In *Diagnostic and statistical manual of mental disorders*. IV-TR, ed. American Psychiatric Association, 424-29. Washington, DC: American Psychiatric Association.

Andrews, B., C.R. Brewin, and S. Rose. 2003. Gender, social support, and PTSD in victims of violent crime. *Journal of Traumatic Stress* 16(4): 421-27.

Aneshensel, C.S., and C.A. Sucoff. 1996. The neighborhood context of adolescent mental health. *Journal of Health and Social Behavior* 37(4): 293-310.

Astin, M.C., S.M. Ogland-Hand, E.M. Coleman, and D.S. Foy. 1995. Posttraumatic stress disorder and childhood abuse in battered women: Comparisons with maritally distressed women. *Journal of Consulting and Clinical Psychology* 63(2): 308-12.

Avison, W.R., J. Ali, and D. Walters. 2007. Family structure, stress, and psychological distress: A demonstration of the impact of differential exposure. *Journal of Health and Social Behavior* 48(3): 301-17.

Avison, W.R., L. Davies, A. Willson, and K. Shuey. 2008. Family structure and mothers' mental health: A life course perspective on stability and change. *Advances in Life Course Research* 13: 233-55.

Bandura, A. 2001. Social cognitive theory: An agentic perspective. *Annual Reviews in Psychology* 52(1): 1-26.

Banyard, V.L., C. Cross, and K.L. Modecki. 2006. Interpersonal violence in adolescence: Ecological correlates of self-reported perpetration. *Journal of Interpersonal Violence* 21(10): 1314-32.

Benight, C.C., and A. Bandura. 2004. Social cognitive theory of posttraumatic recovery: The role of perceived self-efficacy. *Behaviour Research and Therapy* 42(10): 1129-48.

Berg, S.H. 2002. The PTSD diagnosis: Is it good for women? *Affilia* 17(1): 55-68.

Bradley, R., A.C. Schwartz, and N.J. Kaslow. 2005. Posttraumatic stress disorder symptoms among low-income, African American women with a history of intimate partner violence and suicidal behaviors: Self-esteem, social support, and religious coping. *Journal of Traumatic Stress* 18(6): 685-96.

Breslau, N. 2002. Gender differences in trauma and posttraumatic stress disorder. *Journal of Gender-Specific Medicine* 5(1): 34-40.

Breslau, N., H.D. Chilcoat, R.C. Kessler, and G.C. Davis. 1999. Previous exposure to trauma and PTSD effects of subsequent trauma: Results from the Detroit area survey of trauma. *American Journal of Psychiatry* 156(6): 902-7.

Breslau, N., H.D. Chilcoat, R.C. Kessler, E.L. Peterson, and V.C. Lucia. 1999. Vulnerability to assaultive violence: Further specification of the sex difference in post-traumatic stress disorder. *Psychological Medicine* 29(4): 813-21.

Brewin, C.R., B. Andrews, and J.D. Valentine. 2000. Meta-analysis of risk factors for post-traumatic stress disorder in trauma-exposed adults. *Journal of Consulting and Clinical Psychology* 68(5): 748-66.

Briere, J., and D.M. Elliott. 2003. Prevalence and psychological sequelae of self-reported childhood physical and sexual abuse in a general population sample of men and women. *Child Abuse Neglect* 27(10): 1205-22.

Burke, J.G., P. O'Campo, and G.L. Peak. 2006. Neighborhood influences and intimate partner violence: Does geographic setting matter? *Journal of Urban Health: Bulletin of the New York Academy of Medicine* 83(2): 182-94.

Burstow, B. 2005. A critique of posttraumatic stress disorder and the DSM. *Journal of Humanistic Psychology* 45(4): 429-45.

Carr, E.S. 2003. Rethinking empowerment theory using a feminist lens: The importance of process. *Affilia: Journal of Women and Social Work* 18(1): 8-20.

Coker, A.L., P.H. Smith, M.P. Thompson, R.E. McKeown, L. Bethea, and K.E. Davis. 2002. Social support protects against the negative effects of partner violence on mental health. *Journal of Women's Health and Gender-Based Medicine* 11(5): 465-76.

Coker, A.L., R. Weston, D.L. Creson, B. Justice, and P. Blakeney. 2005. PTSD symptoms among men and women survivors of intimate partner violence: The role of risk and protective factors. *Violence and Victims* 20(6): 625-43.

Crenshaw, K. 1989. Demarginalizing the intersection of race and sex: A black feminist critique of antidiscrimination doctrine feminist theory and antiracist politics. *University of Chicago Legal Forum:* 139-67.

–. 1994. Mapping the margins: Intersectionality, identity politics, and violence against women of color. In *The public nature of private violence: The discovery of domestic abuse,* ed. M.A. Finemann and R. Mykitiuk, 93-120. New York: Routledge.

Cunradi, C.B., R. Caetano, C. Clark, and J. Schafer. 2000. Neighborhood poverty as a predictor of intimate partner violence among white, black, and Hispanic couples in the United States: A multilevel analysis. *Annals of Epidemiology* 10(5): 297-308.

Cyr, M., P. McDuff, and J. Wright. 2006. Prevalence and predictors of dating violence among adolescent female victims of child sexual abuse. *Journal of Interpersonal Violence* 21(8): 1000-17.

Diez Roux, A.V. 2001. Investigating neighborhood and area effects on health. *American Journal of Public Health* 91(11): 1783-89.

Elliott, D.M., D.S. Mok, and J. Briere. 2004. Adult sexual assault: Prevalence, symptomatology, and sex differences in the general population. *Journal of Traumatic Stress* 17(3): 203-11.

Fernandes, F. 2003. A response to Erica Burman. *European Journal of Psychotherapy, Counselling and Health* 6(4): 309-16.

Finfgeld, D.L. 2004. Empowerment of individuals with enduring mental health problems: Results from concept analysis and qualitative investigation. *Advances in Nursing Sciences* 27(1): 44-52.

Finkelhor, D., R. Ormrod, H. Turner, and S.L. Hamby. 2005. The victimization of children and youth: A comprehensive, national survey. *Child Maltreatment* 10(1): 5-25.

Follette, V.M., M.A. Polusny, A.E. Bechtle, and A.E. Naugle. 1996. Cumulative trauma: The impact of child sexual abuse, adult sexual assault, and spouse abuse. *Journal of Traumatic Stress* 9(1): 25-35.

Ford-Gilboe, M., J. Wuest, and M. Merritt-Gray. 2005. Strengthening capacity to limit intrusion: Theorizing family health promotion in the aftermath of woman abuse. *Qualitative Health Research* 15(4): 477-501.

Galea, S., R. Acierno, H. Resnick, M. Tracy, and D. Kilpatrick. 2006. Social context and the psychobiology of post-traumatic stress. *Annals of the New York Academy of Sciences* 1071(1): 231-41.

Galea, S., J. Ahern, A. Nandi, M. Tracy, J. Beard, and D. Vlahov. 2007. Urban neighborhood poverty and the incidence of depression in a population-based cohort study. *Annals of Epidemiology* 17(3): 171-79.

Gavranidou, M., and R. Rosner. 2003. The weaker sex? Gender and post-traumatic stress disorder. *Depression and Anxiety* 17(3): 130-39.

Ginzburg, K., Z. Solomon, R. Dekel, and Y. Neria. 2003. Battlefield functioning and chronic PTSD: Associations with perceived self efficacy and causal attribution. *Personality and Individual Differences* 34(3): 463-76.

Goodman, L., L. Saxe, and M. Harvey. 1991. Homelessness as psychological trauma: Broadening perspectives. *American Psychologist* 46(11): 1219-25.

Henderson, C., A. Roux, D. Jacobs Jr., C. Kiefe, D. West, and D. Williams. 2005. Neighbourhood characteristics, individual level socioeconomic factors, and depressive symptoms in young adults: The CARDIA study. *Journal of Epidemiology and Community Health* 59(4): 322-28.

Herman, J.L. 1992. Complex PTSD: A syndrome in survivors of prolonged and repeated trauma. *Journal of Traumatic Stress* 5(3): 377-91.

–. 1997. *Trauma and recovery: The aftermath of violence – from domestic abuse to political terror.* Rev. ed. New York: Basic Books.

Hobfoll, S.E., D. Canetti-Nisim, and R.J. Johnson. 2006. Exposure to terrorism, stress-related mental health symptoms, and defensive coping among Jews and Arabs in Israel. *Journal of Consulting and Clinical Psychology* 74(2): 207-18.

Humphreys, C., and S. Joseph. 2004. Domestic violence and the politics of trauma. *Women's Studies International Forum* 27(5): 559-70.

Hyman, S.M., S.N. Gold, and M.A. Cott. 2003. Forms of social support that moderate PTSD in childhood sexual abuse survivors. *Journal of Family Violence* 18(5): 295-300.

Johansen, V.A., A.K. Wahl, D.E. Eilertsen, and L. Weisaeth. 2007. Prevalence and predictors of post-traumatic stress disorder (PTSD) in physically injured victims of non-domestic violence. *Social Psychiatry and Psychiatric Epidemiology* 42(7): 583-93.

Kaysen, D., P.A. Resick, and D. Wise. 2003. Living in danger: The impact of chronic traumatization and the traumatic context on posttraumatic stress disorder. *Trauma, Violence, and Abuse* 4(3): 247-64.

Kilpatrick, D., and B. Saunders. 1997. *Prevalence and consequences of child victimization: Results from the National Survey of Adolescents.* Final Report 181028. Charleston: Medical University of South Carolina, National Crime Victims Research and Treatment Centre.

Levendosky, A.A., G.A. Bogat, S.A. Theran, J.S. Trotter, A. Eye, and W.S. Davidson. 2004. The social networks of women experiencing domestic violence. *American Journal of Community Psychology* 34(1): 95-109.

Leventhal, T., and J. Brooks-Gunn. 2003. Moving to opportunity: An experimental study of neighborhood effects on mental health. *American Journal of Public Health* 93(9): 1576-82.

Lloyd, D.A., and R.J. Turner. 2003. Cumulative adversity and posttraumatic stress disorder: Evidence from a diverse community sample of young adults. *American Journal of Orthopsychiatry* 73(4): 381-91.

McMullin, J.A. 2004. *Understanding social inequality: Intersections of class, age, gender, ethnicity, and race in Canada.* Toronto: Oxford University Press.

McNally, R.J. 2004. Conceptual problems with the DSM-IV criteria for posttraumatic stress disorder. In *Posttraumatic stress disorder: Issues and controversies,* ed. G.M. Rosen, 1-14. Chichester, UK: John Wiley and Sons.

Miles-Doan, R. 1998. Violence between spouses and intimates: Does neighborhood context matter? *Social Forces* 77(2): 623-45.

Ozer, E.J., S.R. Best, T.L. Lipsey, and D.S. Weiss. 2003. Predictors of posttraumatic stress disorder and symptoms in adults: A meta-analysis. *Psychological Bulletin* 129(1): 52-73.

Pearlin, L. 1989. The sociological study of stress. *Journal of Health and Social Behavior* 30(3): 241-56.

–. 1999. The stress process revisited: Reflections on conceptions and their interrelationships. In *Handbook of the sociology of mental health,* ed. C. Aneshensel and J. Phelan, 395-416. New York: Kluwer Academic/Plenum.

Resnick, H.S., D.G. Kilpatrick, B.S. Dansky, B.E. Saunders, and C.L. Best. 1993. Prevalence of civilian trauma and posttraumatic stress disorder in a representative national sample of women. *Journal of Consulting and Clinical Psychology* 61(6): 984-91.

Ryles, S.M. 1999. A concept analysis of empowerment: Its relationship to mental health nursing. *Journal of Advanced Nursing* 29(3): 600-7.

Schumm, J.A., M. Briggs Phillips, and S.E. Hobfoll. 2006. Cumulative interpersonal traumas and social support as risk and resiliency factors in predicting PTSD and depression among inner-city women. *Journal of Traumatic Stress* 19(6): 825-36.

Schumm, J.A., S.E. Hobfoll, and N.J. Keogh. 2004. Revictimization and interpersonal resource loss predicts PTSD among women in substance-use treatment. *Journal of Traumatic Stress* 17(2): 173-81.

Silver, E., E.P. Mulvey, and J.W. Swanson. 2002. Neighborhood structural characteristics and mental disorder: Faris and Dunham revisited. *Social Science and Medicine* 55(8): 1457-70.

Symington, A. 2004. Intersectionality: A tool for gender and economic justice. *Women's Rights and Economic Change* 9: 1-7.

Turner, H.A., D. Finkelhor, and R. Ormrod. 2006. The effect of lifetime victimization on the mental health of children and adolescents. *Social Science and Medicine* 62(1): 13-27.

Vranceanu, A.M., S.E. Hobfoll, and R.J. Johnson. 2007. Child multi-type maltreatment and associated depression and PTSD symptoms: The role of social support and stress. *Child Abuse and Neglect* 31(1): 71-84.

Walker, J.L., P.D. Carey, N. Mohr, D.J. Stein, and S. Seedat. 2004. Gender differences in the prevalence of childhood sexual abuse and in the development of pediatric PTSD. *Archives of Women's Mental Health* 7(2): 111-21.

Wuest, J., M. Ford-Gilboe, M. Merritt-Gray, and H. Berman. 2003. Intrusion: The central problem for family health promotion among children and single mothers after leaving an abusive partner. *Qualitative Health Research* 13(5): 597-622.

Wuest, J., M. Ford-Gilboe, M. Merritt-Gray, and S. Lemire. 2006. Using grounded theory to generate a theoretical understanding of the effects of child custody policy on women's health promotion in the context of intimate partner violence. *Health Care for Women International* 27(6): 490-512.

Yuval-Davis, N. 2006. Intersectionality and feminist politics. *European Journal of Women's Studies* 13(3): 193-209.

Part 4
Disrupting Power and
Health Inequities

Edited by Jo-Anne Lee and Olena Hankivsky

15

Addressing Trauma, Violence, and Pain: Research on Health Services for Women at the Intersections of History and Economics

Annette J. Browne, Colleen Varcoe, and Alycia Fridkin

An intersectional lens has great potential for improving the ways in which health care services are organized and provided to individuals. It can foster the development of more equitable services because of its focus on multiple forms of oppression and structural violence, which give rise to inequities, and because it provides direction for addressing multiple sites of oppression versus sites of oppression as singular dimensions. Such a lens can contribute to more effective care by exposing the consequences of fragmentation and divisions in care that fail to address intersecting forms of marginalization. Our research on primary health care services conducted in partnership with two urban Aboriginal health centres – whose mandates are to provide primary health care to Aboriginal and non-Aboriginal people in the inner city areas of two Western Canadian cities – serves to illustrate this potential. The purpose of this chapter is to draw on insights from this research to illustrate the ways in which intersectionality can generate knowledge about how health services could be more responsive, particularly to the needs of women marginalized by poverty, racism, neo-colonialism, and the politics of place, including how rural, urban, and inner city spaces are shaped. We draw on our research with women who attend the health centres to show how an intersectional lens shapes understandings of the intertwining issues of interpersonal and structural violence, chronic pain, and addictions, which often underpin women's experiences of social suffering, and to reveal how such understandings provide direction toward more effective, responsive, and equitable care. Because discussions of how to apply intersectionality have been limited in health research (Hankivsky and Christoffersen 2008; Hankivsky and Cormier 2009), we aim to make visible how we operationalized an intersectional approach to understand how health services might better meet the complex needs of Aboriginal and non-Aboriginal women marginalized by poverty, racism, and colonialism. We consider the analytical "value-added" of using an intersectional perspective informed by post-colonial feminist perspectives, illustrate its concrete implications for women's health research, provide insight into the application of intersectionality to health services research, and thus aim to bridge the gap between intersectional theory and practice.

In drawing on the term "marginalized," we are wary of reifying women's subject-positions as necessarily marginalized or disadvantaged. Indeed, an intersectional interpretation of marginalization or vulnerability directs us otherwise – to acknowledge the fact that social locations are fluid and shifting, depending on context. Caution is warranted whenever labels or classifications are applied – whether pertaining to ethnocultural groupings or health conditions (as in "injection drug user," "addict," or "homeless person"). Because an intersectional approach challenges categories of analysis and how they are used, it forces us to question the language we employ to classify people and the act of categorizing itself – both of which tend to reduce people to labels or constitute them according to single static identities in ways that obscure the complexity of their lives. For example, the women in Canada who identify as Aboriginal, indigenous, First Nations, Métis, or Inuit are tremendously diverse (Native Women's Association of Canada 2007). Aboriginal women's self-identities also intersect with state-defined identities according to the Indian Act, which subcategorizes sociolegal statuses of "Indians" based on a series of exclusionary criteria (Fiske 2006). This is one example of how "the power of the State seeps into the very essence of individual identity and personal well-being," dynamics that intersectional perspectives can help us to better understand (ibid., 248).

In attempting to respond to the challenge inherent in analyzing health or social issues that may be relevant to particular groups of women while at the same time acknowledging diverse and individual social locations, we draw on Leslie McCall's (2005, 1773) notion of intercategorical complexity within intersectionality, in which socially constructed categories (such as "women who experience marginalization" or "Aboriginal women") are provisionally adopted in order to "document relationships of inequality among social groups and changing configurations of inequality along multiple and conflicting dimensions." In this chapter, "marginalization" therefore refers to the processes by which some people and groups are affected by historical, structural, and social inequities in particular ways and in local contexts (Adelson 2005), and is also inclusive of people's agency, resistance, and resilience in the face of structural violence and inequities.

Conceptualizing Intersectionality from a Post-Colonial Feminist Perspective

"Intersectionality" refers to the extent to which differing aspects of social identity, and various forms of structural oppression, are mutually constructed at the level of individuals, organizations, and broader social systems in complex and interdependent ways; consequently, women experience differing constellations of inequities due to their social positioning within hierarchies of power relations (Collins 2000). Beyond these definitional features, there are wide variations in the conceptualization of intersectionality, related methodologies, and analytical tools (Weber and Parra-Medina 2003; Brah and Phoenix 2004; Hulko 2009). For example, intersectional analyses are inherent to research that draws on post-colonial feminist theories. More specifically, these theories focus particular attention on gender, socio-economic status, and ethnocultural identity as key aspects of social identity, and on racialization, historical subjugation, and colonialism as forms of structural oppression (for example, see Gandhi 1998; Narayan and Harding 2000; Reimer-Kirkham and Anderson 2002). In several of our studies, post-colonial feminist perspectives have been particularly useful in examining how historically mediated institutionalized racism has intersected with gender and economic marginalization to shape health for Aboriginal people in Canada (see Browne et al. in press; Browne 2007; Browne, Smye, and Varcoe 2005, 2007; Smith, Varcoe, and Edwards 2005; Varcoe and Dick 2008). We are particularly drawn to the emphasis in post-colonial feminist theorizing on disrupting "race"-based thinking and processes of racialization, and on understanding and responding to ongoing lived experiences of colonialism and neo-colonialism. Intersectionality, informed by post-colonial feminist perspectives, has therefore been relevant in our research, which focused on the consequences of intersecting structural and historical inequities on health and social suffering.

As with any theoretical perspective, it is important for researchers to engage critically with underlying epistemological assumptions, to consider the social locations of scholars affiliated with particular schools of thought, and to avoid theoretical imposition or appropriation of particular perspectives. For example, distinguishing post-colonial feminist theories, as a strand of Western theorizing, from post-colonial indigenous knowledge is critical. The latter is founded on indigenous ways of knowing and indigenous research processes; importantly, indigenous scholars point to the ways in which indigenous voices have long been excluded from academic and research circles (Battiste 2000). Linda Smith (1999, 98) is particularly concerned that the notion of "post-colonial" carries the message that "colonialism is finished business." When working with intersectional and post-colonial feminist perspectives, therefore, we must fully recognize the ways that neo-colonial discourses, policies, and practices intersect to exert their effects in current times.

With these cautions in mind, an intersectional perspective informed by post-colonial feminist perspectives and indigenous knowledges can be useful in understanding how the consequences of racialization, historical injustices, classism, and gendered inequities are inextricably interrelated, particularly as they influence women's lived experiences of health. Our primary analytical goal is to understand the processes through which multiple social inequalities and social locations are simultaneously generated, maintained, and challenged at the institutional, organizational, and individual levels, thus shaping the health of societies, communities, and individuals (Weber 2006). Four features of intersectional scholarship are particularly salient to our research: an intersectional perspective is driven foremost by the pursuit of social justice; the goal of applying an intersectional analysis is to understand and address the multiple dimensions of social and health inequalities manifest at the macro level of institutions, systems, and organizations, and the micro level of individual experiences of women who live at the intersections of multiple inequalities; inequalities are conceived as social constructions situated in social and historical contexts, and in structures beyond the individual – in societies, institutions, communities, and families – and are characterized as power relationships, not simply as resource disparities between dominant and subordinate groups; and broad intersecting systems of inequality become the targets for intervention, including systems outside of the health arena such as the economy, employability, housing, education, and justice systems (ibid.).

The Intersecting Consequences of Health and Social Inequities

The current Canadian context exacerbates the need for intersectional analyses. Following several decades of neo-liberal policies in Canada, social and health inequities are deepening, and social welfare reforms, along with declining social support services, have had detrimental effects (Raphael 2007, 2009). From an intersectional perspective, issues affecting health and health care inequities are viewed in their historical, political, economic, and social contexts. This is salient for women marginalized by poverty, racism, place, violence, ability, and other forms of oppression as they intersect with gender.

For example, using an intersectional approach to consider the high levels of violence and HIV infection experienced by Aboriginal women reveals how health problems are shaped by colonial and ongoing neo-colonial policies, neo-liberal state policies, racism, and urbanization (Brownridge 2008; Varcoe and Dick 2008). Growing evidence reveals how histories of violence and trauma are intertwined with women's experiences of chronic pain and addiction (see Pearce et al. 2008; Salomon, Bassuk, and Huntington 2002; Sullivan and Holt 2008; Wuest et al. 2008). The cumulative effects of poverty, addictions, violence, and racism are also manifested in the very high rates of HIV among Aboriginal women in Canada: women represent nearly half (45.1 percent) of all positive HIV test reports among Aboriginal people, compared to 19.5 percent in the non-Aboriginal population (McKay-McNabb 2006). Despite these disturbing indicators of social suffering, little attention has been given to the causes of vulnerability and overexposure of Aboriginal women to sexual exploitation, violence, and murder that have historically been, and continue to be, the reality in Canadian society (Amnesty International 2004; Razack 2008).

Overview of the Research

Our research, which was conducted in partnership with two urban Aboriginal health centres, provides an opportunity to apply an intersectional perspective to the particular institutional context of health care.[1] The health centres' mandates are to provide primary health care services to Aboriginal and non-Aboriginal people who are most significantly affected by poverty, historical trauma, social exclusion, racialization, and discrimination. Both centres are located in inner city areas – one is in a northern regional city, and the other is in what is recognized as one of Canada's poorest neighbourhoods. Many of the people accessing the health centres are poor or living in poverty, often residing in single-room-occupancy hotels; many live on or near the street and have significant mental health and addictions issues; and many have experienced the interrelated traumas of violence, childhood abuse, and sexual exploitation. The broad aims of our study are to explore *how* health care services are organized to explicitly address the needs of people affected by marginalization and racialization, and to develop primary care "performance" indicators that adequately reflect the impact of such services on people's health and well-being.

Both health centres include a medical clinic staffed by physicians, nurses, and nurse practitioners, and outreach services aimed at supporting people's health and social needs, drug and alcohol counselling services, and social work services. Services vary depending on location, but examples include hot lunch programs for people living with HIV/AIDS, access to elders who are employed part time, and support services for women with small children. One of the health centres has recently attempted to strengthen services for women who are relatively underrepresented there, in part because of the conditions that create vulnerability to violence and exploitation, and also because of their marginal positioning within male-dominated health care settings and community spaces. This took the form of a women's wellness program, which operates one afternoon per week and aims to enhance Aboriginal and non-Aboriginal women's access to primary health care and related health-promoting services. The program offers a safe place for women to rest and interact with other women if they choose; it also provides lunch (many women have not eaten for days when they come) and priority access to physicians, nurses, and elders in the health centre (on afternoons devoted solely to women). Each week, the program is attended by approximately thirty to sixty women from diverse social locations, including older women, those living in poverty, working in the sex trade, raising children or grand-children, living with addictions, and in violent relationships. Unanticipated benefits of the program include increasing and expanding women's social support networks and reducing the stresses and harms associated with pov-erty, addictions, and violence, thus supporting women to respond in con-structive ways to challenges encountered in their everyday lives. Drawing on examples from both health centres, and from the women's wellness program in particular, we highlight the insights that can be gained by ap-plying an intersectional lens to health services research.

Insights Gained from Research: The Value of Drawing on Intersectional Perspectives

In relation to health services research, there are three interrelated analytical advantages to using an intersectional perspective. First, it provides a tool through which to consider how health and social "problems" are framed. Second, it focuses attention on how health and social issues are intricately interrelated – and in the context of this chapter, how "categories of analysis" such as poverty, addictions, violence and trauma, and chronic pain often intersect in ways that compound their effects. Third, intersectional analyses direct us to think critically about the efficacy of conventional approaches to service delivery and prompt us to reimagine how services could be better tailored to meet women's intersecting health and social needs.

Critically Considering What Is Constructed as "the Problem"

> I was put on Tylenol #3 when I was 12 ... I have pain every single
> day ... So, I've been in and out of the hospital lots, you know,
> being addicted to morphine and pills and everything.
>
> – Woman, age thirty-one

An intersectional perspective helps to widen the scope of what is conven-tionally identified as the "problem" in health services delivery and in women's health research. As Jacqueline Oxman-Martinez et al. (2002) have argued, viewing social problems through an intersectional approach funda-mentally alters the ways in which they are identified, understood, and ex-perienced; this also has the potential to alter how health services and health care providers respond.

In constructing problems, intersectionality offers a more useful approach than one that allows problems to be framed by dominant media, public perceptions, and health care discourses, as such discourses are often driven by interests other than concerns for women's health and well-being. For example, writing about Vancouver's inner city, the Downtown Eastside, Dara Culhane (2003, 594-95) argues, "predictably, national and international media ... offer the virtual voyeur disturbing – or titillating – images of emaciated heroin, crack cocaine, and prescription drug users buying, selling, injecting, and smoking," reflecting a "preference for exotic and spectacular representation of drugs, sex, violence, and crime rather than the ordinary and mundane brutality of everyday poverty." Such images bring a certain framing of problems into the foreground – such as drugs, addictions, and sex work. In the process, individual people themselves are constructed as "the problem." This focus on the individual as the source of the problem downplays the root causes of people's issues, including historical trauma, poverty, unemployment, abuse, racism, and medical involvement such as prescribing practices, and further ignores the ultimate causes of these, such as global economics, ideologies of racial superiority, capitalist priorities, ongoing clawbacks to social welfare systems, welfare colonialism, and state policies regarding resource distribution.

Through the dynamic relations among media, public opinion, and policy (see Chapter 17 of this volume), such a framing of problems is reflected in policy priorities and health services delivery. The wider health services sector in both inner cities include needle exchanges, HIV treatment programs, addictions treatment, and so on, but little is done at the municipal, regional, or provincial policy levels to address poverty, lack of safe and affordable housing, violence and trauma, or racism, particularly as they intersect. Thus, health care providers in the two health centres expend considerable energy on addressing these root causes of addiction but often as an "add on" to the program work for which they are funded. An excerpt from fieldnotes recorded at a "clinical rounds" meeting at one of the health centres is illustrative:

> Throughout the clinical rounds meeting I was struck by the emphasis on housing. For 9 of the 15 patients discussed, the quest for housing was a key focus. The workers were all strategizing how to get housing or improve the housing for each person, sometimes to help them get out of hospital, sometimes to avoid having the patients "discharged to the street" from hospital. The clinic staff waited until their counterparts from other agencies left to discuss some possibilities. Housing is at such a premium that healthcare agencies have to compete with each other to get the best possibilities for their clients. (Fieldnotes 2008)

Problems such as addictions, HIV, or hepatitis C are prioritized in health care funding, policy, and service delivery structures, challenging leaders within the health centres to find ways to fund programs that address the intersecting issues of violence and trauma, chronic pain, and the backdrop of poverty in which these are experienced. Consequently, service providers contend with very limited resources to address underlying problems, such as histories of trauma – and issues related to poverty and housing are structured by the health care system (and in funding arrangements) as falling outside of dominant conventional notions of health programming.

By pointing to underlying intersecting factors, an intersectional lens reminds us that problems such as addictions, HIV, or hepatitis C are highly stigmatized; when these health issues are understood in ways that are decontextualized from their underlying causes, people who experience them are often blamed or held responsible for engaging in problematic behaviours (such as unprotected sex and injection drug use). Such a decontextualized understanding fuels the perception held by many Canadians that those who are affected by these health conditions are the source of the problem. Women who participated in our research were well aware of these wider public perceptions and discourses; one woman, who identified as First Nations, explained her sense of trepidation about being identified as "one of them": "I've heard comments on the bus, like when we're driving by and you see people waiting outside for the clinic to open 'oh my god, look at all those junkies, ooooh.' Like, 'I wonder how often they bathe,' and 'oh, it must just stink there where they're waiting'" (Woman, age forty).

Whereas popular discourses tend to construct people with cancer and other less stigmatizing health conditions as heroes fighting for their lives, strength and courage are underplayed in depictions of people contending with the intersecting challenges of violence and trauma, poverty, and substance use. Representations of disease, self-destruction, and despair dominate, and media, public, or health care discourses pay little attention to the agency and resistance of those who, despite profound constraints on life opportunities, struggle daily to survive and thrive (Culhane 2003). The hyper-visibility of people in inner cities who are living in poverty, affected by addictions, or involved as sex workers fuels this narrow, fixed view of people's social locations and identities. In contrast, an intersectional perspective prompts us to scrutinize taken-for-granted assumptions that categorize particular neighbourhoods as essentially destitute or residents of such neighbourhoods as singularly despairing. Rather, intersectional perspectives remind us that inner cities are often sites of activism, anti-poverty movements, and organizations that provide safe spaces for women such as social housing, shelters, and transition houses (Benoit, Carroll, and Chaudhry 2003). Similarly, our fieldwork and interviews at both health centres show another side to those vilified by media and public discourses – people who offer support and friendship to one another in spite of the most harrowing of life circumstances. An intersectional approach therefore challenges how particular groups and individuals are problematized, critically questions how problems are framed, and draws attention to broader social issues underlying and intersecting with health problems.

Intersections among Poverty, Addictions, Violence and Trauma, and Chronic Pain

Just as intersectional perspectives enable us to challenge what becomes constructed as the problem in health services settings, they further enable us to dispute assumptions about which categories of analysis are relevant to understanding women's health needs. This area of critique is particularly important given the predominance of biomedical perspectives in health care and the tendency to view issues such as poverty, violence and trauma, addictions, and chronic pain as fairly separate entities. In contrast, we are particularly concerned with understanding the intersecting effects of these issues on people's lives and well-being; this understanding also sheds light on the limitations of conventional health care responses and the tendency in health care to address these categories of analysis in isolation from each other and from broader social and political contexts.

Health researchers using an intersectional lens have typically focused on how various "categories of analysis" and social locations (such as race/gender/class, and more recently, age, immigrant status, disability/ability, religion, and sexual orientation) intersect to affect health outcomes (see, for example, Donaldson and Jedwab 2003; Collins, von Unger, and Armbrister 2008; Purdie-Vaughns and Eibach 2008). Intersections among health issues such as addictions, violence and trauma, and chronic pain are emblematic of the intersections of systemic oppressions yet have received less attention. For Aboriginal women in particular, the cumulative experiences of racism, intergenerational trauma, colonization, and poverty compound such intersections. Further, the health care system's response to these intersecting issues warrants analysis. Interventions aimed at addressing the intersecting issues of violence and trauma, chronic pain, and substance use are not well integrated, particularly in ways that are meaningful in the context of women's lives. For example, poverty is rarely analyzed as a factor that *fosters* and exacerbates addictions or as a condition that gives illicit drug use in inner cities its "public" character (Culhane 2003). Rather, the prevailing tendency in health care is to reduce and medicalize multiple intersecting issues to the singular problem of "addictions." This is consistent with dominant legal and medical discourses, which tend to locate the problem of addictions within the individual psyches of those affected by mental illness or those involved in criminal activity.

The medicalization of addictions also comes with an implicit assumption that there are known treatments for addictions. The evidence showing the extensive co-occurrence of addictions with trauma, violence, and chronic pain suggests that addictions are unlikely to be treatable without addressing underlying histories of trauma and pain. However, addiction is often treated in isolation from such histories. It is assumed that solutions or treatments exist for addictions but not for the poverty, racism, and historical or personal trauma that often underlie patterns of addiction. Therefore, if treatment for addiction fails, the individual, not the original definition of the problem, is faulted. From an intersectional perspective, we are prompted to see the limitations of these dominant approaches to addiction, to turn our attention to how multiple problems intersect and compound each other, and to further consider their complex and intersecting root causes.

The health services policy environment also influences the framing of addictions as the primary focus of treatment. For example, the assumption that addictions can be treated in isolation from the wider contexts of people's lives is perpetuated by the process of diagnosing and referring patients for addiction treatment (as opposed to treating the root causes of addiction) and also by the process in which health care agencies must identify separate and distinct billing codes for singularly defined health problems. Although staff at the health centres recognized that addictions cannot be decontextualized from the realities of women's lives, dominant biomedical approaches to diagnosing and treating addictions tend to prevail. In response, staff expend considerable energy on negotiating with patients regarding drug use and approaches to harm reduction, and women are often referred for addiction treatment in settings outside the inner city (informally referred to as "geographic treatment"). Thus, women are supported to contend with their addictions but not with the effects of trauma, ongoing exposure to violence, chronic pain, and the consequences of living in dire poverty.

Because the health care system tends to medicalize addictions and underlying issues, health care interactions often focus on negotiating contracts for methadone use, managing people's frequent requests for opiate and other prescription drugs, and referring them for addictions treatment. Consequently, addiction becomes the primary entry point for addressing women's complex health and social issues. When chronic pain is treated, it is primarily through pharmacological means, with health care providers aiming to balance pain management with concerns about the possible misuse of narcotic medications, the potential for pain medications to fuel addictions, and the potential for "drug seeking" or diversion of drugs. In the process, as is consistently the case with biomedical perspectives, non-pharmacological approaches to pain management, strategies for addressing the violence and trauma, and associated grief and loss that often underpin chronic pain receive less attention. From an intersectional perspective, the co-constructed factors that contribute to addictions are understood as requiring a range of strategies aimed at helping women address these intersecting issues. However, the health care system, as it is currently designed, has few tools at its disposal to do so.

Responding to the Needs of Women Who Are Marginalized and Racialized

> They want me to go off [narcotic medications], but what am I supposed to do about my pain?
>
> – Woman, age thirty-two

As we continue to argue, intersectional perspectives can illuminate the ways in which health services might be structured to be more responsive to women's intersecting needs. Specifically, an intersectional analysis draws attention to the individualistic ideologies underlying health services and to structural and funding constraints. Thereby, it points to two key features of more responsive health care: addressing both the social conditions and determinants shaping women's lives and women's need for safety.

Intersectional analyses call into question the individualistic ideologies that underpin the biomedical focus of most health services. For example, if an elderly woman with osteoporosis who is living in poverty breaks her hip, the fracture may be dealt with competently, but her need for safe housing, nutritional support, transportation, and assistance with the activities of daily living may be ignored, often with further cost to both the health care system and the woman herself (Varcoe, Hankivsky, and Morrow 2007). Similarly, as we have argued, health care tends to focus too narrowly on substance use or addiction; even when health care providers and researchers acknowledge the importance of macro-social forces on women's health, responses within the health care system focus on the more "proximate issues" such as health behaviours (the need to reduce or quit using substances), cultural values (supposed cultural barriers to accessing care), or the need to develop better ways of coping (Weber 2006, 24). These proximate issues become the primary targets for health interventions – leaving broader systems of social inequality underanalyzed and unaddressed.

An intersectional perspective prompts us to look further, to consider *what possibly could be done* to be more responsive to the wider contexts of women's lives and the intersecting factors that exacerbate and mitigate the health effects of social suffering. Such consideration requires an examination of what supports the enactment of individualistic ideologies. For example, broader funding structures and budgetary-reporting requirements are organized in ways that oblige the health centres to "streamline" their services to fit conventional notions of essential health services – often narrowly defined in accordance with biomedical conceptualizations of what counts as legitimate. Residential school healing programs, mental health services (other than psychiatric services, which are very limited), dental care, and violence prevention are not viewed as eligible core-funded programs by the existing funding structure. Despite these limitations, the health centres have become adept at piecing together short-term funding from a variety of sources and arguing for flexibility in how they use their funds, so that they can treat the issues that often underlie women's presenting health or illness concerns. For example, time is devoted not only to treating the physical manifestations of illness but to helping women complete social welfare applications, disability forms, and social housing applications, and to access meal programs and food banks. One woman, who described herself as First Nations, HIV positive, and "clean for the past 3 months," described the profound effect that obtaining stable housing had on her overall health and sense of self:

> I got the subsidy from them [the nurse and social worker at the health centre] for housing and I got the kids back now ... That really made me look in the mirror at myself ... I knew that I wanted to go to rehab. I've been thinking about it for a whole year since I got the subsidy ... [Other people] don't realize the vacancy rate, the homelessness, living in the inner city hotels, the infestations of bugs. [With] the subsidy, I thought, I've really got to smarten up, pull up my socks and start really watching the company I keep and start getting my life on track. And it's getting there. (Woman, age forty)

Although these strategies and programs for supporting women's health are essential features of the work at the health centres, they are supported on shoestring budgets or implemented within unstable one-time funding sources and are often coordinated or managed "off the sides of the desks" of staff.

Attending to women's needs for safety begins with acknowledging that most of the women who use the health centres have experienced violence, historical and/or emotional trauma, and often childhood sexual abuse; this stance underpins concerted efforts to ensure that the spaces created inside and outside the health centres are safe for women. In one of the centres, this has involved creating a separate area for women and children to sit while they wait for a clinic appointment. In the other centre, the space and activities offered as part of the women's wellness program are provided in ways that are welcoming to diverse groups of women. For example, women who are actively using drugs are treated with respect and welcomed rather than turned away, as might happen in other health care settings. There is an intentional use of unconditional positive regard to foster both emotional and cultural safety for women who are routinely exposed to violence, discrimination, racism, and dismissal. Staff and volunteers also make a concerted effort to connect respectfully, non-judgmentally, and safely with women through the use of activities such as music therapy, art projects, manicures, haircuts, and shoulder or hand massages. Although at first glance such activities might seem to fall outside the health care jurisdiction, a closer look reveals that they permit staff to listen therapeutically to women's discussions about their lives and intertwining health and social needs, and to use touch in ways that are safe, accepting, and comforting – experiences that many of the women rarely have. Some women partake in the women's wellness activities while waiting to see a health care provider at the medical clinic, and others come specifically for the health-promoting aspects of safe and accepting social contact. One woman who described herself as struggling with addictions and unstable housing explained how the extreme challenges of life on the inner city streets made the simplest of caring acts invaluable:

> Because you're missing so much on that connection, not connected to anybody. Those kinds of just simple gestures, just that little bit of, you know, good human touch, you know, once in a blue moon, can really help somebody get to the next step, right? Good human interaction and connections ... That's life saving, life changing, literally, it's that valuable. It's life changing because when I was out there it was not good, it was always for something, you know, you were selling your body or you're giving up a piece of yourself daily, right? And then to have somebody want to do something for you just to help you, like oh my god, it's like, "oh shit there's still people like that out there, you know?" And then it just gives you a whole new perspective. (Woman, age thirty-eight)

Operating from a stance that problematizes social structures, structural violence, and social suffering, rather than locating the source of problems within the psyches of individual people, allows the health centre staff to create a sense of belonging and community, and to actively convey non-judgmental acceptance to those accessing services.

Providing health care from a stance informed by intersectional perspectives, staff at the health centres recognize that many women – because of their experiences of being exploited, marginalized, and racialized, and because many struggle with addictions – encounter dismissal on many levels: in the health care system, the justice system, and the social services sector, as well as with child welfare authorities to negotiate access to their children, and so on. Receiving health care that is philosophically committed to conveying unconditional positive regard is particularly powerful, as a First Nations woman who frequently accessed one of the health centres described: "Well if you judge them [patients], then they go back out ten times worse, right? Because they feel like they're nothing. And I've felt like that. I know how it feels. You feel lost, empty and that you have no one" (Woman age, 37).

Using an intersectional lens, staff view people who attend the health centres, and people from the surrounding community, in ways other than those provoked by the ubiquitous negative media and public portrayals commonly assumed to accurately represent people living in both inner city areas. As a nurse at one of the health centres explained, "I see other parts of their life other than the street life, and that helps me [in my work with people who access the centre] ... I see despair, I see hopelessness, but on the other side of things. I see a community; I see that this is their community."

Because disconnection from self, family, and community is common among women who have experienced multiple forms of violence and trauma (McKeown et al. 2002), and because social inclusion is a key determinant of health, facilitating women's connections to others is critical to their health and well-being. An intersectional approach thus brings the complexity of women's lives into view and frames the facilitation of social inclusion as a legitimate health care priority and health-promoting service.

Implications for Health Services Research: Research as Praxis and Practice

Patricia Hill Collins (quoted in Hankivsky and Cormier 2009, 3) has argued that an intersectional analysis is fully realized only "when abstract thought is joined with concrete action." Basing health services research on an intersectional understanding of the lives of women affected by marginalization and racialization has implications for how research is conducted: it must be normatively oriented toward praxis, with fluid and permeable boundaries between research and practice. This emphasis on socially transformative research calls on researchers to be conscious of their power and positionality, and to use their positions of privilege in ways that directly advance social justice (Harding and Norberg 2005).

In the case of our research, the commitment to "give back" to the two Aboriginal health centres takes various forms. At the policy level, members of our research team collaborate with leaders within the centres to lobby for improvements to policy and funding arrangements. At the organizational level, team members responded to the continual need to piece together funding by using their academic resources to write funding proposals for the women's wellness program. At the micro level of interactions, our engagement with the women's wellness program involves a long-term commitment to developing relationships with women who attend and to doing volunteer work that helps to support the services provided.

In the context of health services, future research is needed to better understand how intersectional and biomedical perspectives can connect to generate new knowledge in complementary ways. Biomedical research, informed by intersectional analyses, is needed to apply emerging understandings of the neurophysiologic basis of associations among, for example, childhood trauma, chronic pain, and addictions (Wuest et al. 2008), in order to design responses to health problems that intersect both with one another and with wider forms of oppression. Research is required at numerous levels (Edwards, Mill, and Kothari 2004) to study the impact of multiple interventions on intersecting health and social issues. Social epidemiological research will continue to be important to show the linkages between experiences of racism/discrimination/stigma and health conditions such as hypertension or cardiovascular disease (Krieger and Davey Smith 2004). Within these paradigms of research, intersectional perspectives will help to expand the depth and complexity of evolving knowledge. Knowledge development focused on expanding our understanding of the interrelatedness of health issues, social locations, and structural factors will in turn help us to improve responsiveness to these issues in health services, policy, and research.

Research is also needed to explore ways of incorporating intersectional perspectives into policies that shape the structure and organization of health care systems and the delivery of health care services. The intersectional literature identifies the importance of including intersectional perspectives in policy (Hankivsky and Christoffersen 2008), but more analyses are needed to explore how policies intersect to structure the organization and delivery of health care services in ways that profoundly affect health and access to responsive health services.

In summary, using an intersectional perspective in health services research aimed at analyzing and improving health care draws attention to the following: how health problems are framed; why particular problems are prioritized, and thus legitimized, over others; how multiple health and social issues such as violence and trauma, chronic pain, addictions, and poverty intersect; and the importance of structuring health services in ways that address the intersecting realities of people's lives. These areas of analysis will be critical to developing strategies for mitigating the ongoing marginalizing and racializing inequities that shape the lives and health of many women in Canada.

Note

1 This study, which is still in progress, uses an ethnographic mixed-methods research design. To date, we have collected the following data: in-depth interviews and focus groups with seventy-two patients (fifty-five of whom self-identified as Aboriginal and seventeen as non-Aboriginal); interviews with forty-four health centre staff; over 850 hours of participant observation at both health centres, including observations of clinical encounters between patients and staff, interdisciplinary staff meetings, the waiting room environments, and the general milieus; and analyses of the health centres' organizational and policy environments. The excerpts we present in this chapter are taken from interviews with women who attended the health centres and our fieldnotes recorded as part of participant observation.

References

Adelson, N. 2005. The embodiment of inequity: Health disparities in Aboriginal Canada. *Canadian Journal of Public Health* 96(Suppl. 2): S45-S61.

Amnesty International. 2004. *Stolen sisters: A human rights response to discrimination and violence against indigenous women in Canada*. Ottawa: Amnesty International.

Battiste, M. 2000. Introduction: Unfolding the lessons of colonization. In *Reclaiming indigenous voice and vision*, ed. M. Battiste, xvi-xxix. Vancouver: UBC Press.

Benoit, C., D. Carroll, and M. Chaudhry. 2003. In search of a healing place: Aboriginal women in Vancouver's Downtown Eastside. *Social Science and Medicine* 56(4): 821-33.

Brah, A., and A. Phoenix. 2004. Ain't I a woman? Revisiting intersectionality. *Journal of International Women's Studies* 5(3): 75-86.

Browne, A.J. 2007. Clinical encounters between nurses and First Nations women in a Western Canadian hospital. *Social Science and Medicine* 64(10): 2165-76.

Browne, A.J., V. Smye, P. Rodney, S. Tang, B. Mussell, and J. O'Neil. 2010. Access to primary care from the perspective of Aboriginal patients at an urban emergency department. *Qualitative Health Research* (prepublished 12 November 2010. DOI: 10.1177/1049732310385824).

Browne, A.J., V. Smye, and C. Varcoe. 2005. The relevance of postcolonial theoretical perspectives to research in Aboriginal health. *Canadian Journal of Nursing Research* 37(4): 17-37.

–. 2007. Postcolonial-feminist theoretical perspectives and women's health. In *Women's health in Canada: Critical perspectives on theory and policy*, ed. M. Morrow, O. Hankivsky, and C. Varcoe, 124-42. Toronto: University of Toronto Press.

Brownridge, D.A. 2008. Understanding the elevated risk of partner violence against Aboriginal women: A comparison of two nationally representative surveys of Canada. *Journal of Family Violence* 23: 353-67.

Collins, P.H. 2000. *Black feminist thought: Knowledge, consciousness, and the politics of empowerment*. New York: Routledge.

Collins, P.Y., H. von Unger, and A. Armbrister. 2008. Church ladies, good girls, and locas: Stigma and the intersection of gender, ethnicity, mental illness, and sexuality in relation to HIV risk. *Social Science and Medicine* 67(3): 389-97.

Culhane, D. 2003. Their spirits live within us: Aboriginal women in Downtown Eastside Vancouver emerging into visibility. *American Indian Quarterly* 27(3-4): 593-606.

Donaldson, I., and J. Jedwab. 2003. Intersections of diversity: Policy research and identity issues. Editorial. *Canadian Ethnic Studies Journal* 35(3): 1-9.

Edwards, N., J. Mill, and A.R. Kothari. 2004. Multiple intervention research programs in community health. *Canadian Journal of Nursing Research* 36(1): 40-54.

Fiske, J. 2006. Boundary crossings: Power and marginalization in the formation of Canadian Aboriginal women's identities. *Gender and Development* 14(20): 247-58.

Gandhi, L. 1998. *Postcolonial theory: A critical introduction*. New York: Columbia University Press.

Hankivsky, O., and A. Christoffersen. 2008. Intersectionality and the determinants of health: A Canadian perspective. *Critical Public Health* 18(3): 1-13.

Hankivsky, O., and R. Cormier. 2009. *Intersectionality: Moving women's health research and policy forward*. Vancouver: Women's Health Research Network.

Harding, S., and K. Norberg. 2005. New feminist approaches to social science methodologies: An introduction. *Signs: Journal of Women in Culture and Society* 30(4): 693-707.

Hulko, W. 2009. The time- and context-contingent nature of intersectionality and interlocking oppressions. *Affilia: Journal of Women and Social Work* 24(1): 44-55.

Krieger, N., and G. Davey Smith. 2004. "Bodies count," and body counts: Social epidemiology and embodying inequality. *Epidemiologic Reviews* 26(1): 92-103.

McCall, L. 2005. The complexity of intersectionality. *Signs: Journal of Women in Culture and Society* 30(3): 1771-1800.

McKay-McNabb, K. 2006. Life experiences of Aboriginal women living with HIV/AIDS. *Canadian Journal of Aboriginal Community-Based HIV/AIDS Research* 1: 5-16.

McKeown, I., S. Reid, S. Turner, and P. Orr. 2002. *Sexual violence and dislocation as social risk factors involved in the acquisition of HIV among women in Manitoba*. Winnipeg: Prairie Women's Health Centre of Excellence.

Narayan, U., and S. Harding, eds. 2000. *Decentering the center: Philosophy for a multicultural, postcolonial, and feminist world.* Bloomington: Indiana University Press.

Native Women's Association of Canada. 2007. *Social determinants of health and Canada's Aboriginal women: Submission by the Native Women's Association of Canada to the World Health Organization's Commission on the Social Determinants of Health.* Ottawa: Native Women's Association of Canada.

Oxman-Martinez, J., J. Krane, N. Corbin, and M. Loiselle-Léonard. 2002. *Competing conceptions of conjugal violence: Insights from an intersectional framework.* Montreal: Centre for Applied Family Studies, McGill University, and Immigration and Metropolis.

Pearce, M.E. (for the Cedar Project Partnership), W.M. Christian, K. Patterson, K. Norris, A. Moniruzzman, K.J.P. Craib, M.T. Schechter, and P. Spittal. 2008. The Cedar Project: Historical trauma, sexual abuse and HIV risk among young Aboriginal people who use injection and non-injection drugs in two Canadian cities. *Social Science and Medicine* 66(11): 2185-94.

Purdie-Vaughns, V., and R.P. Eibach. 2008. Intersectional invisibility: The distinctive advantages and disadvantages of multiple subordinate-group identities. *Sex Roles* 59(5-6): 377-91.

Raphael, D. 2007. *Poverty and policy in Canada: Implications for health and quality of life.* Toronto: Canadian Scholars' Press.

–. 2009. *Social determinants of health: Canadian perspectives.* 2nd ed. Toronto: Canadian Scholars' Press.

Razack, S. 2008. Gendered racial violence and spatialized justice: The murder of Pamela George. In *Daily struggles: The deepening racialization and feminization of poverty in Canada,* ed. M.A. Wallis and S. Kwok, 249-61. Toronto: Canadian Scholars' Press.

Reimer-Kirkham, S., and J.M. Anderson. 2002. Postcolonial nursing scholarship: From epistemology to method. *Advances in Nursing Science* 25(1): 1-17.

Salomon, A., S.S. Bassuk, and N. Huntington. 2002. The relationship between intimate partner violence and the use of addictive substances in poor and homeless single mothers. *Violence against Women* 8(7): 785-815.

Smith, D., C. Varcoe, and N. Edwards. 2005. Turning around the intergenerational impact of residential schools on Aboriginal people: Implications for health policy and practice. *Canadian Journal of Nursing Research* 37(4): 38-60.

Smith, L.T. 1999. *Decolonizing methodologies: Research and Indigenous peoples.* New York and Dunedin: Zed Books and University of Otago Press.

Sullivan, T.P., and L.J. Holt. 2008. PTSD symptom clusters are differentially related to substance use among community women exposed to intimate partner violence. *Journal of Traumatic Stress* 21(2): 173-80.

Varcoe, C., and S. Dick. 2008. The intersecting risks of violence and HIV for rural Aboriginal women in a neo-colonial Canadian context. *Journal of Aboriginal Health* 4(1): 42-52.

Varcoe, C., O. Hankivsky, and M. Morrow. 2007. Introduction: Beyond gender matters. In *Women's health in Canada: Critical perspectives on theory and policy,* ed. M. Morrow, O. Hankivsky, and C. Varcoe, 3-30. Toronto: University of Toronto Press.

Weber, L. 2006. Reconstructing the landscape of health disparities research: Promoting dialogue and collaboration between feminist intersectional and biomedical paradigms. In *Gender, race, class and health: Intersectional approaches,* ed. A.J. Schulz and L. Mullings, 21-56. San Francisco: Jossey-Bass.

Weber, L., and D. Parra-Medina. 2003. Intersectionality and women's health: Charting a path to eliminating disparities. In *Advances in gender research.* Vol. 7, *Gender perspectives on health and medicine,* ed. M.T. Segal, V. Demos, and J.J. Kronenfeld, 181-230. Oxford: Elsevier.

Wuest, J., M. Merritt-Gray, M. Ford-Gilboe, B. Lent, C. Varcoe, and J. Campbell. 2008. Chronic pain in women survivors of intimate partner violence. *Journal of Pain* 9(11): 1049-57.

16

Intersectional Frameworks in Mental Health: Moving from Theory to Practice

Katherine R. Rossiter and Marina Morrow

Research and practice in mental health have typically emphasized biomedical paradigms, where the social contexts of people's lives are seen as ancillary to the "disease" afflicting the individual rather than as interrelated factors central to mental wellness. Feminists and those allied with critical psychology have long attempted to disrupt the hegemony of biomedicine in mental health (see, for example, Burstow 2005; Burstow and Weitz 1988; Caplan 1987; Chesler 1972; Morrow 2008; Ussher 1991) by exposing sexist bias in research and the ways in which the disciplines of psychiatry and psychology have pathologized femininity and women. This research has documented differences between women and men with respect to how they experience mental illness, signal distress, and access services (Gold 1998; Harris and Landis 1997; Kornstein and Clayton 2002; Morrow 2003; 2007; Rhodes et al. 2002). Although some scholars have introduced analyses that examine sex and gender in their intersections with sexual orientation or race and ethnicity (for example, Ad Hoc Working Group 2006; Boyer, Ku, and Shakir 1997; Caplan and Cosgrove 2004; Chan, Chunn, and Menzies 2005), feminist scholars have not made a consistent attempt to better understand how the intersections of multiple structural social factors affect mental health.

Likewise, although there is a burgeoning literature examining the legacies of colonialism and racism, and how these have resulted in high rates of suicide, addictions, and mental health problems for Aboriginal people (Health Canada 2000; Kirmayer, Brass, and Tait 2000), and on how racialized immigrant groups experience specific challenges related to the stresses of acculturation (Boyer, Ku, and Shakir 1997; Canadian Task Force 1988), much of this literature does not integrate an analysis of gender.

The research literature does demonstrate that socially marginalized groups have particular difficulty in accessing appropriate mental health care and that they experience the stigma of mental illness and the accompanying discrimination in varying ways (Alvidrez and Azocar 1999; Collins, von Unger, and Armbrister 2008; Gary 2005; Mill et al. 2007; Ship and Norton 2001).

However, very little scholarship addresses the theoretical and methodological challenges of utilizing intersectional approaches in mental health, and even less gives attention to how these approaches might be operationalized in practice and policy. Further, the transformational potential of intersectional approaches remains untapped with respect to what it would mean to fully introduce analyses of power into mental health research, policy, and practice.

Although there are some emerging intersectional scholars in mental health research (Burman 2004; Burman and Chantler 2003; Kohn and Hudson 2002; Smye and Browne 2002), the literature suffers from several shortcomings. First, the literature that focuses on mental health disparities tends to treat social processes as variables (such as gender, race, class) that can be separated from each other and used as discrete categories of analysis. This literature is typically preoccupied with concerns related to higher rates of certain "mental illnesses" in specific populations and/or with the underuse of mental health services by certain groups. This type of research runs the risk of reinforcing social inequities, by reifying conceptual categories such as gender, race, and culture or by propping up negative stereotypes associated with already disenfranchised groups. Waqar Ahmad (1994) usefully describes this as the "racialization of health research."

Another shortcoming in the literature is that certain kinds of analytic categories have been more studied than others: thus, ethnicity, culture, and gender are examined more frequently than sexual orientation, gender identity, and physical disability in their intersections with mental illness. This has resulted in an undertheorization of how these social processes operate in mental health. Laura Kohn and Kira Hudson (2002, 178) argue that the mental health field needs to "move beyond standard models and methods of inquiry" – that is, that "intersectionality requires a move toward alternative methodologies in order to incorporate measures that take into account multiple facets of individuals, dynamic contextual influences, and multiplicative effects on outcomes." Further, we would argue that intersectional analyses should be used to inform policy and practice in ways that challenge both the dominance of biomedicine in mental health and more progressive emerging paradigms, to include structural analyses of oppression in order to bolster the development of supports that move well beyond symptom management and truly sustain the active citizenship of people with mentally ill health.

To this end, in this chapter we investigate two arenas where Canadian mental health policy and practice have been particularly active in recent years: the development of programs to address stigma/discrimination against people with mental illnesses, and the development of recovery models of care. In our thinking, anti-stigma/discrimination practices are integrally linked to the aims and goals of recovery as this has been articulated in mental health (see Mental Health Commission of Canada 2009a, Ontario Ministry of Health 1993). That is, treating people with dignity and respect as full citizens is foundational to recovery. A number of significant developments in mental health in Canada warrant our focus on these two domains.

The first is the release of the results of a three-year study that extensively examined the state of the mental health care system in Canada – the report of the Standing Senate Committee on Social Affairs, Science and Technology (Kirby 2006). The second is the subsequent establishment of the Mental Health Commission of Canada (MHCC), which is giving mental health an unprecedented political profile (see www.mentalhealthcommission.ca). Among the plans for the commission are the development of a ten-year anti-stigma and discrimination reduction campaign and the development of a framework for a mental health strategy for Canada, which puts recovery at the centre of its focus (MHCC 2009a).

The MHCC thus provides an important political moment in Canadian history for discussing and debating how best to meet the diverse mental health needs of the population. In this regard, there are some encouraging signs: for example, the commission has recently attempted to address service development to meet the needs of ethnocultural groups, immigrants, refugees, and racialized groups (see, for example, MHCC 2009b). Indeed, the MHCC is in its early stages of development. Because it continues to encourage public participation and comment on its activities, it has opened a space for the useful engagement of critiques. In our work, we show how the application of intersectional analyses can reveal critical dimensions of policy and practice that can be enhanced to better address and respond to the diverse needs of the population.

Overview of Intersectionality: Theory, Method, and Application in Mental Health

Intersectional approaches have not been widely adopted in mental health research, but there is growing evidence that scholars are interested in exploring the relationships among social identity categories and mental illness. We take the term "intersectionality" to mean the social, political, and economic processes through which oppression and privilege are experienced by individuals who have the added stigma and discrimination associated with a mental illness diagnosis. That is, intersectionality "is not the intersection itself, but what the intersection reveals about power" (Dhamoon 2008, 9). Like Olena Hankivsky and Renee Cormier (2009) and others (Burgess-Proctor 2006; Collins 1990), we see intersectionality as necessarily coupled with a social justice framework, which understands social and health inequities to be about differential access to power and resources. Thus, intersectionality can be seen as a critical tool for theory and practice, which advances our understanding of how individuals' social locations affect their experiences of mental illness and their access to mental health care. Intersectionality also has the potential to help realize the broader goals of reducing inequities and enhancing citizenship for people with mental illness.

For example, despite the variety of mental health services and supports available in the United States and Canada, many women, particularly those who are economically disadvantaged, are unable to access appropriate treatment to meet their complex and diverse needs (Groh 2007; O'Mahony and Donnelly 2007). Understanding the intersections of mental health status, poverty, gender, and race within the context of diminishing funding for mental health care in the United States reveals a need for mental health policy reform that will improve the response to the needs of diverse populations (Groh 2007). Canadian research has reported similar barriers to mental health treatment for immigrant women with serious mental illness, due to limited financial resources, English-language competency, education, and mobility (Chiu et al. 2005). Self- and social stigma have also been found to play an important role in women's access to social support and their decisions to seek mental health treatment (ibid.).

Intersectional scholarship across disciplines has typically emphasized gender, race, ethnicity, and class, to the exclusion of other categories, such as sexual orientation, gender identity, physical disability, and age. In analyses of race and ethnicity, intersectional mental health scholarship in Canada and the United Kingdom has often focused on women from South and East Asia (see Acharya and Northcott 2007; Burman and Chantler 2003; Chiu et al. 2005) whereas in the United States, the focus has been on African American women (see Kales et al. 2005; Kohn and Hudson 2002). Although much of this scholarship acknowledges the role of socio-economic status, age, education, language, culture, religion, and spirituality (Acharya and Northcott 2007; Chiu et al. 2005; Jarvis et al. 2005), these and other social categories are not typically fully analyzed in their intersections with race and ethnicity.

Similarly, whereas intersectional mental health research in Canada has explored mental health broadly, along a continuum from psychological distress to serious mental illness, much of the research in the United States and the UK has focused specifically on depression (see Hussain and Cochrane 2004; Kales et al. 2005; Kohn and Hudson 2002). This emphasis on select social categories and processes, ethnocultural groups, and mental illnesses has resulted in limited knowledge about a broad range of social categories and mental health problems, which are relevant to mental health policy and service delivery.

From an anthropological perspective, cultural differences pose conceptual and methodological challenges for researchers measuring the prevalence of certain mental illnesses among culturally diverse groups (Kleinman 1987).

Culturally specific meanings of mental health and illness may exert a powerful influence on if, when, and how individuals seek mental health treatment services (Shin 2004). However, an uncritical acceptance of research findings about the underutilization of mental health services among ethnic minority and immigrant populations blinds us to more critical analyses of how these services sometimes fail to respond to the diverse cultural, linguistic, and religious needs of individuals (Hussain and Cochrane 2004; Wilson 2001). Intersectional approaches seek to unpack social categories such as culture to explore their intersections with other powerful categories. In the words of Jennifer Burr and Tom Chapman (1998, 431), a cultural relativism approach, where differences between cultural groups are emphasized, "operates as a smokescreen for the impact of poverty and racism," obscuring the intersections of social categories and processes, and absolving mental health policy makers and practitioners of the responsibility for improving access to mental health services that are responsive to the needs of diverse populations.

Despite growing interest in intersectional approaches to mental health research, practice, and policy, few scholars have moved beyond analyses of social categories to analyses of social processes of discrimination and oppression. We argue that attention to structural processes is critical in overcoming the limitations inherent in the treatment of social categories as static and unchanging variables, an approach that artificially simplifies complex phenomena by categorizing individuals according to broad group membership (Warner 2008). Intersectional scholarship exploring multiple interlocking forms of oppression challenges the assumptions that result from simplistic categorization of individuals, thereby helping researchers, policy makers, and practitioners to better understand the complexity of lived experiences of mental health and illness, and to determine the implications of these intersections for service delivery (Burman 2004).

Despite the complexity and challenges involved in intersectional scholarship, this approach is particularly well suited to understanding the diverse experiences of mental illness among multiply disadvantaged groups, with the goal of reducing psychiatric stigma and discrimination, and increasing opportunities for recovery, inclusion, and citizenship.

Critique of Existing Approaches

Stigma/Discrimination Education Campaigns

Stigma and discrimination resulting from a mental illness diagnosis act as significant barriers to mental health services and acceptance into the community (Health Canada 2002; Martin and Johnston 2007). Additionally, socially marginalized groups (such as women, Aboriginal people, substance users, the poor, individuals living with HIV or AIDS, ethnic minorities, immigrants, individuals with disabilities, GLBTQ, criminalized populations) may experience stigma and discrimination in ways that compound the impact. For example, Faye Gary (2005, 990) suggests that "given the lower socioeconomic status ..., the public and private stigma influences, and the distrust of the mental health system, ethnic minority people are at risk for not receiving adequate mental health care." Mental illness in some cultures is highly stigmatized, resulting in the underutilization of mental health services (Hussain and Cochrane 2004), and low-income, less educated women are more likely than other women to report stigma-related barriers to accessing mental health services (Alvidrez and Azocar 1999). In short, individuals report the layering of stigma associated with physical and mental health conditions, and marginalized group membership (Collins, von Unger, and Armbrister 2008; Hankivsky and Cormier 2009; Mill et al. 2007; Ship and Norton 2001; Walkup, Cramer, and Yeras 2004), which has important implications for access to services, such as mental health care and housing (Reutter et al. 2009).

Anti-stigma programs in Canada have historically developed locally, in isolation from one another, and have been poorly funded and evaluated (Martin and Johnston 2007). Those based in a biomedical model of mental illness have sought to reduce the stigma associated with mental illnesses by drawing parallels to physical forms of illness (Everett 2006). Yet, approaches grounded in a medical model tend to individualize and decontextualize mental health issues, thereby reinforcing negative stereotypes that people with mental illness have impaired judgment and limited control over their behaviour, and may pose a danger to others (Read et al. 2006). The continued dominance of the biomedical paradigm in mental health is thus a significant barrier to understandings of mental illness that move past representations of persons with psychiatric disabilities as "sick" and "dangerous," and toward critical perspectives that focus on the context of individuals' lives and their recovery, inclusion, and citizenship.

More progressive stigma/discrimination awareness campaigns have been limited by tokenistic representations of diverse populations, which often reflect only visible dimensions of difference, such as gender, age, and race. Although these anti-stigma campaigns underscore the universality of mental illness, they fail to communicate the layered stigma and discrimination experienced by socially marginalized groups, and to raise awareness about the intersections of other social identity categories, such as sexual orientation, education, and religion. For example, research suggests that some groups (such as women and Aboriginal people) are more stigmatized than others, yet when they are treated as distinct groups, the intersections of gender and ethnicity in experiences of stigma and discrimination become obscured (Canale and Munn 2005). Thus, even more progressive anti-stigma

campaigns face challenges in communicating how the stigma and discrimination associated with mental illness and addiction are experienced
uniquely by diverse groups, how these are not only quantitatively but also
qualitatively different for various populations, and how they may be compounded by other forms of discrimination.

An intersectional framework requires that anti-stigma and discrimination
campaigns move beyond tokenism toward more meaningful representation
of diverse populations and the delivery of nuanced messages about the
complex intersection of multiple social categories and the layering of stigma
and discrimination. From an intersectional perspective, we argue that efforts
to reduce psychiatric stigma will have limited success if the stigma associated
with poverty and other dimensions of difference is ignored and seen as
separate from the experience of psychiatric stigma. For example, Michael
Kirby (2006, 169) calls for greater attention to the "double-whammy of
mental illness and aging" in the development of a national anti-stigma
campaign. The stigma associated with mental illness and aging must be seen,
from an intersectional perspective, not as independent and additive but as
inextricably linked. The adoption of an intersectional perspective and anti-
oppression framework in anti-stigma and discrimination work will allow for
greater understanding and awareness of intersecting social identities and
the layering of stigma and discrimination.

Furthermore, anti-stigma and discrimination initiatives must address not
only self- and social stigma but also structural or institutional equivalents,
which are reflected in practices and policies that systematically restrict the
rights of persons with mental illness and limit their social, economic, and
political power (Corrigan, Markowitz, and Watson 2004; Corrigan and Watson
2002; Link and Phelan 2001). These initiatives require sustained political
leadership and the targeting of *processes* that perpetuate discrimination (for
example, via constitutional challenges against discriminatory social policies).
We argue that the adoption of an anti-oppression and social justice framework is critical to the success of the MHCC's anti-stigma and discrimination
campaign to increase public awareness of the barriers faced by those with
mental illness, decrease inequities, and increase opportunities for citizenship
(Morrow and Chappell 1999).

Recovery Models of Care

Recovery and anti-stigma/discrimination practices are integrally linked: that
is, the full recognition of the personhood of those with mental illness and
their right to be integrated into society and access resources like all other
citizens is critical to recovery. Indeed, it has been well documented that
barriers to recovery include social isolation and active discrimination against
people with mental illness who try to access services and supports, and/or

Interact with their communities (Corrigan, Markowitz, and Watson 2004; Link and Phelan 2001). At a systemic level, discrimination is codified in policy and the practice of psychiatry through legislation that allows people's rights to be removed; they can be forcibly confined and treated without their consent.[1] Discrimination is also active in social policy, which has, until very recently, ignored the experiences and needs of people with psychiatric disabilities, such as access to disability assistance and the lack of federal and provincial housing strategies that take their specific needs into consideration (Morrow, Frischmuth, and Johnson 2006; Morrow et al. 2009).

Definitions and understandings of recovery differ: some focus more at the individual level, whereas others adopt a social model of recovery. The former are more popularly deployed and typically emphasize individual autonomy, empowerment, hope, and choice. For example, in the Canadian context, the most recent articulation of the components of recovery can be found in the Mental Health Commission of Canada's framework for a mental health strategy (MHCC 2009a). In this document, which was subject to significant public consultation, recovery is described as "a process in which people living with mental health problems and illnesses are empowered and supported to be actively engaged in their own journey of well-being" and one that "builds on individual, family, cultural and community strengths and enables people to enjoy a meaningful life in their community while striving to achieve their full potential" (ibid., 122). Likewise, William Anthony (1993, 15), one of the leaders of the recovery movement in the US, suggests that "recovery involves the development of new meaning and purpose in one's life as one grows beyond the catastrophic effects of mental illness."

Social models of recovery, on the other hand, explicitly recognize the impact of stigma and discrimination on people with mental illness and emphasize social supports, such as the need for housing and economic security (Jablensky et al. 1992; Jacobson and Greenley 2001). For example, the social model most utilized in Canada, the Canadian Mental Health Association's Framework for Support, distinguishes between necessary and unnecessary constraints for those with mental illnesses (Trainor, Pomeroy, and Pape 2004). Necessary constraints are those inherent to the illness, and unnecessary constraints often "reflect a combination of negative attitudes and the absence of needed supports in the community" (ibid., 23). Likewise, the Tidal Model developed in the UK also recognizes the social context within which recovery occurs as well as the barriers to its realization (Barker 2003). These definitions of recovery are consistent with what some refer to as the second order of change in recovery – that is, systemic or political change and an emphasis on ecological perspectives that "shifts the focus away from recovery solely being the responsibility of the individual to one that makes equally strong demands of the environment" (Onken et al. 2007,

18). The emphasis here is on social justice or change that is politicized and encompasses the mitigation of oppression, exclusion, discrimination, and the deviant status of mental illnesses (ibid.).

However, even in these progressive articulations of recovery, systemic and structural understandings of the role of social inequities in mental health, based on factors such as gender, race, culture, ethnicity, income, and sexual orientation, continue to be overlooked. Further, in practice, the degree to which social models of recovery can gain traction is hindered by structural barriers such as the lack of community-based mental health resources, including housing, income security, and employment, as well as the ongoing dominance of the biomedical paradigm in mental health (Morrow 2004; Teghtsoonian 2008; Walker 2006).

The lack of an intersectional analysis in its application to recovery has meant that structural factors and forms of systemic discrimination that affect mental health recovery have largely been ignored. Two examples, from the emerging literature on gender and intersectionality in mental health and addictions in Canada, help to make this point; we discuss these examples in the following section.

Intersectional Theory into Practice

Intersectional scholars have highlighted the importance of moving intersectional theory into practice (Burgess-Proctor 2006; Collins 1990) and yet have struggled with how best to do so. Most argue that an intersectional approach must be grounded in lived experience, or what Evelyn Simien (2007) describes as an "experience-based" epistemology. In recent years, guidelines on how to employ intersectionality have been developed especially for health researchers and policy makers (Canadian Research Institute 2006; Hankivsky and Cormier 2009; Morris and Bunjun 2007). Hankivsky and Cormier (2009) provide a primer on intersectionality designed to assist researchers and policy makers in applying intersectional approaches; it includes health-related examples that have been carefully worked through. Mental health researchers and policy makers would benefit from the utilization of such tools and from sharing across sectors and disciplines the strategies that have thus far been successful.

Here we briefly explore two examples from emerging work on intersectionality in Canada as it is relevant to recovery and anti-stigma/discrimination work in mental health. These examples are shared for discussion purposes and to illustrate the ways in which using intersectionality can enhance our understanding of complex issues in mental health.

The first is drawn from one of the authors' own studies, which examined South Asian and Chinese women's narratives about their experiences of post-partum depression in Canada and what would be most useful for their recovery (Morrow et al. 2008). In this study, women's detailed descriptions of their experiences of depression revealed the importance of psychosocial stresses, particularly those associated with the migration experience, as significant contributors to depression. Migration was shown to disrupt women's relationships with their immediate families (especially their mothers and female relatives), which in turn had an impact on how they experienced the peri-natal period. Careful attention was paid to the particular migration experiences of each woman and how they differed according to class and country of origin. For example, women from India were more likely to have come as family class immigrants and to have better family and social supports than those from China, who were less likely to have joined relatives in Canada (ibid.). This resulted in differing experiences for the women and also the need for different kinds of supports. In this instance, the intersections of ethnicity, culture, and migration experiences that, in turn, are shaped by historical and economic factors, were critical for understanding the mental health needs of women.

In the second example, evidence from research that focused on the experiences of mothers with substance-use problems illustrated the very particular ways in which these women are stigmatized and discriminated against as women (Boyd 2007; Salmon 2007) and also showed the compounding effects that racialization has on Aboriginal mothers (Salmon 2007). In one study (ibid.), focus groups were conducted with six young Aboriginal mothers whose lives had been affected by fetal alcohol spectrum disorder (FASD). Their stories revealed the need for FASD prevention efforts that included both harm reduction and abstinence-based approaches to better reflect the complexity of Aboriginal women's lives and reduce the shame and stigma associated with substance use during pregnancy. Further, the study reinforced that policy makers and practitioners must recognize the diversity of Aboriginal women to avoid applying a "one-size-fits-all" approach to Aboriginal, Inuit, and Métis women in urban and rural settings (British Columbia Centre of Excellence for Women's Health 2009).

In both of these examples, more than one social category was investigated, and the researchers examined the relationship between the categories and the interaction between individual and institutional factors, all considered important elements of an intersectional approach (Hankivsky and Cormier 2009). These brief examples show how the utilization of intersectional theoretical approaches can reveal social and structural factors of relevance to recovery that have typically been ignored by policy makers and practitioners and/or used in ways that have stigmatized certain groups. We argue that intersectionality might also be achieved through the use of innovative knowledge exchange practices that bring together academics, people with lived experience, policy makers, and mental health practitioners for extended dialogues. Two approaches, in particular, might be useful here: participatory action research and arts-based approaches.

Critical feminist and intersectional scholars have found that participatory action and community-based research approaches that seek to challenge dominant discourses of health and illness are particularly valuable in health research with socially marginalized and vulnerable populations (Guruge and Khanlou 2004). Community-based participatory action research approaches have the potential to bring academics, community partners, and policy makers together for interactive dialogue and participation in defining research questions and approaches, and in analyzing and interpreting data (Ristock and Pennell 1996). Participatory action research is premised on the belief that a more open recognition of power differentials between researchers and the communities they research can result in a democratization of the research process, whereby community members actively define the issues of importance to them (Morris and Bunjun 2007; Wallerstein et al. 2003). Although in and of itself, participatory action research will not guarantee the emergence of a more complex understanding of the role of power and privilege in its many intersections, it is the research paradigm best suited to accomplish this. The work of Barbara Schneider (2003), in which people with schizophrenia diagnoses looked at their experiences of housing and homelessness, and which resulted in theatre performances and a film, is an excellent example of participatory research that was able to get at the intersections of mental illness, homelessness, and poverty.

This example also points to the growing interest, nationally and internationally, in arts-based approaches in health research and knowledge translation/exchange (Nisker et al. 2006; Rossiter et al. 2008; Kontos and Poland 2009). Arts-based approaches connect researchers and artists who, together, traverse a "rocky cross-disciplinary terrain" (Rossiter et al. 2008, 278), translating social science research data, through various media (theatre, film, music), into knowledge that can be taken up in mental health policy and practice. The active participation of consumers/survivors in translating research knowledge, based on their experiences, to the public and to policy makers may be particularly beneficial to individuals with mental illness, both by supporting their recovery and providing them with opportunities to challenge and overcome the layered experiences of stigma and discrimination.

For example, theatre has been used in Australia to educate the public about the experience of schizophrenia and psychosis, and to give voice to people with mental illness diagnoses, who may be socially marginalized and disempowered (Keen and Todres 2007; Rolfe, Mienczakowski, and Morgan 1995). In Canada, we have also seen the development, by people with mental illnesses, of a number of comedy troupes (such as Stand Up for Mental Health) that work to dispel myths about mental illness and bring the public in closer contact with people who experience it. Researchers employing theatre to engage citizens in democratic discussions of health policy development in Canada conclude that "theatre has the potential to be a powerful and effective tool for engaging members of the public in regard to a health-policy issue that is scientifically and morally complex, emotionally charged, and controversial" (Nisker et al. 2006, 266). We assert that arts-based approaches may be particularly effective in moving intersectional theory into practice in the area of mental health, particularly if consumers/survivors themselves are involved in the process of knowledge translation.

Discussion

Our analysis of recovery models and anti-stigma work in the mental health field leads us to conclude that one of the greatest barriers to applying critical and intersectional approaches in mental health research, policy, and practice is the continued dominance of a biomedical paradigm in the mental health field. Within this paradigm, mental illness is defined as an objective condition that can be accurately measured and diagnosed across diverse populations (Burr and Chapman 1998). Furthermore, this paradigm supports the use of positivist methodologies that may fail to capture and interpret differences between groups, thereby perpetuating myths and stereotypes about racialized individuals with mental illness. Feryad Hussain and Ray Cochrane (2004, 265) assert that "the widespread use of traditional, positivist research methods has meant that current models of mental health developed on one population, have been held up as a standard by which the mental health of people of differing ethnic origin have been 'measured.'" They call for alternative approaches that, unlike traditional positivist approaches, explore mental illness within a cultural and social context, and avoid "distorting" or "dismissing" culturally relevant factors in the understanding and interpretation of psychological distress (Burr and Chapman 1998; Hussain and Cochrane 2004). We echo this call but argue for the adoption of intersectional approaches, which seek to address the shortcomings both of biomedical paradigms and their attendant positivist methodologies, and more progressive feminist and critical approaches to mental health research, policy, and practice.

The adoption of intersectional perspectives in mental health research, policy, and practice is also difficult given the barriers rooted in systemic racism, sexism, and other forms of discrimination that persist in Canadian society, generally, and in the mental health care system, specifically. However, research examining the intersections of social identity categories reveals not only processes of subordination and oppression but also experiences of advantage and privilege. For example, culture may be a strength for women who adopt culturally specific strategies to cope with mental distress (Acharya and Northcott 2007). Identification with, or membership in, multiple groups may serve to exacerbate or minimize the impact of stigma for individuals with mental illness, depending on whether or not those other groups are also stigmatized (Walkup, Cramer, and Yeras 2004; Watson and Larson 2007). In cases where those groups exert a positive influence, intersectional scholars should explore the positive aspects of diversity and emphasize the strength and resiliency of women from marginalized and vulnerable populations who experience mental illness (Kinnon 1999; O'Mahony and Donnelly 2007).

For example, a study exploring the experiences of Latina women with severe mental illness in the United States revealed that "women internalize and resist the stigma attached to mental illness in their communities by aligning themselves with identities that bestow dignity and respect" (Collins, von Unger, and Armbrister 2008, 395). Intersectional mental health scholarship must continue to challenge the dominance of biomedical approaches and avoid framing positive cultural perspectives and religious practices as sources of treatment non-compliance and denial of mental illness. Doing so only serves to undermine culturally diverse perspectives of health and illness, reinforce negative stereotypes about Canadian immigrants, and strengthen the dominance of biomedical approaches. Additionally, intersectional scholars must move beyond the exploration of single categories, such as gender or race, which have been the focus of much feminist and anti-racist scholarship, to explore various interlocking social categories and processes, and the impact of these intersections on experiences of mental illness and health, stigma, and recovery.

The dominance of a biomedical approach has important implications not only for research but also for mental health practice, where it has supported a "scientist-practitioner" model that does not easily allow for the integration of traditional approaches to healing and recovery, even though integrated treatment models may be preferred among immigrant and racialized women (Chiu et al. 2005; Hussain and Cochrane 2004). Indeed, Michael Walker (2006, 78) argues that "the belief that the medical and psychological vocabularies represent scientifically 'discovered truths' is the biggest obstacle for traditional community mental health programs transitioning to recovery-based services." Intersectional approaches in mental health challenge us to recognize the importance of contextual factors not only in our understanding of how mental illness is understood, experienced, and expressed but also in the way it is treated. However, fundamental shifts in the treatment of mental illness require changes in the training and education of mental health professionals.

Canadian research suggests that many health care providers are attuned to the difficulties that socially marginalized populations face when seeking mental health services, and to the socio-political context within which the mental health system operates (O'Mahony and Donnelly 2007). However, though some mental health care providers may recognize these individual challenges and the systemic discrimination that pervades the mental health care system, there is an ongoing need for professional training that draws attention to the intersections of various axes of inequity and the ways in which experiences of stigma and recovery are intricately linked to social categories and processes of domination and oppression.

In Canada, the training of mental health professionals has focused on cultural sensitivity and competency, which naively suggests that if providers come to understand the cultural differences of their clients, they will be able to provide better care. In response to this, the concept of "cultural safety" has been utilized, which emphasizes the systemic and damaging impact of racism and colonialism, particularly on indigenous populations (Ball 2008; Papps and Ramsden 1996; Smye and Browne 2002). Cultural safety is closely tied to the quality of health care and the health status of minority cultural groups, and can be useful in promoting a social justice framework in health policy analysis and reform (Papps and Ramsden 1996; Smye and Browne 2002). Vicki Smye and Annette Browne (2002, 53) have adopted the notion of cultural safety in Canadian Aboriginal health research to illustrate how "we can better critique issues of institutional racism and discrimination that continue to shape the provision of health care for aboriginal people in Canada." Cultural safety has recently been identified as a necessary component of a mental health strategy and transformed mental health system in Canada (MHCC 2009a). We argue that the concept of cultural safety may be valuable in the training of mental health professionals but also in the analysis of mental health policy and critical exploration of the role of racism and discrimination in experiences of psychiatric stigma and recovery.

Barriers and challenges notwithstanding, intersectional frameworks in mental health are emerging and beginning to show potential for more nuanced and accurate assessments of the lived experiences of individuals with mental illness. The application of intersectionality to a wide range of issues in mental health is necessary, but we especially urge researchers to focus on issues of key policy and practical relevance in the current context. It is encouraging that the MHCC (2009a, 51) has begun to acknowledge the value of an intersectional perspective in mental health policy and practice, recognizing that "we are all multi-faceted individuals, and our individual identities are shaped by the many intersecting dimensions of our lives." Intersectional analyses of recovery models and anti-stigma/discrimination work will be particularly valuable as Canada struggles to define itself and lead other countries in its important national endeavours with respect to developing a mental health strategy that is recovery-based, and an anti-stigma/discrimination campaign that is meant to inform both professionals and the public. We suggest that these initiatives will have greater impact and relevance if they move beyond biomedical and the current more progressive approaches to better respond to the complex recovery needs of diverse populations and promote the active engagement and citizenship of individuals with mental illness. Finally, we assert that intersectionality has the potential to provide the tools and means to reduce inequities, disrupt the existing power relationships in mental health, and move the social justice agenda forward.

Note

1   In Canada, Mental Health Acts, which differ from province to province, constitute the legislative vehicle for involuntary committal. There is an ongoing debate concerning the degree to which people who are mentally ill should be allowed to make decisions about treatment, with a specific focus on their right to refuse it.

References

Acharya, M.P., and H.C. Northcott. 2007. Mental distress and the coping strategies of elderly Indian immigrant women. *Transcultural Psychiatry* 44: 614-36.

Ad Hoc Working Group on Women, Mental Health, Mental Illness and Addiction. 2006. *Women, mental health, mental illness and addiction: An overview.* Winnipeg: Canadian Women's Health Network.

Ahmad, W.I.U., ed. 1994. *"Race" and health in contemporary Britain.* Philadelphia: Open University Press.

Alvidrez, J., and R. Azocar. 1999. Distressed women's clinic patients: Preferences for mental health treatments and perceived obstacles. *General Hospital Psychiatry* 21(5): 340-47.

Anthony, W.A. 1993. Recovery from mental illness: The guiding vision of the mental health service system in the 1990s. *Psychosocial Rehabilitation Journal* 16(4): 11-23.

Ball, J. 2008. Cultural safety in practice with children, families and communities. Poster session presented at the "Early Years Inter-Professional Research and Practice Conference," Vancouver, BC, 30 January-2 February.

Barker, P. 2003. The tidal model: Psychiatric colonization, recovery, and the paradigm shift in mental health care. *International Journal of Mental Health Nursing* 12: 96-102.

Boyd, S. 2007. Women, drug regulation and maternal/state conflicts. In *Women's health in Canada: Critical perspectives on theory and policy,* ed. M. Morrow, O. Hankivsky, and C. Varcoe, 327-54. Toronto: University of Toronto Press.

Boyer, M., J. Ku, and U. Shakir. 1997. *The healing journey: Phase II report – Women and mental health: Documenting the voices of ethnoracial women within an anti-racist framework.* Toronto: Across Boundaries Mental Health Centre.

British Columbia Centre of Excellence for Women's Health. 2009. Preventing FASD through providing addictions treatment and related support for First Nations and Inuit women in Canada. http://www.coalescing-vc.org/virtualLearning/section5/documents/Cmty5_InfoSheet1.pdf.

Burgess-Proctor, A. 2006. Intersections of race, class, gender, and crime: Future directions for feminist criminology. *Feminist Criminology* 1(1): 27-47.

Burman, E. 2004. From difference to intersectionality: Challenges and resources. *European Journal of Psychotherapy, Counselling and Health* 6(4): 293-308.

Burman, E., and K. Chantler. 2003. Across and between: Reflections on researching "race," gender and mental health. *Feminism and Psychology* 13(3): 302-9.

Burr, J.A., and T. Chapman. 1998. Some reflections on cultural and social considerations in mental health nursing. *Journal of Psychiatric and Mental Health Nursing* 5(6): 431-37.

Burstow, B. 2005. Feminist antipsychiatry praxis – Women and the movement(s): A Canadian perspective. In Chan, Chunn, and Menzies 2005, 245-58.

Burstow, B., and D. Weitz, eds. 1988. *Shrink resistant: The struggle against psychiatry in Canada.* Vancouver: New Star.

Canadian Research Institute for the Advancement of Women. 2006. *Intersectional feminist frameworks: An emerging vision.* Ottawa: Canadian Research Institute for the Advancement of Women.

Canadian Task Force on Mental Health Issues Affecting Immigrants and Refugees. 1988. *After the door has been opened.* Ottawa: Minister of Supply and Services.

Canale, M.K., and E. Munn. 2005. The Stigma of Addiction Project: Turning voices into action. *Visions: BC's Mental Health and Addictions Journal* 2(6): 13-14.

Caplan, P. 1987. *The myth of women's masochism.* Scarborough: New American Library of Canada.

Caplan, P., and L. Cosgrove. 2004. *Bias in psychiatric diagnosis.* New York: Rowman and Littlefield.

Chan, W., D. Chunn, and R. Menzies. 2005. *Women, madness and the law: A feminist reader.* London: Glasshouse.

Chesler, P. 1972. *Women and madness.* New York: Avon Books.

Chiu, L., M. Morrow, S. Ganesan, and N. Clark. 2005. Spirituality and treatment choices by South and East Asian women with serious mental illness. *Transcultural Psychiatry* 42(4): 630-56.

Collins, P.H. 1990. *Black feminist thought: Knowledge, consciousness, and the politics of empowerment.* Boston: Unwin Hyman.

Collins, P.Y., H. von Unger, and A. Armbrister. 2008. Church ladies, good girls, and locas: Stigma and the intersection of gender, ethnicity, mental illness, and sexuality in relation to HIV risk. *Social Science and Medicine* 67(3): 389-97.

Corrigan, P.W., F.E. Markowitz, and A.C. Watson. 2004. Structural levels of mental illness: Stigma and discrimination. *Schizophrenia Bulletin* 30(3): 481-91.

Corrigan, P.W., and A.C. Watson. 2002. Understanding the impact of stigma on people with mental illness. *World Psychiatry* 1(1): 16-20.

Dhamoon, R. 2008. Considerations in mainstreaming intersectionality as an analytic approach. Paper presented at the Western Political Science Association, San Diego, 20-22 March.

Everett, B. 2006. Stigma: The hidden killer – Background paper and literature review. Mood Disorders Society of Canada. http://www.mooddisorderscanada.ca.

Gary, F.A. 2005. Stigma: Barrier to mental health care among ethnic minorities. *Issues in Mental Health Nursing* 26: 979-99.

Gold, J.H. 1998. Gender differences in psychiatric illness and treatments: A critical review. *Journal of Nervous and Mental Disease* 186(12): 769-74.

Groh, C.J. 2007. Poverty, mental health, and women: Implications for psychiatric nurses in primary care settings. *Journal of the American Psychiatric Nurses Association* 13(5): 267-74.

Guruge, S., and N. Khanlou. 2004. Intersectionalities of influence: Researching the health of immigrant and refugee women. *Canadian Journal of Nursing Research* 36(3): 32-47.

Hankivsky, O., and R. Cormier. 2009. *Intersectionality: Moving women's health research and policy forward.* Vancouver: Women's Health Research Network.

Harris, M., and C. Landis. 1997. *Sexual abuse in the lives of women diagnosed with serious mental illness.* Amsterdam: Overseas Publishers Association.

Health Canada. 2000. *A statistical profile on the health of First Nations in Canada for the year 2000.* Ottawa: Health Canada.

–. 2002. *A report on mental illnesses in Canada.* Ottawa: Health Canada.

Hussain, F., and R. Cochrane. 2004. Depression in South Asian women living in the UK: A review of the literature with implications for service provision. *Transcultural Psychiatry* 41(2): 253-70.

Jablensky, A., N. Sartorius, G. Emberg, M. Anker, A. Korten, J.E. Cooper, R. Day, and A. Bertelsen. 1992. Schizophrenia: Manifestation, incidence and course in different cultures. A World Health Organization ten-country study. *Psychological Medicine* Monograph Suppl. 20: 1-97.

Jacobson, N., and D. Greenley. 2001. What is recovery? A conceptual model and explication. *Psychiatric Services* 52(4): 482-85.

Jarvis, G.E., L.J. Kirmayer, M. Weinfeld, and J. Lasry. 2005. Religious practice and psychological distress: The importance of gender, ethnicity and immigrant status. *Transcultural Psychiatry* 42: 657-75.

Kales, H.C., H.W. Neighbors, F.C. Blow, K.K.K. Taylor, L. Gilon, D.E. Welsh, S.M. Maixner, and A.M. Mellow. 2005. Race, gender, and psychiatrists' diagnosis and treatment of major depression among elderly patients. *Psychiatric Services* 56(6): 721-28.

Keen, S., and L. Todres. 2007. Strategies for disseminating qualitative research findings: Three exemplars. *Forum, Qualitative Social Research* 8(3): Art. 17.

Kinnon, D. 1999. *Canadian research on immigration and health: An overview.* Ottawa: Health Canada.

Kirby, M. 2006. *Out of the shadows at last: Transforming mental health, mental illness and addiction services in Canada.* Final Report of the Standing Senate Committee on Social Affairs, Science and Technology. Ottawa: Senate Committee on Social Affairs, Science and Technology.

Kirmayer, L., G.M. Brass, and C.L. Tait. 2000. The mental health of Aboriginal peoples: Transformations of identity and culture. *Canadian Journal of Psychiatry* 45(7): 607-17.

Kleinman, A. 1987. Anthropology and psychiatry: The role of culture in cross-cultural research on illness. *British Journal of Psychiatry* 151: 447-54.

Kohn, L.P., and K.M. Hudson. 2002. Gender, ethnicity and depression: Intersectionality and context in mental health research with African American women. *Perspectives* 8(1): 174-84.

Kontos, P.C., and B.D. Poland. 2009. Mapping new theoretical and methodological terrain for knowledge translation: Contributions from critical realism and the arts. *Implementation Science* 4(1): 1-10.

Kornstein, S., and A. Clayton, eds. 2002. *Women's mental health: A comprehensive textbook.* New York: Guilford Press.

Link, B.G., and J.C. Phelan. 2001. Conceptualizing stigma. *Annual Review of Sociology* 27: 363-85.

Martin, N., and V. Johnston. 2007. A time for action: Tackling stigma and discrimination. Report to the Mental Health Commission of Canada. Mental Health Commission of Canada. http://www.mentalhealthcommission.ca/SiteCollectionDocuments/Anti-Stigma/TimeforAction_Eng.pdf.

MHCC (Mental Health Commission of Canada). 2009a. *Toward recovery and well-being: A framework for a mental health strategy for Canada.* Ottawa: Mental Health Commission of Canada.

–. 2009b. *Improving mental health services for immigrant, refugee, ethno-cultural and racialized groups: Issues and options for service improvement.* Ottawa: Mental Health Commission of Canada.

Mill, J., et al. 2007. *The influence of stigma on access to health services by persons with HIV illness.* Canadian Aboriginal AIDS Network. http://caan.ca/new/wp-content/uploads/2010/03/The-Influence-of-Stigma-on-Access-to-Health-Services-by-Persons-with-HIV-Illness.pdf.

Morris, M., and B. Bunjun. 2007. *Using intersectional feminist frameworks in research.* Ottawa: Canadian Institute for the Advancement of Women.

Morrow, M. 2003. *Mainstreaming women's mental health: Building a Canadian strategy.* Vancouver: British Columbia Centre of Excellence for Women's Health.

–. 2004. Mental health reform, economic globalization and the practice of citizenship. *Canadian Journal of Community Mental Health* 23(2): 39-50.

–. 2007. Women's voices matter: Creating women-centred mental health policy. In *Women's health in Canada: Critical perspectives on theory and policy,* ed. M. Morrow, O. Hankivsky, and C. Varcoe, 355-79. Toronto: University of Toronto Press.

–. 2008. Women, violence and mental illness: An evolving feminist critique. In *Global science/women's health,* ed. C. Patton and H. Loshny, 147-74. New York: Cambria Press.

Morrow, M., and M. Chappell. 1999. *Hearing women's voices: Mental health care for women.* Vancouver: British Columbia Centre of Excellence for Women's Health.

Morrow, M., with S. Frischmuth and A. Johnson. 2006. *Community based mental health services in BC: Changes to income, employment and housing supports.* Vancouver: Canadian Centre for Policy Alternatives.

Morrow, M., J. Smith, Y. Lai, and S. Jaswal. 2008. Shifting landscapes: Immigrant women and post partum depression. *Health Care for Women International* 29(6): 593-617.

Morrow, M., A. Wasik, M. Cohen, and K.M. Perry. 2009. Removing barriers to work: Building economic security for people with mental illness. *Critical Social Policy* 29(4): 655-76.

Nisker, J., D.K. Martin, R. Bluhm, and A.S. Daar. 2006. Theatre as a public engagement tool for health-policy development. *Health Policy* 78: 258-71

O'Mahony, J.M., and T.T. Donnelly 2007. Health care providers' perspective of the gender influences on immigrant women's mental health care experiences. *Issues in Mental Health Nursing* 28: 1171-88.

Onken, S.J., C.M. Craig, P. Ridgeway, R.O. Ralph, and J.A. Cook. 2007. An analysis of the definitions and elements of recovery: A review of the literature. *Psychiatric Rehabilitation Journal* 31(1): 9-22.

Ontario Ministry of Health. 1993. *Putting people first: The reform of mental health services in Ontario.* Ottawa: Ontario Ministry of Health.

Papps, E., and I. Ramsden. 1996. Cultural safety in nursing: The New Zealand experience. *International Journal for Quality in Health Care* 8(5): 491-97.

Read, J., N. Haslam, L. Sayce, and E. Davies. 2006. Prejudice and schizophrenia: A review of the "mental illness is an illness like any other" approach. *Acta Psychiatrica Scandinavica* 114: 303-18.

Reutter, L.I., M.J. Stewart, G. Veenstra, R. Love, D. Raphael, and E. Makwarimba. 2009. "Who do they think we are, anyway?": Perceptions of and responses to poverty stigma. *Qualitative Health Research* 19(3): 297-311.

Rhodes, A., P. Goering, T. To, and J. Williams. 2002. Gender and outpatient mental health service use. *Social Science and Medicine* 54(1): 1-10.

Ristock, J., and J. Pennell. 1996. *Community research as empowerment: Feminist links, post-modern interruptions.* New York: Oxford University Press.

Rolfe, A., J. Mienczakowski, and S. Morgan. 1995. A dramatic experience in mental health nursing education. *Nurse Education Today* 15: 224-27.

Rossiter, K., J. Gray, P. Kontos, M. Keightley, A. Colantonio, and J. Gilbert. 2008. From page to stage: Dramaturgy and the art of interdisciplinary translation. *Journal of Health Psychology* 13(2): 277-86.

Salmon, A. 2007. Beyond shame and blame: Aboriginal mothers and barriers to care. In *Highs and lows: Canadian perspectives on women and substance use,* ed. N. Poole and L. Greaves, 227-35. Toronto: Centre for Addiction and Mental Health.

Schneider, B. 2003. Narratives of schizophrenia: Constructing a positive image. *Canadian Journal of Communication* 28(2): 185-201.

Shin, S. 2004. Effects of culturally relevant psychoeducation for Korean American families of persons with chronic mental illness. *Research on Social Work Practice* 14: 231-39.

Ship, S.J., and L. Norton. 2001. HIV/AIDS and Aboriginal women in Canada. *Canadian Woman Studies* 21(2): 25-31.

Simien, E.M. 2007. Doing intersectionality research: From conceptual issues to practical examples. *Politics and Gender* 3(2): 264-71.

Smye, V., and A. Browne. 2002. "Cultural safety" and the analysis of health policy affecting Aboriginal people. *Nurse Researcher* 9(3): 42-56.

Teghtsoonian, K. 2008. Managing workplace depression: Contesting the contours of emerging policy in the workplace. In *Contesting illness: Processes and practices,* ed. P. Moss and K. Teghtsoonian, 69-89. Toronto: University of Toronto Press.

Trainor, J., E. Pomeroy, and B. Pape. 2004. *A framework for support for people with serious mental illness.* 3rd ed. Toronto: Canadian Mental Health Association.

Ussher, J. 1991. *Women's madness: Misogyny or mental illness?* Amherst: University of Massachusetts Press.

Walker, M. 2006. The social construction of mental illness and its implications for the recovery model. *International Journal of Psychosocial Rehabilitation* 10(1): 71-87.

Walkup, J., L.J. Cramer, and J. Yeras. 2004. How is stigmatization affected by the "layering" of stigmatized conditions, such as serious mental illness and HIV? *Psychological Reports* 95(1): 771-79.

Wallerstein, N., B. Duran, J. Aguilar, J. Belone, F. Loretto, and R. Padilla. 2003. Built and social-cultural environments and health within a rural American Indian community in the Southwest. *American Journal of Public Health* 93(9): 1517-18.

Warner, L.R. 2008. A best practices guide to intersectional approaches in psychological research. *Sex Roles* 59: 454-63.

Watson, A.C., and J.E. Larson. 2007. Personal responses to disability stigma: From self stigma to empowerment. *Rehabilitation Education* 20(4): 235-46.

Wilson, M. 2001. Black women and mental health: Working towards inclusive mental health services. *Feminist Review* 68: 34-51.

17
Intersectionality, Justice, and Influencing Policy

Colleen Varcoe, Bernadette Pauly, and Shari Laliberté

Intersectional analyses are inherently oriented to fostering social change that is grounded in social justice and equity (Weber 2006). As health, social, and environmental policies, and the decision-making processes that underpin them, shape the distribution of health resources in complex and multi-faceted ways, one pathway to social change is through the process of influencing policy and policy decision-making processes. Thus, researchers committed to engaging in intersectional analyses oriented to fostering social justice and equity must seek to influence policy. In this chapter, we argue that in order to do so, researchers need to understand the nature of policy processes, the varied values underpinning policy making and policy, and the extent to which the policy contexts they wish to influence are aligned with intersectional analyses. Specifically, we argue that intersectionality is aligned with understanding social justice as a critical-relational concept in which any notion of "justice is coextensive with the political" (Young 1990, 9). More specifically, such analyses of health and social policies must be grounded in a critique of the functional and pluralist theories that underpin the current "welfare corporate societies" (Knuttila 2007; Young 1990) that have depoliticized public life. This means that any analyses of health and social policies start with differences between subgroups and specifically the relations of power among them, with particular attention to the socio-historical context of the policies and structural conditions that shape the varied ways in which such groups differently participate and influence social life (Young 1990).

Such an understanding of social justice stands in sharp contrast to distributive conceptions of justice that tend to dominate Western capitalist societies and shape their formal policy-making processes. From a distributive perspective, state actors are positioned as the primary political decision makers in hierarchical and representative-democratic political structures. The capacity to foster justice is placed within state actors who focus on distributing material goods on behalf of the larger collective in a fair way. Social groups in this larger collective are assumed to be equal and to have equal capacity to influence the state actors. Although grounded in moral and ethical intent, this perspective does not take into account the varied relations of power and how they are formed by structural systems of power.

In order to influence policy effectively, it is thus important that intersectional researchers explore the tensions between these conceptions of justice and how they influence policy processes and specifically the roles and positions of the state, civil society, and various social groups as they interact in addressing collective needs. The purpose of this chapter is therefore to draw on literature and a study of policy makers in one Canadian province, so as to propose strategies that might assist researchers to influence policy more effectively. First, we outline an understanding of social justice that we see as integral to intersectional analysis. Second, we present findings of a study that explored how policy processes work and the role of evidence in policy making, highlighting the varied understandings of social justice and equity operating in the formal policy-making context. Finally, we use insights from this study to reflect on the relationship between intersectional research and policy, and to propose strategies for influencing policy through intersectional research.

Intersectional Analysis, Inequity, and Social Justice

Despite variation in definitions and approaches, intersectional scholarship is concerned with the nature and consequences of systems of social inequity (Collins 2000; Weber 2006). Intersectionality involves examining how different forms of structural oppression are constructed with effects at the level of individuals, organizations, and broader social systems in complex and interdependent ways. Intersectional scholarship is oriented beyond descriptive analyses toward eradicating inequities, driven foremost by the pursuit of social justice (Weber 2006). Lynn Weber argues that with respect to health inequities, intersectional approaches contrast to the biomedical paradigm. Whereas within the biomedical paradigm, inequities are conceived of as resource differences among individuals, intersectional scholarship considers inequities as socially constructed consequences of structures beyond the individual and as the consequences of power differences between dominant and subordinate groups. Whereas the biomedical paradigm aims at intervention into the proximate causes of inequities – such as health behaviours, ways that health services are offered, and other factors that mediate between social inequities and individual health outcomes – intersectional scholarship targets for change in the organization of societal institutions, political decision-making structures, cultural production mechanisms, and the relations of power and inequity that emerge out of such social systems.

Intersectional scholarship, with its understanding of inequity as constructed by social structures, is closely aligned with an understanding of social justice that begins with the analysis of differences between subgroups, particularly the distribution of power and the structural conditions that shape inequities (Young 1990, 2001). This critical relational approach stands in contrast to the more dominant understandings of justice that focus on fair distribution of resources in society. Distributive Justice, although informed by a range of theoretical perspectives, focuses on the redistribution of material goods in society (Beauchamp and Childress 2001) but not on the processes that shape this distribution (Young 2001). For example, whereas distributive justice would draw attention to fair distribution of health care resources such as whether a psychiatrist is available to each community, critical-relational approaches to social justice draw attention to how certain groups are disadvantaged from accessing psychiatric care and to the ways that decision-making processes are depoliticized in relation to health care resource allocation, such as the distribution of practitioners.

This process of depoliticization has developed within the emergence of the "welfare corporate society" (ibid., 67) and the separation of the state and civil society through the emergence of bureaucratic state structures that have served to advance capitalism. After the Second World War, such structures emerged within the New Deal in which "business and government would accede to demands for collective bargaining rights, more leisure time, more pay, social security and unemployment benefits and similar measures to improve the material life and security of working people. In return, workers forfeit demands to restructure production, to control the goals and direction of enterprises or the whole economy, or to have community control over administration of services" (ibid., 70). This has served to foster a tendency to view policy as primarily about distributing goods or more specifically determining "the best way to allocate the surplus for individual or collective consumption rather than the more central question of the best way to control the process to realize social needs and the full potentialities of human beings" (Smith and Judd 1984, quoted in ibid.). In this context, the citizen is positioned passively as consumer of state services, and the government is positioned as the arbiter of the competing interests in which it is situated. Both of these conceptions serve to perpetuate pluralist notions of government in which government is demarcated from the public, and policy decision making is done in private by "experts" who impartially mediate in a competitive context of interest groups. Iris Marion Young (ibid., 75) argues that distributive notions of justice are predicated on an individualist conception of human nature that serves an ideological function and specifically that "operating within the confines of distributive issues, interest group pluralism ... perpetuates a depoliticized public life that fragments social life and privatizes citizens' relationship to the state. It discourages public deliberation about collective decisions, especially about the goals of government, or the organization of institutions and relations of power. The depoliticized process of policy formation in welfare capitalist society thus makes it difficult to see the institutional rules, practices, and social relations that support domination and oppression, much less to challenge them."

Working toward redressing social and health inequities, and toward social justice, thus requires social change. Health inequities cannot be resolved without addressing the structural conditions that produce the inequities in the first place (Farmer et al. 2006). Weber (2006, 22) has argued that "if we hope to significantly change the landscape that constitutes health science and policy on health disparities, merely identifying the contributions to be made by intersectional and related scholarship is not enough. To produce a deeper understanding of the ways that differentials of power perpetuate health disparities and to effect change in the practice of science and policy, these approaches also must be in a position to engage in critical exchange with dominant paradigms on a more equal footing." Intersectional health researchers thus need to engage critically with biomedicine and distributive understandings of equity and justice, and they must seek to understand and work toward transforming hierarchical and depoliticized policy-making processes that dominate to produce and sustain inequities.

The Health Policy Ethics Study

As researchers using intersectional approaches to study inequity in the areas of violence against women, rural Aboriginal women's health and health care experiences, mental health care for youth, health care for people marginalized by poverty and homelessness, and "voice" in health care and policy for children and youth, we were concerned about the limited uptake of our work in policy. We joined with policy makers also concerned with social justice and interested in ethics to examine how the explicit use of an ethical lens, enlisting concepts such as equity and social justice, might better inform the policy-making process.

We posed the following questions:

- How can policy makers, researchers, and those most affected by policy work together to enhance equity?
- How is equity currently addressed in policy? What equity lenses are currently in use?
- What concepts of equity are used to inform these lenses? What concepts of social justice are embedded within these equity lenses?
- How can evidence be used in policy making to enhance equity? How is evidence currently used in policy? What values underpin the use of evidence? How should evidence be used?

In recognition that the relationship between evidence and policy is messy, complex, ambiguous (Greenhalgh and Russell 2005), and not well understood (Burton 2006), we oriented our research toward learning about how the use of an ethics lens and evidence about health inequities might better inform policy. Research evidence is far from the primary consideration that policy makers must take into account. Policy making is a highly political, complex endeavour, where evidence is weighed within the context of multiple competing demands (Muir Gray 2004), and where values related to equity may or may not have significant influence. Caitlin Hughes (2007) argues that the relationship between evidence and policy may take many forms: policy decisions may be made in the absence of evidence, evidence may be one of many factors taken into account, or evidence may be selectively recruited to support preferred policy directions.

Despite repeated and extensive acknowledgment of the non-linear relationship between evidence and policy, we have little empirical study regarding how evidence is specifically used by policy makers or how values inform policy work (Jewell and Bero 2008). Social policy research has tended to focus on analyzing public policies themselves, to the neglect of analyzing governance systems in which policy processes are embedded (Clarke and Newman 1997), therefore underestimating how features of political processes affect the incorporation of the best evidence into decision making (Jewell and Bero 2008). Extant empirical work in the United Kingdom and the United States emphasizes the influence of context (Bullock, Mountford, and Stanley 2001), especially the structural and values context of policy making (Jewell and Bero 2008). The importance of the political, structural, and values context became increasingly clear as our team, comprising researchers and provincial policy makers, began working together. Repeatedly, the policy makers on the team pointed out that the researchers were not taking into account the complexities of context and policy processes in our quest to understand how evidence and values operated. Thus, we elected to use ethical inquiry within a qualitative participatory methodology to explore the perspectives of health and social service policy makers in the government of one Western Canadian province, by focusing on policy processes, values, and evidence.

Ethical inquiry entails the identification of values and value tensions, clarifying concepts and analyzing arguments, questioning what is valued, determining how different values complement or contradict one another, and elucidating the tensions between different values, and between espoused and enacted values (Monmeyer 1990). As taken up by Nuala Kenny and Mita Giocomini (2005), ethical analysis has particular relevance to intersectional scholarship – oriented to analyzing power differences between groups and a relational conception of justice – in that it attends to analyzing both the substance of policies and underlying structures. According to Kenny and Giocomini (ibid.), ethical inquiry can address *substantive* and *procedural* policy concerns using descriptive, normative, and theoretical analytic approaches.

Substantive ethical dimensions focus on the criteria, reasons, or rationale informing policy; procedural dimensions highlight how policies come to be, including the structural and governance systems in which policy processes are embedded. Descriptive ethics is concerned with "what is," whereas normative ethics is concerned with "what ought to be" (ibid.). Theoretical ethics focuses on the various philosophical perspectives that provide a rationale or justification for decisions or actions. We interviewed policy makers in order to examine their perspectives regarding what rationales, processes, values, and philosophies currently underlie and should underlie policy.

After obtaining ethical approval from the universities with which the academic researchers were affiliated, we interviewed eleven people identified by the policy makers as government "thought leaders" who might have an interest in equity. Through these discussions, we recruited and interviewed twenty-four policy makers in both group and individual interviews. Those interviewed were from different ministries in health and social service areas, and represented different levels of government, including assistant deputy ministers, departmental directors, and consultants. Importantly, all people interviewed worked within the bureaucratic levels of government – they were neither politicians nor lobbyists. The interviews were taped and transcribed. Using qualitative analytic techniques, the core research team reviewed all the transcripts in their entirety, coded the transcripts individually, and compared their analyses within and across transcripts. Each member of the core research team initially coded a few transcripts, and together we developed the initial coding scheme. All data were coded using this scheme, each code was examined in more depth, and an overall analysis was developed. Preliminary analyses were shared with the larger research team and refined.

Findings

Using an ethics lens to explore policy making highlighted the complex political nature of policy processes, provided insights regarding the role of values and evidence in policy making, and illustrated how various understandings of social justice and equity operate in the formal policy-making context. The analysis underscored the importance of understanding the multiple systemic and structural factors that shape complex policy issues and influence policy-making processes. In keeping with literature arguing that the relationship between evidence and policy must be understood as non-linear, the analysis suggested a range of important input points at which evidence might be used.

Conceptions of Equity and Social Justice in Policy Processes

All research participants espoused equity as a value (at least in part because it was the focus of our research), but there were differences in how equity was understood, ranging from strictly distributive understandings to concern with access to the social determinants of health and to an appreciation of the nature and cycle of oppression. Participants' understandings were shaped by multiple influences, particularly the dominance of economic values and biomedicine. For many, equity was primarily focused on access to health care rather than on equitable health outcomes. For others, access to health care was understood as an issue of *equality* – that is, having equal and available services in all communities. Frequently, equity and equality were conflated with differences grounded in different perspectives regarding what is just and fair. Such differences are illustrated in the following quotation, which highlights how a dominant focus on access to biomedical services prevails in discussions of equity and equality:

> One of our key pillars is that we have sustainable, timely, and appropriate access to medical services for ... citizens ..., but nowhere in our strategy or statement does it say "and it will be equitable," because we realize across the province it's not an equitable system ... In [urban centres] you're probably going to have access to different diagnostic testing, higher levels of doctor-to-patient ratios, different specialists that are within an hour's drive of your home, whereas if you live in the north or in a more rural area we understand that there are going to be inequities. So what we're looking at trying to do is identify what the barriers are and trying to get the barriers to access to services as low as possible.

Although this example highlights geography as a determinant of access to health care, other participants emphasized income, age, or disease status as potential barriers to service. One example offered related to HIV and the fact that the primary focus in policy is on people who use injection drugs, thus ignoring barriers to health care access (such as stereotyping and racism) for other relevant groups such as Aboriginal women. Conceptions of fairness in access that emphasize equality are rooted in distributive notions of social justice, which focus on ensuring equal access to health care, not on redressing unjust conditions that shape access. Understanding equity as equal access for all groups is premised on the assumption that all groups are the same and deserve to be treated equally; it does not consider the socio-historical contexts and decision-making structures that shape allocation of resources (including those beyond health care) across various groups of people. This predominant focus on equality of access is congruent with the bureaucratic structures and proceduralism that evolved in the twentieth century in order to foster equality of access in welfare capitalist systems (Young 1990). Within this context, underpinned by a functionalist and pluralistic perspective of the state, "interest-group politics" prevail, which "effectively locks individual citizens out of direct participation in public decision-making and also keeps them ignorant of the proposals deliberated and decisions made." Further, "citizens cannot voice their demands or participate in policy discussions except as constituencies organized around some specific government program or interest" (ibid., 73). For health care leaders who are interested in equality and who work at regional and local levels, this perspective also serves to focus on adding resources such as transportation and child care costs to address the unequal material circumstances that pose barriers to access for some groups. This focus of intervention has been identified as a more distal intervention, and Paul Farmer et al. (2006) argue for the importance of both distal and proximal interventions in order to address the structural roots of health outcomes.

In contrast to this distributive perspective of equality/equity (and social justice), other participants' reflections hinted toward equity from a relational social justice perspective. Some viewed equity as removing barriers such as racism that might act as a deterrent to accessing services. In the following example, the focus is on barriers that, if removed, might increase access for Aboriginal people to all treatment services: "For example, for ... adult residential addictions treatment ... we're taking a look at in terms of access ... That was one place where we looked at ... what capacity is there in our system to accept people who are Aboriginal aside from, you know, the residential treatment centres that are Aboriginal [specific]."

Some participants with population or public health backgrounds understood equity from both a distributive perspective and a population health perspective with a focus on health outcomes. For some, this meant improving or achieving overall population health by reducing disease through improving the health of certain groups, such as those with disabilities, the elderly, or those with mental illnesses. For example, one participant argued, "Coming from the world of population and public health, what we're looking at is what determines people's health when they get to the system, and certainly reducing inequities is a big part of what we're doing. There's lots of mechanisms ... to improve people's income and education and the social conditions in the community, to reduce disparities, and that's basically what we're talking about because we know the people in the north have poorer health outcomes than in the south, and Aboriginals are worse, and lower-income families have worse outcomes, so that's definitely a way of reducing inequities."

Others expressed an understanding of equity that extended beyond achieving similar health outcomes for groups to include concern for structural factors that create and sustain health differences. One participant debated the criteria on which equity might be judged:

What equity are we talking about? So just equity of disease outcomes? Or health outcomes? Or some countries have happiness indexes. Is that the equity that we're looking for? Or should we look at something that is more Western, which is Maslow's Hierarchy of Needs and say the equity we really want is for everyone to have their optimal chance of self-actualization given the determinants of health, the biological issues, the genetic issues, all that stuff but ... If you put money into this level, say, food, shelter, clothing, a lot of that involves education, right, education, getting jobs, etc., otherwise you can't put a roof over your head. So what proportion of money should we distribute to education versus health, versus other things, to actually allow those people to have an equitable chance of self-actualizing? Like, is that what we really want as opposed to, you know, we want to increase your life expectancy?

This understanding, which is more consistent with those that highlight equity as a moral concern about potentially remedial systematic differences embedded in social structures (Whitehead and Dahlgren 2006), begins to draw attention to the role that procedural values, including financial decision making, play in addressing equity.

The emphasis on equality and equity of access to health care in policy – rather than on equity in relation to social determinants of health or health outcomes or, more critically, to equity in access to decision-making processes that structure such distributive patterns – was consistent with the importance of the Canada Health Act in Canada. Our analysis suggests that this emphasis was sustained by several interrelated influences: the mandate established by the Canada Health Act for Canadian health care to provide access to hospital, physician, and surgical-dental services (Department of Justice Canada 1985), the ascendancy of biomedicine, and the dominance of economic concerns without analysis of values or with equity considered in a post hoc fashion, in what Stephen Birch and Amiram Gafni (2002, 2004) call "equity after the fact."

The Canada Health Act was not the only factor that shaped participants' understandings of the meaning of equity as "equality of access to services." Ideological and discursive dynamics inherent in the current representative democratic decision-making structure also played a critical role. Some participants argued that notions of equity and social justice, reflective of a left-leaning political ideological perspective, were tacitly avoided in government. One explained that in policy processes, "we generally would shy away from the term 'equity,' although we would use proxies for that." This participant suggested that the Canada Health Act was one such proxy. Another participant reflected that mention of equity in policy-making processes was acceptable in "actual philosophical ideas of what equity is, and what it means. And we speak of it and I hear it often mentioned at meetings and such, but it's, it's not addressed so precisely. It's more about, okay, let's try and get something that is equal, but we don't speak of equity itself." This avoidance of the overt usage of equity and social justice was confirmed by policy makers on the research team who recognized that such terms were too reflective of a left-leaning political perspective and thus best avoided.

These discursive dynamics make sense in the context of the current representative democratic system in which policy making operates. Reflecting on the political decision-making structures, one participant shared the following perspective:

> There's sort of a dissonance between ... what we should be doing, and what I have to do. The other thing is I'm, you know, we're in a democracy here, right, I'm here as a servant to the minister to try and provide [the minister] the best advice of what we should be doing and so, but it's the minister's decision. My job is to actually lay it all out and say, okay, I think we need to go this way, you know, and here's the reason why, here's all the reasons, other options and, you know, to bring that, bring that awareness to the government, right. That's what my role is as a public servant, right, so I mean that's what my job is, my job is not to, to, um, champion justice per se ... I can speak truth to that and say this is where I'm coming from and this is why and this is what should be there, but I'm not the elected official, right, and so I would be sort of in a way running a little mini-tyranny here if I was actually running policy based on what I think and subverting the democratic system, right?

Such reflections attest to the current hierarchical and representative democratic system in which policy making is grounded in a technical approach to rationality and in which values are separated from decision-making processes (Dallmayr 1980; Hartrick Doane and Varcoe 2005; Holmes, Perron, and O'Byrne 2006). In this context, where values are separated from technical decision-making processes, justice and equity are but one of many ways of framing and addressing issues. This stands in contrast to Young's (1990, 9) argument that "when people say a rule or practice or cultural meaning is wrong and should be changed, they are usually making a claim about social justice." In this case, rather than making claims about social justice, public servants as well as citizens are depoliticized because decision-making power and the values and perspectives embodied within that power are seen as being at the political, ministerial level.

Finally, the concept that government plays a key role in mediating and distributing resources generated in broader economic systems was reflected in participants' concern for costs, which seemed in tension with their concern for equity, and shaped how they understood equity. This dominant influence was readily evident in often-used phrases such as "value for money," "biggest bang for the buck," "the economic argument," and "making a business case," as well as in the participants' emphasis on economic-costing as an important form of argumentation or evidence. As one participant explained,

> Government – they can just do three things: it can tax, it can spend, it can regulate. Equity and social justice [are] actually beneficial for the economy. At least certainly in the current climate of the more right wing sort of governments [it is important to have] research on that link. I think one thing that we've been asked more and more for, is a lot around that economic argument ... I think we're starting to need it now, even in the early childhood population ... Before, it was like okay well, it will help their learning ... and now it's like, okay, this is the cost, if you don't do it, this is what's going to happen – so changing the strategy to more of an economic argument than just because it's a good thing to do.

Importantly, many recognized that addressing health equity as disease reduction means that policy issues can be framed within the mandate of health ministries, whereas using a social determinants of health framework (for example, to address poverty) would raise the greater challenge of collaboration across ministries with attention to how financial decisions are made. Despite varied understandings, there was a strong explicit valuing of equity and an interest in dialogue about equity; however, these values and interests must be considered in light of the realities of extant policy processes.

How Policy Processes "Really" Work: Public Outcry, Course Corrections, and Evidence

From the perspective of people engaged in the everyday work of policy, policy making is a complex process of negotiating multiple tensions. Although policy makers saw equity as relevant, and possibly a goal of policy, it was not the primary goal. Rather, they described working continuously to support politicians and to manage "public outcry." Repeatedly, those we interviewed described their roles in monitoring public opinion and emphasized how powerful such opinions were in shaping policy decisions. Although the participants worked on strategic initiatives within their areas of concern (such as particular aspects of health, housing, income assistance), they were aware of wider political and social influences that would create both opportunities and constraints on their work. Thus, "evidence" was seen as useful insofar as it aligned with multiple other factors. For example, one participant explained, "Decision making ultimately rests with folks who kind of are going to look at how many media clippings and at other proxies for public concern line up with the evidence, with the policy advice, with all those ingredients that flow into decision making at the end of the day."

Evidence was valued and sought, but rather than driving policy change, it was seen as a source of direction to which policy makers turned when public outcry drew attention to a particular issue:

> [Public outcry] can also be people who decide to speak out to the media who aren't particularly part of an advocacy group, it can be concerned parents who are meeting with their MLAs, it can be what the *Vancouver Sun* decides to do in terms of a series for a week. I mean I think it's a whole lot of factors pressuring from a whole lot of different angles, but at the end of the day if you ask a decision maker, be that a politician or a really senior bureaucrat, "What is a public priority around this?" people are immediately going to default to this or that or the other because they've been hearing about it constantly, and then the question is, "Well what does the evidence say?"

Thus, the policy-making process was described primarily as one of responding to public outcry in a series of "course corrections." As a result, issues for groups who are less influential in generating public outcry tend to be of lower priority:

> Folks who make decisions about dollars when faced with umpteen things that have been nudged through [the policy priority queue] are going to inevitably lean to the things that there is the greatest public outcry about. Government is very good at focusing its attention on fixing problems, and what we're talking about in terms of equity is trying to use evidence to say ... we need to tackle this range of things in order to prevent problems or, or deal with what is less visible because the inequity ... is inevitably going to rest in populations that to a certain extent aren't as visible or aren't on the public agenda in the same way [as other problems].

Public-outcry-driven and problem-driven policy-making processes lead to policies dealing with single issues as they arise in the public view. The participants described policy processes as primarily a complaint-driven series of course corrections. In the following, focus group participants used methadone programs as an example of this process:

> *Participant A:* [Policy is] complaint-driven, so we end up with a group of physicians in Vancouver, in the Downtown Eastside complaining and eventually complaining to the media about aspects of the methadone program. We end up with other people complaining about physicians and what they may or may not be doing around billing practices, so we end up with this sort of series of complaints.

Participant B: And we engage in, as a result, information gathering in whatever way we can to facilitate building the evidence that we might need
in order to help foster that course correction.

Participant A: But ... the methadone program has now years of complaints
and years of government work-around to deal with this complaint and
that complaint and the other complaint, which ... in case after case have
been very legitimate issues that have been brought forward. But you end
up with the work-around here and the work-around there and let's put
this payment thing because the pharmacists are saying this is such a challenge, let's do this because this and, you know, the health authority and
on and on and on, so we end up with this series of work-arounds without
having that systems overview.

Participants described policy processes from a pluralist perspective, in
which the role of government is to impartially mediate between competing
interests, which are assumed to be equal. According to Young (1990), the
two core principles of equality and proceduralism inherent in such political
systems are oriented to using large bureaucratic organizations to conduct
collective activity in private and impartial ways that are driven by procedural
rules. Bureaucratic structures in liberal democratic systems have been critiqued for the way in which they position citizens as consumers and clients
of government services and in depoliticized spaces (Young 1990). Further,
research participants' comments on the role of public outcry, and how it is
managed in government, are reflective of the emergence of "interest group
politics," which in turn results in a fragmented public life (ibid.). Within
such a fragmented public life, "there is no forum within the public sphere
of discussion and conflict where people can examine the overall patterns
of justice or fairness produced by these processes" (ibid., 73). Indeed, participants in this study contrasted their observations of policy processes as
a series of course corrections with what they called "system overview,"
"whole government," and "broad landscape." They ultimately saw these
approaches, which share decision making both horizontally (across sectors)
and vertically (across publics), as more compatible with the pursuit of equity.
They described such broad approaches as necessary to redress inequities,
but as rarely enacted. Thus, participants had an interest in, but diverse
understandings of, equity and were positioned within systems and processes
that were not oriented toward social justice and the contributions of intersectional research.

Policy and Intersectional Research

In contrasting the course correction approach to policy development with
what they referred to as "full landscape" approaches, the study participants

drew attention to intersecting systems of social inequity and thus implicitly to the compatibility between intersectional research and such an approach. This alternative reflected the preferred ideal and was referred to as a "whole systems," "whole of government," "comprehensive and equitable," and "integrated" approach to decision making in which all stakeholders and issues (such as funding, relationships, locations of services, rural/urban contexts) were considered important in decision-making processes. This approach was identified as more deliberative, integrated, intersectoral, and preventative: "Let's look at the whole big picture and then see the systemic interrelationship between all of those various decisions we've made all through the years: what that turns up in terms of the overall program rather than yet again responding to – and we're going to have to respond to – what's on the television."

Within this whole landscape approach, the quest for choosing strategic directions for the greatest impact was less oriented to economic factors and more concerned with systemic ones: "How do you consider the range of issues that intersect and choose those strategic areas for action three or four or five or six that are going to have the biggest sort of nudging system impact beyond what you're doing ... What are the things we can try and tackle that are going to create the most change on a systems level?"

Further, participants emphasized the importance of drawing attention to the intersections among health issues:

> In the case of hepatitis C we actually had a [political leader] ... who was quite prepared to stand up and talk at great length in public in front of hundreds and hundreds of people living in downtown hotels in Vancouver about the sentinel nature of hepatitis C, how it was drawing attention to a range of other linked and related kinds of [problems] ... if you think of it as something that needs attention for its own sake but also something that needs attention because it's drawing your attention to groups who are vulnerable to all sorts of other health things.

Drawing attention to the intersections of multiple problems is ideally compatible with research using intersectional approaches. Inequities related to structural conditions such as poverty, racism, place, gender, ableism, and political voice are invariably intertwined with one another and manifest themselves in myriad health and social problems. Not only did interviewees advise exploiting intersections to draw attention to inequities, they noted that researchers could help policy makers identify where they might get "the biggest bang for the buck," through policies that would have broad and multiple effects. More specifically, throughout the interviews the policy makers identified types of research that were lacking: research at the policy/

practice interface, research at a systems level, research on models for shared governance and accountability, and research regarding programs and services, particularly those to address inequities.

Discussion and Implications

Understanding policy processes as complex negotiations of multiple tensions in order to manage public outcry suggests that, rather than focusing primarily on getting evidence "in front" of policy makers, researchers may more effectively influence policy when they seek multiple entry points for evidence into the policy-making process. These findings suggest that researchers need to expand the range of processes through which evidence is brought to bear on policy. Participants pointed to the broad and pervasive influence of public opinion in ways that suggest the need for strategies to influence public opinion that extend beyond involvement with public media. For example, almost all interviewees identified particular researchers or research units with whom they had relationships. Thus, they were able to turn to known sources when evidence was required and access, not single studies, but a more complex wealth of information, a necessity identified by others considering the evidence-policy relationship (see, for example, Waddell et al. 2005). Thus, early involvement of multiple stakeholders, including citizens, those most affected by policies, advocacy groups, and policy makers, will allow researchers to identify and use numerous points of influence – creating public outcry through multiple stakeholders and offering evidence produced through intersectional analyses at each turn.

Rather than seeing policy makers as ideologically opposed to equity and social justice, researchers might consider the diverse values held by those doing policy work, their social locations as policy makers, and the particular policies and policy contexts within which they work. Our findings echo Alex Stevens's (2007) contention that although evidence is used selectively to further the interests of powerful social groups, this reflects wider social organization rather than the deliberate connivance of policy makers. Researchers would benefit from recognizing that policy makers' values and the values framing policy are underpinned by various conceptions of justice and shaped by particular governance (decision-making) systems. Making values explicit and understanding how various conceptions of justice are operating in public and policy discourse are key to critically analyzing and reframing policy. Given the espoused social justice orientation of intersectional research, it is imperative that researchers make explicit the particular conception of justice being employed in intersectional research. We argue that those doing intersectional research should draw on conceptualizations of social justice founded on addressing both material (distributive) and non-material (social) questions of justice rather than presupposing dichotomies or problematizing the efforts of policy makers aimed at distributive issues. Nancy Fraser (2007) describes a three-dimensional theory of justice that brings together the political dimension of who is represented in making policy, the economic dimension of distribution, and the cultural dimension of who is recognized or counts in policy. She argues that neither dimension alone can provide an adequate understanding of what is needed for justice in a capitalist society. Thus, intersectional researchers seeking to redress structural injustices that produce inequities can play an important role in drawing attention to and reframing questions of justice in ways that account not only for concerns about distribution but also for *processes* that inform distribution, including representation in policy making, recognition of who suffers injustices, and the sources of and dynamics that sustain injustice. This can be achieved through focusing attention on different sources of evidence that highlight intersecting injustices, research related to policy making, and research processes that foster participatory democracy.

Further, researchers might identify where value for social justice is held and align with those people/opportunities. For any research working with intersectional approaches, early analysis of the diverse values operating in public discourse and policy will permit researchers to take those values into account and to explicitly use attention to values as way of encouraging uptake of evidence. Given the dominance of economic values, researchers should not ignore or avoid economic arguments: instead, they should attend to economics while drawing attention to values such as equity. Researchers can build on policy and public concern for economics and efficiency but with clear social goals (equity goals) in mind.

In concert with current literature on knowledge translation (Lavis 2006), our analysis suggests that researchers doing intersectional work should foster relationships with policy makers and those most affected by targeted policies over time, engage both policy makers and the publics in identifying policy questions relevant to their research from the inception of research, design research to address policy problems and provide evidence regarding the impact of structural changes, design research that seeks to evaluate structural reforms that serve to increase public voice in core political decision-making processes, and seek multiple ways to use evidence to inform public opinion, including, but not limited to alignment with advocacy and interest groups, shaping research agendas and funding, and media engagement. Each of these strategies would contribute to fostering alignment of interests in the current system and serve to orient researchers, publics, and policy makers toward reforming current representative-democratic systems toward social justice and equity. Or as one of our participants aptly noted, "[When] the evidence is really intelligent that comes from community meetings and newspaper articles and letters to the minister and letters to MLAs, and a whole mass of intelligence comes forward in a very pointed way to government ... when it's clear like that, government can turn around and say, okay ... pay attention to this."

References
Beauchamp, T., and J. Childress. 2001. *Principles of biomedical ethics*. 5th ed. New York: Oxford University Press.
Birch, S., and A. Gafni. 2002. On being NICE in the UK: Guidelines for technology appraisal for the NHS in England and Wales. *Health Economics* 11(3): 185-91.
–. 2004. The "NICE" approach to technology assessment: An economics perspective. *Health Care Management Science* 7(1): 35-41.
Bullock, H., J. Mountford, and R. Stanley. 2001. *Better policy making*. London: Cabinet Office, Centre for Management and Policy Studies.
Burton, P. 2006. Modernising the policy process. *Policy Studies* 27(3): 173-95.
Clarke, J., and J. Newman. 1997. *The managerial state*. London: Sage.
Collins, P.H. 2000. *Black feminist thought: Knowledge, consciousness, and the politics of empowerment*. 2nd ed. New York: Routledge.
Dallmayr, F.R. 1980. Critical theory and public policy. *Policy Studies* 9(4): 522-34.
Department of Justice Canada. 1985. *Canada health act*.
Farmer, P.E., B. Nizeye, S. Stulac, and S. Keshavjee. 2006. Structural violence and clinical medicine. *PLoS Medicine* 10(3): 1686-91.
Fraser, N. 2007. Re-framing justice in a globalizing world. In *(Mis)recognition, social inequality and social justice: Nancy Fraser and Pierre Bourdieu*, ed. T. Lovell, 17-35. New York: Routledge.
Greenhalgh, T., and J. Russell. 2005. Reframing evidence synthesis as rhetorical action in the policy making drama. *Health Care Policy* 1(1): 31-39.
Hartrick Doane, G., and C. Varcoe. 2005. *Family nursing as relational inquiry: Developing health-promoting practice*. Philadelphia: Lippincott Williams and Wilkins.
Holmes, D., A. Perron, and P. O'Byrne. 2006. Evidence, virulence, and the disappearance of nursing knowledge: A critique of the evidence-based dogma. *Worldviews on Evidenced-Based Nursing* 3(3): 95-102.
Hughes, C.E. 2007. Evidence-based policy or policy-based evidence? The role of evidence in the development and implementation of the Illicit Drug Diversion Initiative. *Drug and Alcohol Review* 26(4): 363-68.
Jewell, C.J., and L.A. Bero. 2008. Developing good taste in evidence: Facilitators of and hindrances to evidence-informed health policy making in state government. *Millbank Quarterly* 86(2): 177-208.
Kenny, N., and M. Giocomini. 2005. Wanted: A new ethics field for health policy analysis. *Health Care Analysis* 13(4): 247-60.
Knuttila, M. 2007. The state and social issues: Theoretical considerations. In *Power and resistance: Critical thinking about Canadian social issues*, ed. L. Samuelson and W. Antony, 16-49. Halifax: Fernwood.
Lavis, J.N. 2006. Research, public policymaking, and knowledge-translation processes: Canadian efforts to build bridges. *Journal of Continuing Education in the Health Professions* 26(1): 37-45.
Monmeyer, R.W. 1990. Philosophers and the public policy process: Inside, outside, or nowhere at all? *Journal of Medicine and Philosophy* 15: 391-409.
Muir Gray, J.A. 2004. Evidence based policy making. *British Medical Journal* 329(7473): 988-89.
Stevens, A. 2007. Survival of the ideas that fit: An evolutionary analogy for the use of evidence in policy. *Social Policy and Society* 6(1): 25-35.
Waddell, C., J.N. Lavis, J. Abelson, J. Lomas, C.A. Shepherd, T. Bird-Gayson, M. Giocomini, and D.R. Offord. 2005. Research use in children's mental health policy in Canada: Maintaining vigilance amid ambiguity. *Social Science and Medicine* 61(8): 1649-57.

Weber, L. 2006. Reconstructing the landscape of health disparities research: Promoting dialogue and collaboration between feminist intersectional and biomedical paradigms. In *Gender, race, class and health: Intersectional approaches,* ed. A. Schulz and L. Mullings, 21-59. San Francisco: Jossey-Bass.

Whitehead, M., and G. Dahlgren. 2006. *Levelling up (part 1): A discussion paper on concepts and principles for tackling social inequities in health.* WHO Collaborating Centre for Policy Research on Social Determinants of Health, University of Liverpool. Copenhagen: WHO Regional Office for Europe.

Young, I.M. 1990. *Justice and the politics of difference.* Princeton: Princeton University Press.

18

Intersectional Feminist Frameworks in Practice: CRIAW's Journey toward Intersectional Feminist Frameworks, Implications for Equity in Health

Jo-Anne Lee

Intersectionality, Governance, and CRIAW

The Canadian Research Institute for the Advancement of Women (CRIAW), one of Canada's oldest national feminist organizations, was begun by feminist academics in the 1970s to meet the publishing needs of mainly white academic women and bring feminist knowledge to a wider audience. This chapter examines CRIAW's tumultuous shift away from a gender-based analysis (GBA) approach toward intersectional feminist frameworks (IFFs) as an approach for analyzing social relations and social categories (Hankivsky 2005). I interrogate intersectionality as a material process and practice, not solely as a promising theoretical framework and category for analysis. I see intersectionality as an emergent practice that is constitutive of, and constituted by, social relations and identities. Exposing tensions within CRIAW as it moved toward an intersectional approach in its work may reveal some of the difficulties that organizations, especially women-centred community health organizations funded by state agencies, might confront in attempting to adopt IFFs in research and practice (Harding 2005).

This chapter also argues that viewing intersectionality as a form of material everyday practice linked to power will help alert anti-racist feminist practitioners to the possibility that structural power at the heart of organizations may stall the adoption of intersectional approaches. When organizations shift from a gender-only focus to an intersecting or interlocking view of social inequality, such a move will invariably expose structures and operations of privilege that previously went undetected. This exposure is likely to trigger a painful backlash within the organization.

Few empirical studies have examined intersectionality as a form of practice linked to governance (MacDonald, Osborne, and Smith 2005). However, women scholars of colour have long documented their battle for inclusion in Canadian national and regional women's organizations under other rubrics (see Fitzgerald, Guberman, and Wolf 1982; Carty 1993). Much feminist research on governance has focused on women's relationship to the formal state (Vickers, Rankin, and Appelle 1993). As yet, feminist scholars have paid little scholarly and critical attention to governing structures, laws, policies, regulations, procedures, and discourses operating within non-profit NGOs. Although feminist activists of colour have written about their exclusion from decision-making positions within national women's organizations and within the women's movement more broadly, little attention has been given to the relationship between excluded "others" and organizational governance within community-based women's associations. My use of the word "governance" refers not only to the politics of representation but also to the policies, procedures, and regulations that govern the selection, election, roles, and responsibilities of women elected to boards of non-profit groups. These factors influence the appearance of bodies that occupy these seats. I want to draw attention to those invisible policies and procedures that are written in legal documents but that seem to receive attention only when the organization holds its annual general meetings and election of officers. At those moments, regulatory power is most uncovered. This exposure often surprises and dismays "othered outsiders" who wish to bring about change.

The internal representational structures and practices of non-profit community-based feminist organizations are ideal for investigating intersectionality, since criteria or eligibility for representation explicitly and implicitly select for particular social identities in preference to others. Such an analysis pays attention to the changing contexts in which particular social identities gain meaning. Usually, social identities of individuals involved in governance are taken for granted or assumed to be male. Researchers tend to portray such actors as neutral subjects occupying roles emptied of socially ascribed identities. Furthermore, organizational routines, procedures, policies, and discourses are often not subjected to critical analysis, intersectional or otherwise; they are merely assumed as the backdrop to action. Some feminist scholars have analyzed the gendering of organizational structures, but intersectional lenses have not yet been applied to the same degree.

I would like to make several caveats before proceeding. First, I draw mainly on personal observations and experiences; I do not claim to speak on behalf of CRIAW. Because I am an insider, my views are necessarily partial and incomplete. Second, I write from a situated standpoint as a racialized minority feminist activist scholar from the western edge of Canadian national geopolitical space. I am aware that these positions accent my perspectives and my relations with others, and cannot be separated and bracketed out in this narrative.

The Context for CRIAW's Shift to Intersectionality

In the past decade, CRIAW has moved from a mainly white, middle-class, professional academic organization that offered a publishing venue to university-based researchers to an organization that translates and brings policy-relevant research to community-based social justice organizations working for change and, more recently, to one that partners with grassroots community-based organizations in undertaking research. CRIAW's mission remains broadly within the field of knowledge production, translation, and communication (www.criaw-icref.ca). Recently, the organization has been engaged in a process of reconsidering mainstream approaches to questions of social and economic justice, particularly the ways that feminist lenses are applied to government policies (Morris and Bunjun 2007). Previously, CRIAW had championed the adoption of gender-based analysis (GBA) of government policies and programs (Hankivsky 2005). Stemming from the second-wave women's movement in Canada and implemented by the state, GBA has helped to push the Canadian government and many women's and social justice organizations to address the differential impact of policies and programs on women and men. Although GBA brought greater awareness of women's inequality relative to men, a gender-only lens failed to account for the complexity of diverse women's lives (Collins 1990). As many writers have observed, prioritizing one identity entry point (such as gender) or one relation of power (such as patriarchy) to the exclusion of others (race, class) misrepresents the full diversity of women's lived realities.

When I first joined CRIAW in 2000, I entered into an organization at war with itself. Tensions were flying over whether English should continue to dominate CRIAW. Because CRIAW is a national organization headquartered in Ottawa, its political agenda and structure were shaped by its proximity to the federal government bureaucracy and to Quebec-Canada constitutional politics. Any claims to represent women as a "national" women's organization were quickly challenged by French-speaking academics from Quebec. National debates over Quebec's struggle for recognition and self-determination that challenged Anglo-national hegemony also filtered into and delimited the kinds of issues that were included in CRIAW's agenda (Rankin and Vickers 2001). Anglo-Franco language tensions dominated in the 1970s and 1980s, and they continued to haunt CRIAW. Today, they take other forms, but they are still discussed within a historic context of French-speaking women (of colour, now) feeling excluded and marginalized in a national feminist research organization. Other authors have described internal conflicts within CRIAW as class tensions between grassroots activists and academic feminists (Christiansen-Ruffman 1991).

When women of colour, indigenous, and disabled women began to ask ourselves why the work of articulating IFF and applying it within CRIAW did not feel empowering – why we always felt as if we were at war – we began to identify and name CRIAW's governance structure as a systemic and invisible barrier that operated silently to privilege the voices of Anglo women from particular regions. Despite our stated intent, year after year, the faces on the board, those sitting at the table, were predominantly white, English speaking, middle class, and of a particular age – second-wave activists who had broken the ground on gender discrimination. Although each year a minority of board members, such as myself, came from marginalized backgrounds, we were never present in sufficient numbers to make much difference.

Although many mainstream board members also saw the need for IFF at an intellectual level, they did not apply this understanding to CRIAW's representational and governance structures. For many, this would have meant giving up their seat at the table. I saw many women fighting tooth and nail to maintain their position of power. Attempts to include Aboriginal women, francophone women, women of colour, disabled women, and others often ended in tears and rancour. Betrayal and mistrust were always just under the surface, erupting at the least expected times. As risk- and conflict-averse as many women are, the easiest thing to do was to wait out terms of appointment while moving on another flank: constitutional reform. As a strategy of change, the executive of the board, of which I was a member, decided to hire external planning consultants, with the support of Status of Women funding, so that staff and board volunteers could participate in civil dialogue. These were painful conversations that were very difficult and tense, even with outside assistance.

Naming the white, middle-class, and able-bodied leadership of the feminist movement in Canada is nothing new; many minority feminist activists have written about their exclusion from mainstream women's organizations for at least four decades (see Lachapelle 1982; Ng 1982; Thornhill 1985). If mainstream feminist organizations have resisted more inclusive practices for so long, what hope is there for mainstream public health policy organizations – male dominated and chronically resistant to gender mainstreaming – to embrace an even more complex and inclusive intersectional feminist perspective (Hankivsky 2005)? I ask this question less out of irony than from a sense of pragmatic urgency. The rush among theorists to embrace intersectionality and its academic success as a concept may amount to very little if it cannot be implemented in practice due to hegemonic resistance to sharing power. A first step is to name practices of power (Fellows and Razack 1998).

Confronting CRIAW's Governance Structure

CRIAW's shift toward intersectional approaches began in 1992 when it held a feminism and anti-racism conference that started to address some intersecting issues, including connections between sexism and other equally oppressive barriers to social and economic equity. One of the first of its kind in Canada, the conference brought together over a thousand participants.

CRIAW conducted a study documenting how national women's organizations were making strides to become more inclusive and diverse. But the organization itself had not examined its own governing structures of exclusion and inclusion. Twelve years later, in 2004, CRIAW adopted a new board structure requiring representation from diverse regions and social groups. This small change opened up the possibility that CRIAW could recruit board members based on a matrix of categories: these included regional representation (BC, the Prairies, Ontario, Quebec, Atlantic, and territories), representation from four equity groups (Aboriginal women, racialized women, women with disabilities, and lesbian, bisexual, or transgendered women), language, skills, issue focus, community- and university-based researchers, and expressed level of commitment. In addition, the board's nominating committee looked for members with the following skills:

- knowledge of women's economic security and social justice issues
- experience with poverty issues
- experience in working within intersectional feminist frameworks
- connections to key communities
- policy development expertise
- fundraising expertise
- front-line hands-on skills.

Without making these constitutional and programmatic changes, CRIAW could not have fully implemented intersectional analytical approaches in every aspect of its work, a goal that was identified as central to its strategic plan.

Like other national non-profit organizations, CRIAW operates under a set of bylaws that follow the requirements set down by the Canada Corporations Act (Industry Canada 2004). Provincial non-profit organizations must comply with acts governing non-profit incorporation in their jurisdictions. The laws governing the rules by which non-profit societies operate reinforce a hierarchical electoral system of governance and accountability that replicates principles of Western capitalist and masculinist top-down colonial administrative bureaucracy. The primary purpose of these bylaws is to ensure financial accountability. One aspect of CRIAW's governance that had a profound determining effect on its operations was the election of officers, as specified in the bylaws. The original founders of CRIAW adopted a system of representation that mirrored provincial representation to the federal government. In this system, the Atlantic region enjoyed a representation that, due to historical happenstance, was out of proportion to its size. Because of its proximity to Europe, it had been colonized and settled before the rest of Canada, a process that produced four small provinces, each of which had parliamentary representation. CRIAW's adoption of this system meant that most board members came from the Atlantic provinces. The fact that every province could elect one or more board representatives depending on population did not alter this situation. These representational practices gave Atlantic region board members a greater influence in setting policy directions than those from other regions. Issues that were not seen as relevant to Atlantic women or were not of interest to Atlantic board members were often unintentionally excluded from CRIAW's agenda for action. This system of representation and decision making remained in place for over thirty years and constrained CRIAW's desires to move toward incorporating intersectionality in its work.

Rational arguments about the complexity of women's lives had not been sufficient to convince several board members and staff to change CRIAW's constitution to include specific criteria for board selection, such as social identities of race, class, and sexuality, among others, and to recognize the limitations that geopolitical criteria alone placed on achieving CRIAW's stated desire for change. External forces were also significant in pushing change, in particular state policies and officials. Status of Women Canada, CRIAW's major funder, demanded that CRIAW demonstrate greater productivity and relevancy, and it threatened significant funding cuts if this could not be demonstrated. At the same time, neo-liberal state policies of downsizing, cutbacks, and privatization were having devastating effects on grassroots women's organizations. Consequently, community-based women's groups were increasingly vocal in demanding accountability from the large national women's groups (called the Big 8) including CRIAW, who were perceived as consuming a disproportionate share of Status of Women's program funding – money that community-based groups, especially women's centres and advocacy organizations, needed because they were no longer receiving funding for advocacy and training. CRIAW was forced to evaluate its programs and priorities. When it was created in the 1970s, few publishing outlets existed for academic feminists, and CRIAW helped fill the gap. Now it was clear that its publications program no longer played the role it once did for academic feminists. Few academics were publishing with CRIAW, because they now had access to higher-valued publishing outlets, such as refereed journals, within their disciplines.

If CRIAW were to remain viable, the board had little choice but to adopt a more relevant issue-focused agenda. It began shifting CRIAW's work away from a general publishing program. It engaged in a strategic planning exercise that identified as its priority and mission economic and social justice through fighting poverty and social exclusion, using an intersectional feminist framework.

During this time of transformation, changing power alliances continually threatened to derail movement. Two presidents failed to fulfill their mandates (for different reasons: one withdrew for health and work reasons, and the other simply was not available to attend meetings). Both were white lesbians who saw the shift in focus from a gender-based framework and a publishing program as a move from issues that had been previously centred. As new voices, new issues, and new directions were identified, individuals invested in the older gender-based inequality (sexuality and language diversity) model simultaneously withdrew commitment to the organization. The withdrawal came from many sources. Some white women voiced resentment at being asked to make room for minority women, some elite women of colour mirrored white elite behaviour, and some marginalized women who had other leadership opportunities refused to accept tokenistic positions. Thus, stable leadership was being withdrawn from CRIAW at the very moment that it was most needed. CRIAW's internal political struggles followed a pattern that was unfolding in other feminist organizations (Carty 1993; Findlay 1993; Gottlieb 1993; Agnew 1996; Rebick and Roach 1996; Srivastava 2005; Khan 2008). Sunera Thobani (Khan 2008, 19), a former president of the National Action Committee on the Status of Women (NAC), describes similar dynamics within the NAC: "Once women of colour emerged in the leadership, many White women left the organization and then blamed the women of colour for the decline in NAC's stature. I think that's leading to another important moment of transformation, and it might be very dangerous for us."

I do not want to suggest that this was the first time that intersecting identity categories influenced CRIAW's operations. Intersecting identity categories beyond gender have always been at work in shaping the context for CRIAW's work. The co-production and co-constitution of identity categories with governing structures and policies is not new (see Clippingdale 1996). What distinguished this moment was the qualitative and substantive difference in the type of categorical intersections involved, as well as the intense resistance to change. Because previous categorical imperatives usually paralleled nationalistic interests, their exclusionary operations had been somewhat masked. In this case, emergent identity categories not linked to dominant interests and power were perceived as irrelevant and disruptive to CRIAW's functioning. White women felt strong in resisting change because they perceived certain identity categories as irrelevant, while simultaneously, and contradictorily, discursively claiming to support the goal of inclusivity and intersectionality.

The Contributions of Racialized Women

Racialized minority women were at the forefront of encouraging the board to shift its focus from publishing the work of feminist academics to taking a more activist intersectional feminist approach that served community-based social justice organizations as well as academic women. Marginalized women standing at the intersection of multiple forces of inequality were instrumental in providing the intellectual content of CRIAW's new agenda. Just as in academic writing, where black, Asian, indigenous, queer, and working-class women were leaders in challenging the universalizing voice of white feminist scholarship, working-class women and those of colour provided leadership in challenging white middle-class dominance in feminist organizations (Combahee River Collective 1977; hooks 1981; Lorde 1984; Collins 1990; Green 2007). For some staff and board members, intersectionality was a vague and imprecise concept. For others, it was intuitively known but difficult to express, whereas others saw little need to move past a gender and diversity perspective that offered them a speaking position from which to access femocratic state power. Staff needed to learn this new framework, but they were also pressed to deliver products to justify Status of Women funding. They lacked the time and energy to read the explosion of research on intersectionality and the new scholarship on social exclusion and poverty. I saw staff – always pressed to do the work without having the time to obtain the prerequisite knowledge – desperately playing catch-up to some of the academic board members who were teaching and researching in this area. These constraints placed a burden on a small number of minority women on the board and in staff to generate research themes, do the research, provide contacts from their own networks, and also do the writing and editing. Writing ourselves into texts, which started as a labour of love, became a form of knowledge appropriation and exploitation.

This knowledge divide was also seen as a class and race divide, which caused further tensions. The knowledge lag was driven in part by Status of Women Canada's demands for performance-based outcomes and deliverables within a one-year time frame. CRIAW found itself pushed to produce "deliverables" in the form of written publications, forums, workshops, and consultations. Documents and events became the measures of worth and value, and feminist principles of collaboration, support, consultation, understanding, and growth were sidelined.

The politics of knowledge production within CRIAW were also observed in how CRIAW generated content about feminist intersectionalities. In keeping with feminist principles, CRIAW approached the question of how to implement intersectionality in policy analysis and research through a participatory consultative process. Ideas generated by women from the global "South" influenced some staff and board members who had participated at international forums where the issues and frameworks confronting women in the South were brought forward. CRIAW carried these ideas to Canada. In February 2004, it held a roundtable with Canadian feminist activists and women from the South on integrated feminist analysis. In March 2005, CRIAW took a draft to the Beijing +10 meetings at the United Nations in New York. In collaboration with the Women's International Coalition for

Economic and Social Justice, it held a workshop on moving beyond GBA, which was attended by eighty women activists from around the world. The workshop confirmed widespread support and recognition of the need for more complex intersectional approaches that did not centre solely on gender inequality between men and women. This consultation was followed, in June 2005, by a think-tank conference held in Ottawa involving twenty academic and community-based participants. One main outcome of these consultations was recognition of the need to move from identity-based analytics toward more structural analysis and to include globalization and colonialism as critical to intersectional analysis. The consultations also underscored the necessity to engage in transnational feminist alliances as a political strategy of intervention. Marginalized women attending the workshop criticized the gathering for remaining centred in Western, modernist frames of thought. They gave several examples of non-categorical identities and the need to be true to the principles of intersectionality as an alternative way of naming the complex realities of marginalized women.

Aboriginal women challenged CRIAW to develop a methodology that would not require divided subject positions of researcher/object of research. "What was the point of intersectional feminist frameworks that could not address the real problems indigenous women face in their lives?" they asked. They pointed out that the Indian Act continues to create discriminatory barriers for indigenous women in Canada. State labels such as Métis and Inuit serve to create and exacerbate divisionary identity politics within indigenous communities. One participant described this "research labelling" process as "disabling." Another argued that the "women most impacted by multiple barriers, women who quite commonly occupy 'subject' status for our methodological enquiries, continue to not be meaningfully present as knowledge producers themselves" (author notes; see also CRIAW 2006).

Another critique referenced refugee women who were without categorical national identities. Their inability to claim a provisional category as a point of departure shed another light on a missing dimension of intersectional theory as it had been conceptualized. Intersectionality cannot be only about already constituted or recognized categories of identity. Men and women who lack legal documents, such as citizenship papers, are literally without categorical homes. Identity categories of gender, race, ethnicity, class, and sexuality are salient and meaningful only when a nation-state recognizes one's personhood. Such categories of identity matter differently for refugee women when they are not embodied subjects holding identity and recognition. CRIAW was challenged to respond to how intersectional analysis would help to advance the rights of these women and men. Unfortunately, those critical views have not yet been fully incorporated in CRIAW's research documents.

Following these consultations, CRIAW adopted the term "intersectional feminist frameworks" (IFFs) to reflect the need to conceptualize intersectional feminist analyses as multiple and plural. This perspective now informs much of CRIAW's work in drawing attention to the experiences of marginalized women.

Erasures of Intellectual Contribution as a Site of Struggle

Texts do not write themselves. Given the complexity, diversity, and changing nature of women's lives in shifting and multiple contexts, IFFs demand a collaborative process to generate new knowledge. Although CRIAW engaged in a consultative and collaborative process to develop its approach to intersectionality, I saw knowledge integrated without full recognition of minority women's intellectual contribution through storytelling, critique, and analysis. The failure to textually acknowledge their original and germinative contributions, and their critiques of established ways of knowing, meant that many marginalized women's important contributions were made to disappear. This erasure gives the impression that these novel insights were generated virginally and emerged fully formed in the thoughts of staff or the clear-language contract writer who "authored" the final document. In reality, grassroots-driven collaborative and consultative processes generate new knowledge through a process of dialogue. Quotidian practices – "it's just the way we do things" – unproblematically reproduce knowledge appropriation with little recognition given to the hard work of generating original thought through marginalized women's intellectual leadership. Even to name and utter an analysis that is opposed to what is assumed as "truth" will generate reactions of pain and anger. Minority women board members had to pay protracted attention to the details of knowledge production to ultimately change authorship practices within CRIAW.

Implications for Intersectionality and Equity in Health

To be useful to anti-racist decolonizing feminists in the women's movement who already refuse dominant explanatory frameworks that do not fully describe their realities (though claiming to do so), feminist intersectional health researchers must also locate themselves in relation to practices of knowledge production (Cole 2008; Hankivsky 2005). As yet, feminist scholars of intersectionality have paid little attention to the specific contexts in which the multiply located subjects of privilege and marginality are situated in the field of practice, much less locate themselves. Ange-Marie Hancock (2007) worries that intersectionality as a concept threatens to immobilize political action. To a certain extent, Hancock is accurate: intersectionality can be used discursively to mask resistance to change and sharing power, but when it is viewed as a form of emergent practice, its ultimate contribution will depend largely on the outcomes of struggles in everyday life. Recognizing the doubled and contingent nature of intersectionality as discourse and practice will help activists to comprehend the contradictions inherent in the glacial pace of meaningful change and the seemingly supportive statements of inclusion of marginalized others who live complex lives.

The Canadian women's health movement has made advances in improving the health standing of mainstream women, but it has also, paradoxically, left those most marginalized behind (Morrow, Hankivsky, and Varcoe 2007; Harding 2005). Aboriginal, immigrant, disabled, poor, and elderly women remain disproportionately represented in those groups demonstrating the greatest health disparities (Varcoe, Hankivsky, and Morrow 2007). Canada's diminishing status as a world leader in population health is in part a consequence of its dismal progress in addressing health disparities of the most marginalized (Hankivsky and Christoffersen 2008). Will employing an intersectional feminist approach in research and theory help reverse this downward slide? There is no clear answer, beyond acknowledging mainstream health organizations' myopic and astigmatic view of what constitutes women's health and well-being and how this is to be achieved, and using intersectional feminist lenses in research and policy analysis. Nonetheless, it is imperative to move beyond merely articulating aspirational statements about health equity and inclusion, and searching for promising analytical frameworks. We must also recognize multiple interactions across and among material and discursive practices of knowledge production, organizational governance, and identity formation that work together to produce the conditions that give rise to health disparities among women.

Furthermore, it is still rare to find minority women as authors, researchers, and analysts of their own realities; they are still viewed as objects and victims on which others act and speak (Harding 2005). One illustration drawn from the field of women's health research that speaks to this need to keep pushing conceptual boundaries is the long-standing and persistent racism, sexism, and classism in the nursing profession and in the workplace that generate negative effects on minority women's health as both workers and health consumers. Although this reality has been repeatedly documented as constitutive of health disparities for minority women as health providers and receivers, little meaningful change has occurred (Anderson 2000; Calliste 1996; Das Gupta 1996; Flynn 2005; Bernard 2005). As previously stated, given that minority and indigenous women, as workers and volunteers, are often simultaneously taking the lead in bringing about change and living the consequences of exclusion and marginalization, achieving equality will be slow and challenging work. This is precisely what I have tried to reveal in my discussion of CRIAW's long and arduous journey toward more inclusive intersectional practice in working for social justice and equality. Making meaningful change is long, complicated, and difficult. Complexifying research and theoretical frameworks to include other strands of women's identities is only one small but necessary step.

Conclusion

In writing this chapter, I have located myself as an interlocutor who stands simultaneously inside and outside. This is a well-known strategy of critical feminist ethnography that asks self-reflexive methodological questions, such as "What did I see?" "What happened here?" "Where am I located?" I have used my multiple subject positions as an insider/outsider, simultaneously privileged and oppressed, located in the community and the academy to provide a view of intersectionality in action. My brief excursion into CRIAW's adoption and implementation of IFFs in all aspects of its work reveals the high demands that intersectionality places on its practitioners. If intersectional perspectives are to be meaningfully operationalized in social justice organizations, their governance structures must be transformed to ensure that those marginalized are included at the decision-making table. Failing to do so simply talks the talk but does not walk the walk.

When viewed as a form of practice, IFFs are emergent and contingent, with outcomes that cannot be predicted a priori. As a mode of knowledge production, IFFs remain inescapably intertwined with power. Although widely embraced for bringing greater complexity and accuracy to understanding the diverse conditions that give rise to inequality and differences among and between women and men, boys and girls, and those who identify across genders, as well as the heterogeneity within social categories, intersectional analytical frameworks have not been subjected to much empirical research (McCall 2005). Although epistemological debates may help to clarify what we mean by feminist intersectional approaches at the level of theory, these debates on their own are insufficient to fully understand and address the overall, multiple, and shifting effects of intersecting structures of inequality in hindering feminist goals of equality and justice. If one is working within an established organization that is struggling to understand gender discrimination, whose governance structure does not reflect principles underlying IFFs, whose research staff might not have the necessary training in IFFs, and where the most marginalized women are not at the decision-making table, then not only will IFFs meet considerable resistance and foot dragging, but any conceptual contributions will be moot. By asking how IFFs are actualized, my intention is to continue to interrogate alternative paradigms and to forestall premature closure. If intersectional theories are too readily and uncritically embraced as alternative heuristic tools for conceptualizing, problematizing, and understanding the diversity of and inequality in people's lives, much of the complexity of women's lives will continue to be erased.

References

Agnew, V. 1996. *Resisting discrimination: Women from Asia, Africa, and the Caribbean and the women's movement in Canada.* Toronto: University of Toronto Press.

Anderson, J.M. 2000. Gender, "race," poverty, health and discourses of health reform in the context of globalization: A postcolonial feminist perspective in policy research. *Nursing Inquiry* 7: 220-29.

Bernard, W.T. 2005. Black women's health in Nova Scotia: One woman's story. In Harding 2005, 47-71.

Calliste, A. 1996. Antiracism organizing and resistance in nursing: African Canadian women. *Canadian Review of Sociology and Anthropology* 33(3): 361-90.

Carty, L., ed. 1993. *And still we rise: Feminist political mobilizing in contemporary Canada.* Toronto: Women's Press.

Christiansen-Ruffman, L. 1991. Bridging the gap between activism and academe: The Canadian Research Institute for the Advancement of Women. In *Women and social change: Feminist activism in Canada,* ed. J.D. Wine and J.L. Ristock, 258-82. Toronto: James Lorimer.

Clippingdale, L., ed. 1996. *Memories and visions: Celebrating 20 years of feminist research with CRIAW/ICREF 1976-1996.* Ottawa: Canadian Research Institute for the Advancement of Women.

Cole, E.R. 2008. Coalitions as a model for intersectionality: From practice to theory. *Sex Roles* 59: 443-53.

Collins, P.H. 1990. *Black feminist thought.* Boston: Unwin Hyman.

Combahee River Collective. 1977. A black feminist statement. Reprinted in *The second wave: A reader in feminist theory,* ed. L. Nicholson, 63-70. New York: Routledge, 1983.

CRIAW (Canadian Research Institute for the Advancement of Women). 2006. Intersectional feminist frameworks: An emerging vision. Ottawa: CRIAW/ICREF.

Das Gupta, T. 1996. Racism in nursing. *Studies in Political Economy* 51(Fall): 97-116.

Fellows, M.L., and S. Razack. 1998. The race to innocence: Confronting hierarchical relations among women. *Journal of Gender, Race and Justice* 1(2): 335-52.

Findlay, S. 1993. Problematizing privilege: Another look at the representation of "women" in feminist practice. In Carty 1993, 207-24.

Fitzgerald, M., C. Guberman, and M. Wolf, eds. 1982. *Still ain't satisfied! Canadian feminism today.* Toronto: Women's Press.

Flynn, K. 2005. Nurses in resistance. In Harding 2005, 3-13.

Gottlieb, A., ed. 1993. What about us? Organizing inclusively in the National Action Committee on the Status of Women. In Carty 1993, 371-86.

Green, J., ed. 2007. *Making space for indigenous feminism.* Blackpoint, NS: Fernwood.

Hancock A.-M. 2007. When multiplication doesn't equal quick addition: Examining intersectionality as a research paradigm. *Perspectives on Politics* 5(1): 63-79.

Hankivsky, O. 2005. Gender vs. diversity mainstreaming: A preliminary examination of the role and transformative potential of feminist theory. *Canadian Journal of Political Science/Revue canadienne de science politique* 38(4): 977-1001.

Hankivsky, O., and A. Christoffersen. 2008. Intersectionality and the determinants of health: A Canadian perspective. *Critical Public Health* 18(3): 271-83.

Harding, G.S., ed. 2005. *Surviving in the hour of darkness: The health and wellness of women of colour and indigenous women.* Calgary: University of Calgary Press.

hooks, b. 1981. *Ain't I a woman? Black women and feminism.* Boston: South End Press.

Industry Canada. 2004. Primer for directors of not-for-profit corporations (rights, duties and practices). Industry Canada. http://www.ic.gc.ca.

Khan, S. 2008. The fight for feminism: An interview with Sunera Thobani. *Upping the Anti: A Journal of Theory and Action* 5. http://auto_sol.tao.ca.

Lachapelle, C. 1982. Beyond barriers: Native women and the women's movement. In Fitzgerald, Guberman, and Wolfe 1982, 257-75.

Lorde, A. 1984. *Sister outsider.* Trumansburg, NY: Crossing Press.

MacDonald, G., R.L. Osborne, and C.C. Smith, eds. 2005. *Feminism, law, inclusion: Intersectionality in action.* Toronto: Sumach Press.

McCall, L. 2005. The complexity of intersectionality. *Signs: Journal of Women in Culture and Society* 30(3): 1771-1800.

Morrow, M., O. Hankivsky, and C. Varcoe. 2007. *Women's health in Canada: Critical perspectives on theory and policy.* Toronto: University of Toronto Press.

Ng, W. 1982. Immigrant women: The silent partners of the women's movement. In Fitzgerald, Guberman, and Wolfe 1982, 249-56.

Rankin, L.P., and J. Vickers. 2001. Women's movements and state feminism: Integrating diversity into public policy. Research Directorate, Status of Women Canada. http://dsp-psd.pwgsc.gc.ca/Collection/SW21-80-2001E.pdf.

Rebick, J., and K. Roach. 1996. Beyond inclusion: Transforming NAC. In J. Rebick and K. Roach, *Politically speaking,* 105-22. Vancouver: Douglas and McIntyre.

Srivastava, S. 2005. You're calling me a racist? The moral and emotional regulation of antiracism and feminism. *Signs: Journal of Women in Culture and Society* 31(1): 29-62.

Thornhill, E. 1985. Focus on black women. *Canadian Journal of Women and the Law* 1: 153-62.

Varcoe, C., O. Hankivsky, and M. Morrow. 2007. Introduction: Beyond gender matters. In Morrow, Hankivsky, and Varcoe 2007, 3-32.

Vickers, J., P. Rankin, and C. Appelle. 1993. *Politics as if women mattered: A political analysis of the National Action Committee on the Status of Women.* Toronto: University of Toronto Press.

Afterword

Olena Hankivsky

As a way to progress toward improved understandings of health inequities, the research in this volume addresses current debates and challenges associated with the operationalization of intersectionality. As noted in the Introduction, although intersectionality frameworks are gaining currency across a number of disciplines, they have yet to be fully tested in the field of health. This volume responds to this lacuna by examining the shared but largely uninvestigated conceptual terrain between intersectionality theory and health research, policy, and practice in Canada.

Because one of the key goals of the collection is to link theory to practice in a way that is largely absent in the field of health inequities, it is important to reflect on how the research featured here relates to the "ideal" framework of intersectionality conceptualized by Dhamoon and Hankivsky in Chapter 1. To quickly summarize, this ideal version includes the following prerequisites for an optimum application of intersectionality: laying out the historical foundations, contestability, and specificity of terms; being clear about what kinds of differences are to be analyzed and focusing on analyzing interactive processes of differentiation that produce and govern subjects; attending to the different levels at which power operates and subject formation occurs and the various degrees and forms of penalty and privilege that shape everyone's lives; transcending unidimensional, additive, and hierarchical models of analysis; and ensuring that research and policy are directed by social justice agendas. It is also important to evaluate how the efforts to operationalize intersectionality yield insights that can inform how the theory of intersectionality may be adjusted or reconceived for future discussions of health inequities.

To begin, all contributors identify the challenges of bridging the distance that exists between theory and practice in a way that more closely reflects the origins of intersectionality, while grappling with the real challenges of extending intersectionality theory to a range of health issues and empirical research. A well-known fact is that the complexity and nuance of theory are not always suited to the clarity and expedience required for practical application. Moreover, as was highlighted in the Introduction of this volume, one of the key challenges facing aspiring intersectionality health researchers is how to undertake work that necessitates the translation of theory to empirical research in a field where there are various interpretations and conceptualizations of intersectionality. Elsewhere, L.S. Weldon (2008) has similarly observed that different versions of intersectionality have differing possibilities in terms of research utility. Although the contributors to this volume utilize differing and unique interpretations of intersectionality, and some even refrain from using the actual terminology of intersectionality, collectively all the featured research does draw on, and satisfies, the tenets of the ideal or optimum model proposed by Dhamoon and Hankivsky at the beginning of this book.

Further, despite the inherent translational challenges, the contributors succeed in providing concrete suggestions regarding how the theory to application translation can be realized. They point toward the richness and diversity of conceptualizations, research methodologies, and interpretations of findings that intersectionality affords. As a result, they directly challenge assertions that an intersectional perspective "does not have any methods associated with it or that it can draw upon" (Phoenix and Pattynama 2006, 189) and that, because its historical roots are in the social sciences and humanities, its currency in the context of health research is limited. As is briefly enumerated and discussed below, these applications not only further legitimate the transformational potential of intersectionality, they point to ways in which this paradigm can be further developed and advanced to improve its utility in the realm of health inequities.

First, contributing researchers provide much evidence that more complex approaches to conventional understandings of health disparities are needed. For instance, they reveal why single category approaches in health research, which may focus on sex, gender, race, or socio-economic status for example, fail to address the actualities of the human condition, including the range of determinants that shape experiences of health. Barbara Clow similarly argues that an intersectionality perspective "reminds us forcibly that the determinants of health are dynamic and changeable and that specific facets of human experience or individual identity may be more or less significant from one illness, issue or context to the next." (Barbara Clow et al. 2009) Accordingly, throughout the collection, one can observe the way in which the authors push against the often used "holy trinity" of race, class, and gender, which binds much intersectionality research, and in so doing, they reveal the importance of considering the full range of health determinants, including religion, spirituality, culture, geography, place, age, and the state of the economy, to people's health and well-being.

In addition, the authors provide concrete suggestions on how to identify the relevance of and determine the relative importance of often-times intersecting social locations related to gender, sex, ethnicity, immigration experience, sexual orientation, religion, age, geography, and socio-economic status. In the process, they caution against essentializing Identity categories and emphasize that an intersectionality framework elucidates the importance of capturing not only the diversity of social locations but also the diversity *within* categories of analysis and the variation within and between social collectivities. They succeed in showing that intersectionality embraces rather than avoids the complexities that are essential to understanding the social inequities that manifest in health inequities.

Significantly, the authors also illustrate how the intersections of multiple, interlocking, and mutually constituted structural arrangements and systems of oppression create and maintain health inequities. Unlike additive models, the research featured in this volume really does focus on the interactive effects of both social relations and structures, and thus it succeeds in revealing new issues and new insights for analysis. The ways in which diversity of difference is woven through this volume underscores how the various interactions that come into play to produce health also become more or less relevant depending on the specific contexts, including temporal contexts, in which they operate. By advancing understandings of the social construction of health, the research also provides a necessary balance and complement to the biomedical, psychosocial, and behavioural models that dominate in the field of health. Erroneously, these models focus either on individual bodies with little consideration of the social forces and contexts that shape health (Weber and Fore 2007, 197), or on harmful individual behaviours and lifestyle choices without adequately interrogating the underlying contexts that actually shape individual health and behaviours.

A second major theme that runs through the collection and adds to our understanding of health and intersectionality analysis is that of power. All the chapters underscore the importance of maintaining a critical analytic eye on relations and discourses of power. In doing this, and by drawing on concrete examples, they disrupt an idealized representation of Canada. Canada is consistently ranked as one of the best places in the world to live and often recognized as an international leader in responding to issues of diversity in research and policy, including developments in the areas of social determinants of health, multiculturalism, and gender-based analyses. In reality, however, policy and health care practices mask dimensions of diversity and create variations in access and treatment according to gender, sex, language ability, ethnicity, religion, social location in the family, and other variables, through the configuration of Canada's socio-political and economic framework. So, in the efforts toward achieving a healthier Canada, a country where health is not so closely aligned with disempowerment and marginalization as an outcome of compromised social justice, the authors demonstrate the hopeful possibility that intersectionality has to offer research and policy as well as transformative health practice.

This explicit focus on power also highlights the pressing need for young and established researchers to reflect on their own privilege and power in order to take responsibility for the kind of knowledge they produce. Ann Russo (2010, 311) puts it well when she states: "What intersectionality taught me is that I consistently need to consider the implications of the research, policies and politics that I am forging in terms of whether they contribute to the perpetuation of any of the interconnected systems of oppression and privilege." Important dimensions of power are at play in the production of knowledge, even among researchers and decision makers who are committed to better understanding and responding to health inequities. For example, one of the ongoing impediments to having intersectionality recognized as a legitimate framework for health research is the resistance of gatekeepers who determine and control research priorities and whose scholarship shapes the thinking of dominant research paradigms (Dill and Zambrana 2009). Not surprisingly, then, the featured research in this collection has emerged within this often challenging environment and thus illustrates the very different stages of research and policy development within this burgeoning field.

Third, the book shows the breadth of ways to adopt an intersectionality framework in a variety of qualitative and quantitative methodological frameworks, thus challenging any pre-existing notions that this approach is suited only for select and narrow methodological translation. At the same time, it is clear that methodological development in the field requires sustained focus and continued efforts. This includes, in the realm of quantitative research, further development of "multilevel," "hierarchical," "ecological," or "contextual" modelling, because it is these types of models that have the most potential for introducing more complexity in research design and data interpretation (McCall 2005, 1788). One of the strongest messages that emerged in the volume, however, was the need for advancement of mixed methods approaches to intersectionality so that the strengths and benefits of both qualitative and quantitative methods can be drawn on to improve the study of the complexities inherent in health inequities.

Each chapter also provides concrete recommendations for ensuring more consistent uptake of intersectionality informed analysis and advancing the field. To begin, though many of the authors interrogate the linkages between intersectionality and a variety of other theoretical and methodological perspectives and tools, including health determinants frameworks, post–colonial theory, transnational theory, sex-and gender-based analyses, community-based and participatory search, and indigenous methodologies, additional research that builds on these preliminary investigations would be a fruitful undertaking. In particular, better delineating areas of overlap, conflict, and difference would ensure a clearer understanding of the distinct features of intersectionality as a normative theory and research paradigm.

In addition, although intersectionality frameworks focus on the importance of addressing historical foundations in examining relationships between interactions that shape human life and experiences, with a few exceptions (Vespa 2009; Hankivsky 2007) little attention has been paid to understanding intersecting experiences over time, such as would be consistent with a life course or lifespan approach. A number of contributions effectively capture different life stages, but in most instances, these only describe specific snapshots in time. Future work could focus on using a longitudinal approach to investigate critical stages of development and important transitions over extended timeframes. This would capture longer-term cumulative effects of dynamic interacting social locations and structural forces, including the trajectories of global and national economic, political, and legal structures, and policy developments and changes that affect health care systems and related social supports and services.

Furthermore, this volume demonstrates the need for more sustained efforts to realize the potential of an intersectionality-based analysis in health across all disciplines and health pillars. In this regard, a particularly fruitful area for development is to examine how intersectional and biomedical paradigms can interface. The potential relationship between intersectionality and biomedical research is only starting to be considered, but as Ursula Kelly has suggested elsewhere, "it is important to articulate new criteria for conducting and analyzing science that incorporate feminist intersectionality and biomedical paradigms in a new epistemology (Kelly 2009, E54)." Similarly, Janneke van Mens-Verhulst and H. Lorraine Radtke (2006, 6-7) argue that

one cannot hope to engage health care researchers without including the body as part of the analysis, and without paying attention to the biological aspects of the body. Bodies as a whole, or broken down into smaller dimensions, can be treated like the identity categories that up until now have been the focus of research on intersectionality. This has the advantage of treating the body category in an equivalent manner to other categories and avoiding the privileging of biology associated with biological reductionism. Moreover, the analysis would focus on the intersection of biology and other forms of difference, thereby avoiding the binary of biology/environment.

Although it is widely acknowledged that biomedical researchers do not focus enough on the ways in which bodies are socially constructed and experienced, intersectionality scholars have not thought enough about *both* systemic and biological aspects of human experience (Einstein and Shildrick 2009). Thus, integrating biological aspects of human experiences and interrogating the creation of intersectional *bodies* has important implications for the theory of intersectionality.

Finally, many of the contributors to the volume share concerns about their ongoing struggles of trying to ensure that their research does not reify the subject positions of populations that are already labelled as vulnerable, marginalized, or stigmatized. On this point, a possible avenue for progressing would be to focus on issues of resilience. The complex interplay between individual agency and social structure in the context of intersectionality is emerging in the wider literature (e.g., Dhanji 2010; Ozbilgin 2009; Chong et al. 2009; Schilling 2008) but is still underdeveloped in examinations of health inequities. At the same time, the reach of intersectionality should be expanded beyond the typical current foci on "marginalized" and "vulnerable" groups. Because intersectionality is an aspect of social organization that shapes all human lives (Weldon 2008), it should also lead to examinations of how privilege is constructed, maintained, and experienced and to investigations of those who fall into the category of "in-between groupings"(Sen et al. 2009). These types of lines of inquiry are developing in other areas (e.g. Jones 2009; Weigt et al. 2008; Hurtado and Sinha 2008) but have yet to be explicitly at the forefront of intersectionality-inspired inquiries of health inequities. To realize its fuller potential, intersectionality should be applied to many different issues, across different settings, and to different groups. Researchers should draw on this paradigm to transform the understandings of experiences and needs of *all* population groups.

Overall, then, the chapters in this volume express pragmatic optimism about intersectional approaches in health research, while realistically acknowledging their partialities, to more fully capture the complex and shifting contexts that construct social injustice and inequality, and thus to more strategically and effectively guide oppositional practices. Broadly, each chapter not only asserts but illustrates, through empirical work, that conceptualizing health in Canada benefits from theories that validate complexity across numerous health experiences, illnesses, and diseases. Through this lens, researchers can create more accurate and inclusive knowledge of human lives and health needs, which can inform the development of systematically responsive and socially just health systems and policy (Hankivsky and Christoffersen 2008). And moreover, both explicitly and implicitly, this body of work provides avenues for further development in terms of intersectionality theorizing in the realm of health. In these ways the contributors both guide and inspire further explorations of the relationship between intersectionality and health among both emerging and established researchers. Although the focus of this book is largely on the application of intersectionality in the context of health research and policy, many of the chapters address gaps, tackle issues, and raise questions that contribute to the ongoing project of refining and clarifying the intersectionality paradigm. This includes working through connections between theory and practice, and furthering the understanding of best practices in intersectional research and practice, all of which hold great promise for extending the widespread applicability of intersectionality, not only in Canada but across the globe.

In sum, intersectionality is burgeoning as both a theory and research paradigm. In the field of health issues and services, however, its transformational potential is only starting to be explored and fully acknowledged. As evidenced by this collection, significant progress is being made in Canada in this "innovative site of inquiry," which has the potential to revolutionize the way in which health research and policy making are undertaken. Indeed, the broad range of interdisciplinary researchers featured in this volume have been stimulated by the possibilities of this perspective and are making great efforts and commitments to apply it in order to expose, better understand, and prioritize inequities that continue to persist at individual and structural levels of society. The foundational work in this volume provides concrete suggestions that are intended to encourage further investigations and chart new directions that will build on these preliminary research efforts. In the final analysis, the knowledge gained from this contribution is intended to inform intersectionality theory and be a catalyst for more inclusive and effective research as well as for policy and practice change that leads to innovative and viable real-world solutions to a range of health inequities.

References

Chong, V., K. Umb, M. Hahn, D. Pheng, C. Yee, and C. Auerswald. 2009. Toward an intersectional understanding of violence and resilience: An exploratory study of young Southeast Asian men in Alameda and Contra Costa County, California. *Aggression and Violent Behavior* 14: 461-69.

Clow, B., A. Pederson, M. Haworth-Brockman, and J. Bernier. 2009. *Rising to the challenge: Sex and gender-based analysis for health planning, policy and research in Canada.* Halifax: Atlantic Centre of Excellence for Women's Health.

Dhanji, H. 2010. Resilience theory as a tool for the promotion of successful cognitive development among high-risk population of children in developing countries. *Attaché: An International Affairs Journal:* 39-50. http://www.theattache.ca.

Dill, B.T., and R.E. Zambrana, eds. 2009. *Emerging intersections: Race, class and gender in theory, policy and practice.* Chapel Hill: Rutgers University Press.

Einstein, G., and M. Shildrick. 2009. The postconventional body: Retheorising women's health. *Social Science and Medicine* 69: 293-300.

Hankivsky, O. 2007. Gender based analysis and health policy: The need to rethink outdated strategies. In *Women's health in Canada: Critical theory, policy and practice,* ed. M. Morrow, O. Hankivsky and C. Varcoe, 143-68. Toronto: University of Toronto Press.

Hankivsky, O., and A. Christoffersen. 2008. Intersectionality and the determinants of health: A Canadian perspective. *Critical Public Health* 18(3): 1-13.

Hurtado, A., and M. Sinha. 2008. More than men: Latino feminist masculinities and intersectionality. *Sex Roles* 59: 337–49.

Jones, S.R. 2009. Constructing identities at the intersections: An autoethnographic exploration of multiple dimensions of identity. *Journal of College Student Development* 50(3): 1-12.

Kelly, U.A. 2009. Integrating intersectionality and biomedicine in health disparities research. *Advances in Nursing Science* 32(2): E42-E56.

McCall, L. 2005. The complexity of intersectionality. *Signs: Journal of Women in Culture and Society* 30: 1771–1802.

Ozbilgin, M.F., ed. 2009. *Equality, diversity and inclusion at work: Theory and scholarship.* Cheltenham: Edward Elgar.

Phoenix, A., and P. Pattynama. 2006. Editorial. *European Journal of Women's Studies* 13(3): 187-92.

Russo, A. 2010. The future of intersectionality: What's at stake. In *The intersectional approach: Transforming the academy through race, class and gender,* ed. M.T. Berger and K. Guidroz, 309-18. Chapel Hill: University of North Carolina Press.

Schilling, T.A. 2008. An examination of resilience processes in context: The case of Tasha. *Urban Review* 40: 296–316.

Sen, G., A. Iyer, and C. Mukherjee. 2009. A methodology to analyse the intersections of social inequalities in health. *Journal of Human Development and Capabilities* 10(3): 397-415.

van Mens-Verhulst, J., and H. Lorraine Radtke. 2006. Intersectionality and health care: Support for the diversity turn in research and practice. http://www.vanmens.info/verhulst/en/wp-content/Intersectionality%20and%20Health%20Care-%20january%202006.pdf.

Vespa, J. 2009. Gender ideology construction: A life course and intersectional approach. *Gender and Society* 23(3): 363-87.

Weber, L., and E. Fore. 2007. Race, ethnicity, and health: An intersectional framework. In *Handbook of the sociology of racial and ethnic relations,* ed. H. Vera and J. Feagin, 191-218. New York: Springer.

Weigt, J.M., and C. Richards Solomon. 2008. Work-family management among low-wage service workers and assistant professors in the USA: A comparative intersectional analysis. *Gender, Work and Organization* 15(6): 621-49.

Weldon, L.S. 2008. Intersectionality. In *Politics, gender, and concepts: Theory and methodology,* ed. G. Goertz and A. Mazur, 193-218. Cambridge: Cambridge University Press.

Contributors

Annette Bailey, RN, is completing her PhD in public health science with specialization in health promotion and education. Her dissertation research examines traumatic stress and resilience among black women who lose children through gun violence. She currently holds a position as lecturer at York University's School of Nursing.

Jennifer Black, PhD, RD, is Assistant Professor of nutrition and dietetics at the University of British Columbia. Her research focuses on the social and contextual determinants of health, food practices, and nutrition. She is interested in how attitudes and behaviours related to health, food security, and dietary choices are influenced by socio-cultural and neighbourhood-level factors. Her research is shaped by her background as a registered dietitian. She holds a PhD from New York University and completed a post-doctoral fellowship in the social determinants of health in the Department of Sociology at the University of British Columbia.

Annette J. Browne, PhD, is Associate Professor at the University of British Columbia in the School of Nursing. She is also a new investigator with the Canadian Institutes of Health Research. Annette's career as a researcher stems from her clinical experience as an outpost nurse who lived and worked in northern First Nations and Inuit communities. Her research focuses on the factors shaping health and health care inequities, with a particular emphasis on implications for indigenous people. Central to Annette's research program is her commitment to working in partnership with clinical agencies, communities, leaders in Aboriginal health, and policy makers. She has a PhD in nursing from UBC and a master's degree as a family nurse practitioner from the University of Rhode Island, USA.

Natalie Clark, MSW, is a PhD candidate in Public Policy through Simon Fraser University and is a member of Faculty in the School of Social Work and Human Service at Thompson Rivers University. She is the director of the Centre for Community Based Youth Health Research at TRU, which examines the impact of a number of factors on youth health within an intersectional framework. Natalie's community-based participatory research projects over the last fifteen years have focused on marginalized and at-risk young women's experiences with issues of sexual exploitation, eating disorders, and addictions; she has also examined youth justice and health, violence, trauma, and the support needs of girls and women. Her most recent research deals with the health and transition of experiences of marginalized youth growing up in small cities and rural communities and with urban Aboriginal youth health in the BC Interior.

Sarah de Leeuw, PhD, is an assistant professor in the Northern Medical Program, the University of Northern British Columbia, the Faculty of Medicine at UBC. She is a human geographer and creative writer whose research focuses on social justice and the workings of power. She is specifically concerned with colonialism, the social and geographic determinants of health, and the role of creative arts in ameliorating socio-cultural disparities. For over fifteen years, she has also worked with feminist organizations, arts centres, and research institutes focused on the health and well-being of indigenous peoples. She has twice won the CBC Literary Award for Creative Non-Fiction, and her writings appear in venues ranging from *The SAGE Handbook of Social Geography* and *The International Encyclopaedia of Human Geography* to *Fiddlehead* and *Riddle Fence* to the *Canadian Family Physician* and the *International Journal of Mental Health and Addiction*.

Rita Kaur Dhamoon, PhD, works in the area of modern and contemporary political theory. Her primary teaching and research interests are in critical social and political thought, including identity/difference politics, multiculturalism, culture, feminist and gender theory, critical race studies, post-colonial and anti-colonial thought, liberalism and its critics, and democratic theory. Before joining the University of the Fraser Valley, Rita held a Grant Notley Memorial Post-Doctoral Fellowship in the Department of Political Science at the University of Alberta (2005-7) and a SSHRC Post-Doctoral Fellowship in the Department of Political Science at the University of Victoria (2007-8). She has worked with and for a number of anti-racist and feminist organizations and networks in Canada and the UK.

Parin Dossa, PhD, is Professor of Anthropology at Simon Fraser University. Her teaching and research interests include migration, gender and health, structural violence in war and peace, aging and culture, and anthropological theory. Her ethnographic work has focused on Muslim women in Canada and abroad. She is the author of *Politics and Poetics of Migration: Narratives of Iranian Women from the Diaspora* (2004) and *Racialized Bodies, Disabling Worlds: Storied Lives of Immigrant Muslim Women* (2009). She is also co-producer of two videos: *New Voices: Ethnic Elders in Canada* and *Out of the Shadows: Narratives of Women with Developmental Disabilities*. Currently, she is exploring how narratives of trauma can inform health and social policy of refugees and internally displaced women in Afghanistan, from homeland to diaspora.

Isabel Dyck, PhD, is a feminist geographer and Professor Emeritus at the School of Geography, Queen Mary University of London. Her theoretical interests relate to the interrelationships among the body, gender, health, and place, including how medical science is implicated in social inequalities. Her research in Canada, using a variety of qualitative methods, has investigated employment issues for women with chronic illness; the home as a site of long-term health care; and various health and settlement issues for international migrants, including the reconstitution of home and family. Recent research with households from diverse minority groups in London, England, examines continuities and transformations of health knowledge and practices in the context of globalization, with a focus on immigration processes and diaspora formation.

Marilyn Ford-Gilboe, RN, PhD, is a professor and faculty scholar in the Arthur Labatt Family School of Nursing (Faculty of Health Sciences) at the University of Western Ontario. Her research program focuses on understanding how personal, social, economic, and structural factors support or undermine the health of vulnerable women and their children, particularly those who have experienced violence. As principal investigator of a Canadian Institutes of Health Research (CIHR) New Emerging Team grant, Marilyn has led an interdisciplinary team in conducting a longitudinal study of women's health and resources in the early years after leaving an abusive partner. She is involved in numerous other funded projects in the areas of intimate partner violence, including studies that address issues faced by Aboriginal and immigrant women, and those that test interventions, including a health intervention for women who have recently left an abusive relationship (the i-HEAL).

Alycia Fridkin is a doctoral student in the Interdisciplinary Studies Graduate Program at the University of British Columbia. She holds a master's of health science in health promotion from the University of Toronto, and she is currently the Student Director of the Canadian Public Health Association. Her goal of reducing health inequities through policy change has led her to focus her doctoral research on what is needed to foster the development of health and social policies that promote equity for indigenous peoples in urban Canadian contexts. Her broader research interests include health inequities, indigenous/Aboriginal health, critical policy analysis, and the involvement of marginalized groups in health policy and decision-making.

Tahira Gonsalves, MA (Sociology), is presently working for the Ontario provincial government. She has previously worked at the International Development Research Centre and at the Canadian Research Institute for the Advancement of Women, both in Ottawa. Most recently, she coordinated a community-academic research project on newcomer youth mental health. She has experience in international development; gender-based policy research; and immigrant, child, and youth mental health.

Margo Greenwood, PhD, is Academic Leader of the National Collaborating Centre for Aboriginal Health and an associate professor in both the First Nations Studies and Education programs at the University of Northern British Columbia. She is an Indigenous scholar of Cree ancestry with more than twenty years' experience in the field of early childhood education. While Margo's focus has been on all children, she is recognized regionally, provincially, nationally, and internationally for her work on Indigenous children. In recognition of her years of work to promote awareness and policy action on the rights and well-being of Indigenous children, youth and families, Margo Greenwood was the recipient of the Queen's Jubilee medal in 2002 and was recently awarded the Confederation of University Faculty Associations' Academic of the Year Award.

Olena Hankivsky, PhD, is Associate Professor in the School of Public Policy at Simon Fraser University, founder and co-director of the Institute for Critical Studies in Gender and Health, and former co-leader of the Women's Health Research Network. Her areas of research are focused on gender and health, and she is recognized for her work on intersectionality and its applications to health research and policy. She is co-editor and leading contributing author of *Women's Health in Canada: Critical Perspectives on Theory and Policy* (2007), one of the first texts on women's health research in Canada. Additionally, she is author of *Social Policy and the Ethic of Care* (2004). In 2008, Olena was awarded a Research Chair in New Perspectives in Gender and Health by the Canadian Institutes of Health Research and a Senior Scholar Career Award in Population Health by the Michael Smith Foundation for Health Research.

Jill Hanley, PhD, is Assistant Professor at the McGill School of Social Work, where she teaches courses on applied research, community practice, and social policy. Her research and publications are focused on organizing access to social rights for migrants with precarious status, particularly labour, housing, and health. She is also co-founder of Montreal's Immigrant Workers' Centre, where she is still very active.

Louise Hara has worked within the women's movement, both community-based and in academe, in order to create or support avenues through which women can explore their experiences of social, economic, legal, and political structures, and formulate collective responses to violence and oppression. As a women's centre representative to numerous local, provincial, and national associations, committees, and working groups, she gained considerable experience and knowledge of the functions and activities that are the underpinnings of feminist organizing initiatives. Louise has also participated in two feminist participatory action research projects, Women Organizing Activities for Women (2000-3) and Women's Employability and Health Project (2005-7). Since 2002, she has contracted her services in community coaching, facilitation, and research to diverse groups and agencies.

Wendy Hulko is an associate professor of social work at Thompson Rivers University in Kamloops, BC, and a qualified health researcher with the Centre for Research on Personhood in Dementia at UBC in Vancouver, BC. She holds a BA hon. in sociology and Spanish (Trent University), a master's in social work (University of Toronto), and a PhD in sociology and social policy (University of Stirling), and has worked in the field of aging since 1993. Wendy's background includes long-term-care nursing, hospital social work, and government policy and planning. Since 2007, she has been collaborating with Secwepemc Nation elders and health authority decision makers to research First Nation views on memory loss in later life and culturally safe dementia care.

Sarah Hunt is a PhD candidate at Simon Fraser University in the Department of Geography and has worked as a researcher, educator, and program coordinator in communities across BC for the past ten years. Sarah's work has focused on issues such as Aboriginal post-secondary education, community responses to violence and trauma, and issues of decolonization in indigenous communities. Her doctoral research uses critical legal and Indigenous geographies to examine how systems of law and governance shape intergenerational violence in rural First Nations reserves. Sarah is a member of the Kwakwaka'wakw First Nation from Tsaxis (Fort Rupert) on Vancouver Island.

Ilene Hyman, PhD, is an assistant professor in the Dalla Lana School of Public Health at the University of Toronto and a research associate at Cities Centre, University of Toronto. She has over twenty years of experience in public health and immigrant research in Canada and overseas. Her expertise is in the area of health and its determinants for immigrant and racialized populations. Ilene has been the principal investigator on numerous CIHR and/or peer-reviewed community-based research projects examining health, chronic disease, mental health, intimate partner violence, and cancer screening among these populations. She is currently the principal investigator for Migration and Diabetes, a study of risk factors associated with diabetes and diabetes management needs in four newcomer communities in Toronto.

Connie Kaweesi, MSW, is chair of the Health and Human Service Programs at Northern Lights College. A social work educator, she teaches social service worker and social work courses at the Northern Lights College and the University of Northern British Columbia. She has worked in the social and health field for the last twenty-six years. Connie has lived in northern British Columbia since 1985 and has worked with clients in the criminal justice system, with First Nations communities, and with marginalized women. Her areas of social work practice include individual and group counselling, clinical supervision, consultation, and research. Connie's clinical practice is based on cognitive-behaviour therapy and feminist counselling. Her specific areas of clinical practice are domestic violence, anger management, and anxiety and trauma.

Nazilla Khanlou, RN, PhD, is Echo's OWHC chair in Women's Mental Health Research in the Faculty of Health at York University and an associate professor in its School of Nursing. Her clinical background is in psychiatric nursing. Her overall program of research is situated in the interdisciplinary field of community-based mental health promotion in general and mental health promotion among youth and women in multicultural and immigrant-receiving settings in particular. She has received grants from peer-reviewed federal and provincial research funding agencies and was the health domain leader of the Centre of Excellence for Research on Immigration and Settlement (2001-8) in Toronto and a visiting scholar (2005-6) at the Wellesley Urban Health Institute. She has published articles, books, and reports on immigrant youth and women, as well as on mental health issues. She is involved in knowledge translation to the public through media.

Karen M. Kobayashi, PhD, is Associate Professor in the Department of Sociology at the University of Victoria. Her research interests include the economic and health dimensions of ethnic inequality in Canada, intergenerational relationships and social support in mid- and later-life families, and the socio-cultural dimensions of dementia and personhood. With funding from the Canadian Institutes of Health Research and the Social Sciences and Humanities Research Council of Canada, her current research programs focus on the relationship between social isolation and health care utilization among older adults, the negotiation of social support and care work in families, and the healthy immigrant effect in mid- to later life. She has recently published in *Ethnicity and Health, Gender, Place, and Culture,* the *Journal of Aging and Health,* and the *Canadian Journal on Aging.*

Shari Laliberté, RN, MN, is a PhD student in the School of Nursing at the University of British Columbia. She is also currently on leave from Thompson Rivers University, where she is an assistant professor. Her research interests centre on the use of critical, participatory, and visual inquiry methods to explore child voice in public policy and political decision-making processes as a root determinant of the socio-environmental determinants of child and youth mental health. Shari has used photovoice to investigate youth perspectives on the meaning and determinants of youth "mental health" and is currently building on this work in her dissertation research, which will focus on exploring ways of supporting youth to engage, inform, and influence child and youth mental health, and the relevant public policies that shape its socio-environmental determinants.

Robin LeDrew gained a BSW with honours from the University of Victoria as a mature student and has been employed as a frontline social worker at Whitevalley Community Resource Centre in Lumby, BC, for eighteen years. She has been involved in the local arts council, social justice issues, and the women's movement at local, provincial, and national levels. As one of the community-based researchers for the Women's Health and Employability research project under Colleen Reid, she wrote the "Lumby Report." She co-presented at the Public Health Association of BC in 2006, the Canadian Research Institute for the Advancement of Women in 2007, CU EXPO in 2008, and two Women's Health Research Network summer institutes. She is co-author of *Our Common Ground: Cultivating Women's Health through Community Based Research* (2009).

Jo-Anne Lee, PhD, is Associate Professor in the Department of Women's Studies at the University of Victoria. After working in grassroots community organizations in Canada and abroad for many years, Jo-Anne returned to school to study sociology. She publishes in the areas of immigrant women, multiculturalism, participatory action research and community organizing and development, urban ethnic minority women's activism, anti-racism, and racialized and indigenous girls' issues. With John Lutz, she is the co-editor of *Situating Race and Racisms in Space, Time and Theory* (2005) and, with Rita Wong, of a special issue of *West Coast Line* (2008) on minority women's activisms on the West Coast. Her published work appears in *Canadian Women's Studies, Gender, Place Culture,* and other feminist journals and anthologies. She is currently working on a book about rethinking girlhoods from intersectional, transnational, anti-racist, and decolonizing perspectives that draw on two participatory action research projects she undertook in the past six years.

Marina Morrow, PhD, is an associate professor with the Faculty of Health Sciences and director of the Centre for the Study of Gender, Social Inequities and Mental Health (CGSM) at Simon Fraser University. The CIHR-funded centre supports collaborative, interdisciplinary, and multi-sectoral teams of researchers and research users from Canada, the United States, Australia, and the United Kingdom. CGSM investigators are involved in developing innovative research, knowledge exchange, and training initiatives that address social inequities and mental health. Marina's research interests are in critical health policy, with foci on mental health reforms, mental health and social inequity, and the impact of neo-liberal reforms on health policy. Her most recent publication (with Wasik, Cohen, and Perry) is "Removing Barriers to Work: Building Economic Security for People with Mental Illness" in the *Journal of Critical Social Policy*.

Jacqueline Oxman-Martinez, PhD (sociology), is a visiting researcher in School of Social Work at University of Montreal. Her research interests include issues of violence against women, child neglect, poverty, and children's well-being, including immigrant and refugee children. She has also analyzed migration policies and issues related to gender disparities and inequalities created by precarious immigration status, examining government policies and human rights of asylum seekers, temporary workers, and trafficked human beings. She was the holder of several research grants (ICRS, FQRSC, SSHRC), has collaborated extensively with researchers across the country and internationally, and has developed effective knowledge exchange partnerships with representatives of community organizations and policy makers at federal and regional levels. Her numerous publications reflect the wide range of her academic production.

Bernadette Pauly is an associate professor in the School of Nursing at the University of Victoria and a scientist in the Center for Addictions Research of British Columbia. Her research interests include inequities in health and access to health care in the context of homelessness and substance use. A primary focus in her work is ethical analysis of health policy through an equity lens. She has completed research on access to health care for street-involved populations in primary health care clinics and needle exchange services and better understanding of ethical practice that reduces inequities. She is currently a co-lead of a CIHR-funded new emerging team grant that includes a focus on the development of an equity lens in public health programs and policy.

Pamela Ponic, PhD, is a post-doctoral researcher jointly at the School of Nursing, University of British Columbia, and the BC Centre of Excellence in Women's Health in Vancouver, BC. She is also a research associate with the BC Non-Profit Housing Association. Her program of research examines the relationships between systemic power inequities and women's access to health-promoting resources, recently with a focus on how housing and related determinants affect women's health after leaving abusive relationships. Most recently, she was principal investigator on a provincial multi-site feminist participatory action and photovoice research project on women's barriers to housing after leaving violent relationships. She is particularly interested in how multi-method community-based research processes can affect policy and community change.

Steven G. Prus, PhD, is Associate Professor in the Department of Sociology at Carleton University. Issues of seniors' well-being underpin his research interests. His current research uses panel data to examine the social causes of healthy aging of individuals and international data to investigate the health-age relationship at the population and country levels of analysis.

Colleen Reid, PhD, is on faculty in Child and Family Community Studies at Douglas College and is adjunct professor at the Institute for Critical Studies in Gender and Health at Simon Fraser University (SFU). She completed her post-doctoral studies in Health Sciences at SFU (2007) where she was principal investigator of the research project that is discussed in Chapter 4. Her areas of interest include the social determinants of health, health promotion and women's health, community development, and community-based research. She has written extensively about the challenges and promises of community-based research in women's health and recently co-wrote a manual titled *Our Common Ground: Cultivating Women's Health through Community Based Research* (2009, with E. Brief and R. LeDrew).

Sheryl Reimer-Kirkham, RN, PhD, is Associate Professor in the School of Nursing at Trinity Western University (TWU), Langley. She is director of the graduate nursing (MSN) program and teaches health care ethics, health policy, and qualitative research. Her research program focuses on pluralism and social justice in health care and nursing education. A current funded research project examines religion, spirituality, culture, gender, and place in home health care. She is a founding member of TWU's Religion in Canada Institute and Institute of Gender Studies.

Katherine R. Rossiter is a PhD Candidate in the School of Criminology, and Associate Director of The FREDA Centre for Research on Violence Against Women and Children, at Simon Fraser University. She holds degrees in Criminology and Psychology and is a graduate of the *Research in Addictions and Mental Health Policy and Services* (RAMHPS) program, a CIHR Strategic Training Program. Her doctoral research focuses on victimization and trauma in the lives of women who are receiving forensic mental health services in British Columbia. Other research interests include the victimization and criminalization of vulnerable populations, ethical and methodological issues in researching sensitive topics, and the development of trauma-informed approaches in the criminal justice and mental health systems.

Joan Samuels-Dennis, PhD, is an assistant professor with the Faculty of Health Science (School of Nursing) at York University in Toronto. Her clinical and research interests include the mental health of women and girls from diverse and marginalized populations, evaluations of interventions for women and children exposed to violence, development of evidence-based practice, and the study of personal, social, and environmental factors that perpetuate the long-term effects of violent and non-violent traumas.

Sonya Sharma, PhD, is a research associate in the Department of Theology and Religion at Durham University, UK. Her research is examining young people's experiences of Christianity while they attend English universities. With a group of Canadian scholars, she is also exploring the negotiation of religious, spiritual, and cultural plurality in home health care. Her doctorate was a qualitative exploration of Christian women's sexuality. Of key interest is how the differences between people and people's identities are negotiated at the intersections of religion, gender, class, race, sexuality, and culture. Other interests include the interrelationship between familial and religious practices and spaces, feminism and religion, and embodiment and research practices. She co-edited *Women and Religion in the West: Challenging Secularization* (2008).

Alison Sum completed her master of arts degree in kinesiology at the University of Victoria in 2008. Her chapter, co-written with her thesis co-supervisor Jo-Anne Lee, is inspired by her graduate interdisciplinary research on health, ethnicity, and identity. After completing her MA, she worked at the BC Ministry of Healthy Living and Sport as a policy analyst. Alison now intends to incorporate her research and policy experience into health care practice, as she is currently completing a second master's degree, in occupational therapy, at the University of British Columbia. She was involved with antidote multiracial girls' and women's network for four years. She continues to strive for social justice, health, and wellness throughout her career and leisure pursuits.

Colleen Varcoe, PhD, RN, is a professor in the School of Nursing at the University of British Columbia. Her research focuses on women's health with emphasis on violence and inequity, and the culture of health care with an emphasis on ethics, and aims to promote ethical practice and policy in the context of violence and inequity. Her recently completed studies include exploration of the interacting risks of violence and HIV infection for rural and Aboriginal women, and rural maternity care for Aboriginal women. She is currently co-leader of a longitudinal study of the effects of violence against women after they have left abusive partners, of a study examining primary health care at urban Aboriginal health clinics, and of a study of Aboriginal women's experiences of leaving abusive partners.

Gerry Veenstra, PhD, is Associate Professor of sociology, associate member of the School of Population and Public Health, and faculty associate of the Peter Wall Institute for Advanced Studies at the University of British Columbia. He currently holds a Senior Scholar Award from the Michael Smith Foundation for Health Research. His current research projects involve quantitative investigations of race and ethnicity, perceived discrimination, and health inequalities in Toronto and Vancouver; intersectionality theory and health inequalities in Canada; loneliness, social capital, poverty, and mortality in Alameda County, California; genetic discrimination and Huntington disease; and the culture of class in Canada.

Bilkis Vissandjée, PhD, is a professor in the School of Nursing at the University of Montreal. She is also a researcher at the Public Health Research Institute of the University of Montreal as well as the Research Centre of the CSSS (Centre de santé et des services sociaux) de la Montagne. The common theme of her work is to better understand the relationship between gender, culture, and migration as social determinants of health. Her research addresses the need for gender- and diversity-sensitive indicators that value and reflect women's lives, work, productivity, and social, cultural, and economic security over the lifespan. As the academic co-director of the Centre d'excellence sur la santé des femmes – Consortium Université de Montréal (1996-2002), she contributed significantly to the research program that addresses the complexities involved with immigrant women's access to health services. Bilkis has also worked with diverse international institutions, in an effort to sensitize people to the life conditions of women living in developing countries. She collaborated with the Shastri Indo-Canadian Institute, the International Development Research Council, the Canadian International Development Agency, the Aga Khan Foundation, and the United Nations Development Program.

Index

Note: "(f)" after a page number indicates a figure; "(t)"after a page number indicates a table